Clinical Handbook of Pediatric Endocrinology

Clinical Handbook of Pediatric Endocrinology

Edited by Jeffery Desmond

hayle
medical

New York

Hayle Medical,
750 Third Avenue, 9th Floor,
New York, NY 10017, USA

Visit us on the World Wide Web at:
www.haylemedical.com

ISBN: 978-1-63241-732-9

Cataloging-in-Publication Data

Clinical handbook of pediatric endocrinology / edited by Jeffery Desmond.
    p. cm.
Includes bibliographical references and index.
ISBN 978-1-63241-732-9
1. Pediatric endocrinology. 2. Endocrine glands--Diseases. 3. Pediatric endocrinology--Diagnosis.
4. Pediatric endocrinology--Treatment. I. Desmond, Jeffery.
RJ418 .C55 2019
618.924--dc23

Table of Contents

Preface

Pediatric endocrinology is a field of medicine that is concerned with the disorders of the endocrine glands. Such disorders manifest as abnormalities in physical growth and sexual development of a child, such as dwarfism and gigantism, intersex, delayed puberty, gonadal dysgenesis, ovarian and testicular dysfunction, etc. Other conditions in children involving disorders of adrenal, pituitary and thyroid glands include underactive or overactive thyroid gland, childhood obesity, multiple endocrine neoplasia, adrenoleukodystrophy, among others. Depending on the condition, pediatric endocrinologists may design treatment modalities involving intensive insulin therapies, radioactive iodine treatment, personalized nutritional evaluation and psychosocial evaluation, parathyroid and thyroid surgeries, etc. This book discusses the fundamentals as well as modern approaches of pediatric endocrinology. It unfolds the clinical aspects of pediatric endocrine disorders, which will be crucial for the progress of this field in the future. In this book, using case studies and examples, constant effort has been made to make the understanding of the difficult concepts of pediatric endocrinology, as easy and informative as possible, for the readers.

The researches compiled throughout the book are authentic and of high quality, combining several disciplines and from very diverse regions from around the world. Drawing on the contributions of many researchers from diverse countries, the book's objective is to provide the readers with the latest achievements in the area of research. This book will surely be a source of knowledge to all interested and researching the field.

In the end, I would like to express my deep sense of gratitude to all the authors for meeting the set deadlines in completing and submitting their research chapters. I would also like to thank the publisher for the support offered to us throughout the course of the book. Finally, I extend my sincere thanks to my family for being a constant source of inspiration and encouragement.

Editor

Identification of factors associated with good response to growth hormone therapy in children with short stature: results from the ANSWER Program®

Peter A Lee[1*], John Germak[2], Robert Gut[2], Naum Khutoryansky[2] and Judith Ross[3]

Abstract

Objective: To identify factors associated with growth in children on growth hormone (GH) therapy using data from the American Norditropin Studies: Web-enabled Research (ANSWER) Program® registry.

Methods: GH-naïve children with GH deficiency, multiple pituitary hormone deficiency, idiopathic short stature, Turner syndrome, or a history of small for gestational age were eligible (N = 1,002). Using a longitudinal statistical approach, predictive factors were identified in patients with GHD for change from baseline in height standard deviation score (ΔHSDS) following 2 years of treatment.

Results: Gradual increases in ΔHSDS over time were observed for all diagnostic categories. Significant predictive factors of ΔHSDS, ranked by significance were: height velocity (HV) at 4 months > baseline age > baseline HSDS > baseline body mass index (BMI) SDS > baseline insulin-like growth factor I (IGF-I) SDS; gender was not significant. HV at 4 months and baseline BMI SDS were positively correlated, whereas baseline age, HSDS, and IGF-I SDS were negatively correlated with ΔHSDS.

Conclusions: These results may help guide GH therapy based on pretreatment characteristics and early growth response.

Introduction

Treatment with exogenous growth hormone (GH) has become a well-accepted therapeutic option for children with growth failure. Since the availability of recombinant human GH (rhGH) in 1985, a wide range of conditions associated with decreased growth, including GH deficiency (GHD), Turner syndrome (TS), Noonan syndrome (NS), children born small for gestational age (SGA), Prader-Willi syndrome (PWS), idiopathic short stature (ISS), and SHOX (short stature homeobox) gene haploinsufficiency have been approved by the United States Food and Drug Administration (FDA) for treatment [1-4].

Treatment with GH has been demonstrated to increase both short-term growth and adult height in pediatric patients with a variety of different growth disorders [5-8]. However, considerable variability in response to this treatment has been reported across and within different diagnostic categories [9-11]. Such variability makes decisions about whether to treat with GH, when to begin treatment, and what dosing to use more difficult [12].

Reports from clinical trials and analyses suggest multiple factors that influence the response to GH treatment. Variables associated with better responses to GH treatment in patients with ISS include first-year growth response, younger age at start of treatment, the difference in height at the start of treatment from target height SD score (HSDS), and GH dose [13,14]. Additional factors may include underlying genetic conditions,

* Correspondence: plee@psu.edu
[1]Department of Pediatrics, Milton S. Hershey Medical Center, Penn State College of Medicine, Hershey, PA, USA
Full list of author information is available at the end of the article

presence of concomitant illness, and compliance with treatment [15].

Formal height prediction models have been developed that combine information regarding patient- and treatment-related factors. Such prediction models of response to GH have been developed for patients with isolated or idiopathic GHD [16-20], SGA [21-23], chronic kidney disease [24], ISS [25], and TS [26]. These models have the potential to aid individualized GH treatment planning and the adjustment of therapy based on early responses [27]. However, even though GH treatment regimens can be based on model-derived predictions of growth response [28], existing models account for only about one-half of the variability in the response to GH. Addition of genetic, biochemical, and other new variables to existing models may improve their accuracy and clinical utility [29,30].

Since 2002, the ANSWER (American Norditropin Studies: Web-enabled Research) Program® registry has collected information on patients receiving Norditropin. Participation within the ANSWER Program is at the discretion of the participating physicians and includes diagnostic categories in which treatment with growth hormone is used. The aim of this paper is to report growth response among different diagnostic categories and to identify factors associated with greater growth response over the first 2 years in children with GHD undergoing treatment with GH.

Methods
Answer program registry
Data for this analysis were obtained from the ANSWER Program registry, a collection of long-term efficacy and safety information from patients treated with Norditropin® (somatropin [rDNA origin] injection, Novo Nordisk A/S, Denmark) [31] in the United States. Patient histories and physical examination data were entered by participating physician investigators using the ANSWER Program registry reporting form, a web-based data entry tool. Informed consent was obtained in all cases. While the registry enrolls GH-treatment-naïve and non-naïve patients, for the purpose of this analysis, only naïve patient data from the following diagnostic categories were included in the current analyses: 1) GHD (isolated/idiopathic), 2) multiple pituitary hormone deficiency (MPHD), 3) TS, 4) SGA, and 5) ISS.

Study description
Patient data collected at the first visit and/or follow-up visits included age, gender, GH dose, HSDS, insulin-like growth factor-I (IGF-I) SDS, body mass index (BMI) SDS, bone age, and annualized height velocity (HV). The maximal stimulated serum GH concentration was also recorded. Height and BMI SDS (z scores) were calculated according to the standard formulas provided by the Center for Disease Control and Prevention [32]. IGF-I SDS scores were calculated using a standard algorithm and reference values provided by Diagnostic Systems Laboratories, Inc. (Webster, TX, USA). Data were collected at baseline and at 4 months, 1 year, and 2 years of GH treatment. Data at 4 months were collected within a 1-month window and data at 1 and 2 years were collected within a 3-month window. To eliminate the potential of erroneous data having been entered, the following rules were used to remove patients from the analysis: lack of height information at baseline, 4 months, 1 year, or 2 years; baseline age 0 or > 18 years; baseline HSDS less than -5 or greater than +2; and baseline height < 35 cm or > 200 cm. Also, patients were excluded when key variables from baseline or subsequent values were deemed physically or chronologically implausible (3.77% of potential subjects were excluded according to this criteria).

Regression model development
In this study, a longitudinal statistical approach was used to identify factors that have significant predictive value for change in HSDS from baseline (ΔHSDS) in a regression model. ΔHSDS data collected following the first and second years of treatment were included in the model. A smoothing procedure was applied for the corresponding mean value curves for first-year HV and baseline age. Due to the limited number of patients in the MPHD, TS, SGA, and ISS diagnostic categories, regression analysis was only performed for patients with GHD. The curves presented were built using polynomial regression. The quadratic polynomial regression, under the assumption that the height SD is not a function of baseline age, provided a sufficient fitting, while higher terms (for example, cubic and fourth degree) were not statistically significant.

Results
Baseline demographics
The ANSWER Program registry (as of November 30, 2009) contained information for over 9,000 patients, of which 1,002 GH treatment-naïve patients from selected diagnostic categories (GHD, MPHD, TS, SGA, and ISS) met the criteria for inclusion in this analysis. Baseline demographic characteristics for the subjects in this study by specific diagnostic category are summarized in Table 1. The study included longitudinal data for 698 patients with GHD, 71 with MPHD, 60 with TS, 50 with SGA, and 123 with ISS. Mean baseline ages were lower for MPHD (6.4 years), SGA (7.1 years), and TS (8.5 years) groups compared to those for GHD (10.9 years) or ISS (11.2 years). Baseline mean peak GH levels were lowest for patients with GHD and MPHD (5.5 and

Table 1 Baseline demographics by diagnostic category

	GHD		MPHD		Turner		SGA		ISS	
	n	Mean (SD)	n	Mean (SD)	n	Mean (SD)	n	Mean (SD)	n	Mean (SD)
Gender										
Male	543	-	53	-	0	-	33	-	91	-
Female	155	-	18	-	60	-	17	-	32	-
Age	698	10.9 (3.46)	71	6.4 (5.23)	60	8.5 (4.17)	50	7.1 (3.41)	123	11.2 (2.88)
HSDS	698	-2.2 (0.86)	71	-2.0 (1.36)	60	-2.5 (0.77)	50	-2.8 (0.97)	123	-2.3 (0.68)
IGF-I SDS	605	-2.5 (1.26)	31	-3.2 (1.54)	34	-2.0 (1.43)	32	-2.1 (1.53)	114	-2.2 (1.11)
BMI SDS	681	-0.1 (1.38)	49	0.5 (1.84)	55	0.5 (0.97)	49	-0.8 (1.35)	123	-0.8 (3.38)
Bone Age, yrs	616	9.4 (3.31)	39	8.0 (4.58)	43	7.8 (3.45)	44	6.1 (3.36)	115	9.7 (2.93)
Peak GH, ng/mL	606	5.5 (2.69)	40	3.6 (3.03)	5	12.5 (8.25)	17	13.8 (10.95)	97	15.2 (8.10)
GH dose, µg/kg/day	697	45.9 (10.1)	71	40.6 (11.2)	60	51.9 (9.0)	50	49.9 (13.5)	123	46.1 (8.6)

BMI, body mass index; GH, growth hormone; GHD, growth hormone deficiency; HSDS, height standard deviation score; IGF-I, insulin-like growth factor I; ISS, idiopathic short stature; MPHD, multiple pituitary hormone deficiency; SD, standard deviation; SDS, standard deviation score; SGA, small for gestational age

3.6 ng/mL, respectively). Baseline mean GH dose (µg/kg/day) for the different diagnostic categories was the lowest for MPHD patients, consistent with their apparently greater degree of GH deficiency and associated GH sensitivity. For all diagnostic categories, the mean and median GH dose did not increase more than 0.007 mg/kg/day over the two years, indicating a very narrow GH dose change over this period.

Height outcomes

The effects of GH treatment on ΔHSDS over 2 years of treatment are shown in Table 2. Gradual increases in ΔHSDS were observed over time and ranged between 0.15 (ISS) to 0.37 (MPHD) at 4 months, and 0.82 (TS) to 1.20 (MPHD) at 2 years, with the largest ΔHSDS observed at year 1 and year 2 in patients with MPHD and SGA. Annualized HV at 4 months was 13.6 cm/year for MPHD, and between 8.33 (TS) and 9.96 (SGA) cm/year for the other indications (Figure 1). Within each diagnostic category, mean annualized HV was the greater during the first year, and generally decreased during the second year. Mean annualized HV at 1 year was greatest for MPHD at 10.74 cm/year, and ranged between 7.97 (TS) and 9.57 (GHD) for the other indications.

Regression analysis

Linear regression was performed on HSDS data for patients with GHD (Table 3). Variables significantly associated with ΔHSDS 1 and 2 years included HV at 4 months, and baseline age, HSDS, BMI SDS, and IGF-I SDS. The ranking of importance of predictive factors as related to ΔHSDS (as determined by the F value, the higher the more influential) was as follows: HV at 4 months > baseline age > baseline HSDS > baseline BMI SDS > baseline IGF-I SDS. HV at 4 months and baseline BMI SDS were positively correlated with ΔHSDS, while

baseline age, HSDS, and IGF-I SDS were negatively correlated with ΔHSDS. Gender was less influential than the above factors (Table 3) and was not detected as statistically significant in this analysis.

Table 2 HSDS and ΔHSDS by diagnostic category

	HSDS		ΔHSDS	
	n	Mean (SD)	n	Mean (SD)
GHD				
Baseline	698	-2.22 (0.86)	-	-
4 Months	698	-2.03 (0.82)	698	0.19 (0.33)
Year 1	698	-1.61 (0.83)	698	0.61 (0.49)
Year 2	697	-1.17 (0.88)	697	1.06 (0.64)
MPHD				
Baseline	71	-1.98 (1.36)	-	-
4 Months	70	-1.62 (1.30)	70	0.37 (0.68)
Year 1	70	-1.13 (1.04)	70	0.85 (0.76)
Year 2	70	-0.79 (1.04)	70	1.20 (1.04)
Turner				
Baseline	60	-2.49 (0.77)	-	-
4 Months	59	-2.32 (0.82)	59	0.18 (0.20)
Year 1	60	-1.99 (0.86)	60	0.50 (0.31)
Year 2	60	-1.68 (0.90)	60	0.82 (0.43)
SGA				
Baseline	50	-2.76 (0.97)	-	-
4 Months	50	-2.48 (0.88)	50	0.28 (0.47)
Year 1	50	-1.96 (0.93)	50	0.80 (0.59)
Year 2	50	-1.59 (1.00)	50	1.18 (0.65)
ISS				
Baseline	123	-2.31 (0.68)	-	-
4 Months	123	-2.16 (0.69)	123	0.15 (0.19)
Year 1	123	-1.77 (0.69)	123	0.54 (0.38)
Year 2	123	-1.41 (0.79)	123	0.90 (0.59)

GHD, growth hormone deficiency; HSDS, height standard deviation score; ISS, idiopathic short stature; MPHD, multiple pituitary hormone deficiency; SD, standard deviation; SGA, small for gestational age.

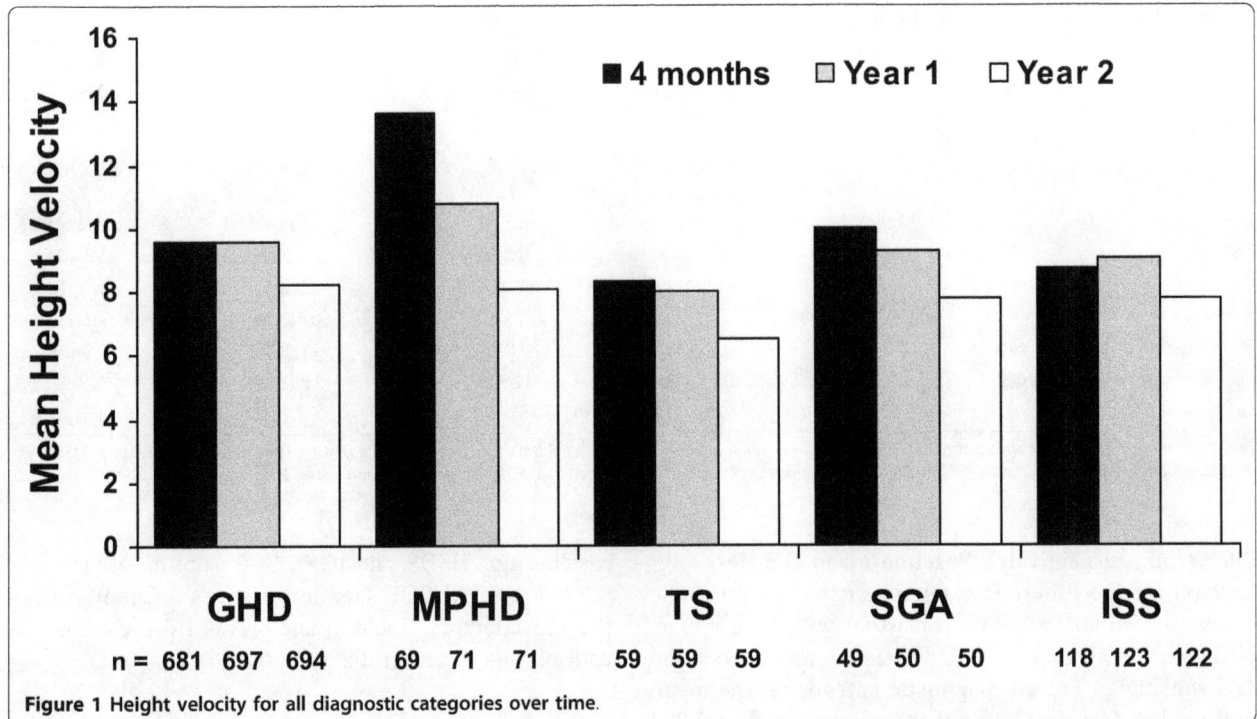

Figure 1 Height velocity for all diagnostic categories over time.

Analysis of the mean values was used to build smoothed curves for demonstration of the relationship between first-year ΔHSDS and baseline age (Figure 2A and 2B), and between first-year HV and baseline age (Figure 2C and 2D) in male and female patients with GHD. Generally, the curves demonstrate that younger baseline age is associated with greater ΔHSDS and HV in these patients. Similar curves were observed with male and female patients for both ΔHSDS and first-year HV.

Discussion
In this longitudinal study of GH treatment in patients with GHD, MPHD, TS, SGA, and ISS, HSDS improved over time. For patients with GHD, several variables were identified that correlated with growth response during the first and second years of GH treatment. HV at 4

Table 3 Regression model for longitudinal ΔHSDS at year 1 and year 2 for patients with GHD (n = 698).

Characteristic	β Estimate	F Value	P Value
Height velocity at 4 months	0.0319	214.31	< .0001
Baseline age	-0.0439	74.17	< .0001
Baseline HSDS	-0.0776	29.11	< .0001
Baseline BMI SDS	0.0398	20.62	< .0001
Baseline IGF-I SDS	-0.0245	5.74	.0169
Gender	-0.0438	2.46	.1175

BMI, body mass index; GHD, growth hormone deficiency; HSDS, height standard deviation score; IGF-I, insulin-like growth factor I; SDS, standard deviation score.

months was the most significant predictor of ΔHSDS observed in the first 2 years of GH treatment. This observation that 4-month HV was such a strong predictor is a novel finding, since many studies do not consistently report growth this early in the treatment cycle. Additional factors that were influential in predicting HSDS outcomes were ranked in order of importance: younger baseline age > lower baseline HSDS > higher baseline BMI SDS > lower baseline IGF-I SDS.

For the GHD patient population, age and baseline HSDS were important determinants of the response to GH treatment, as previously demonstrated [18,20]. However, other reports have also indicated additional significant factors, such as birth weight SDS and GH dose [20]. The present results also indicated that higher baseline BMI was positively correlated with the growth response to GH for patients with GHD. Birth weight SDS and weight SDS were shown to be correlated with growth response to GH in the Pharmacia Kabi International Growth Study, suggesting that the heavier the child was, the greater the expected growth response to GH treatment [20]. The impact of BMI in this study might reflect, at least in part, the importance of nutrition for optimization of outcomes in patients receiving GH [1,33].

In general, the results from this analysis are consistent with previously published results for specific patient populations. A prior prediction study in patients with TS indicated that first-year growth response to GH was

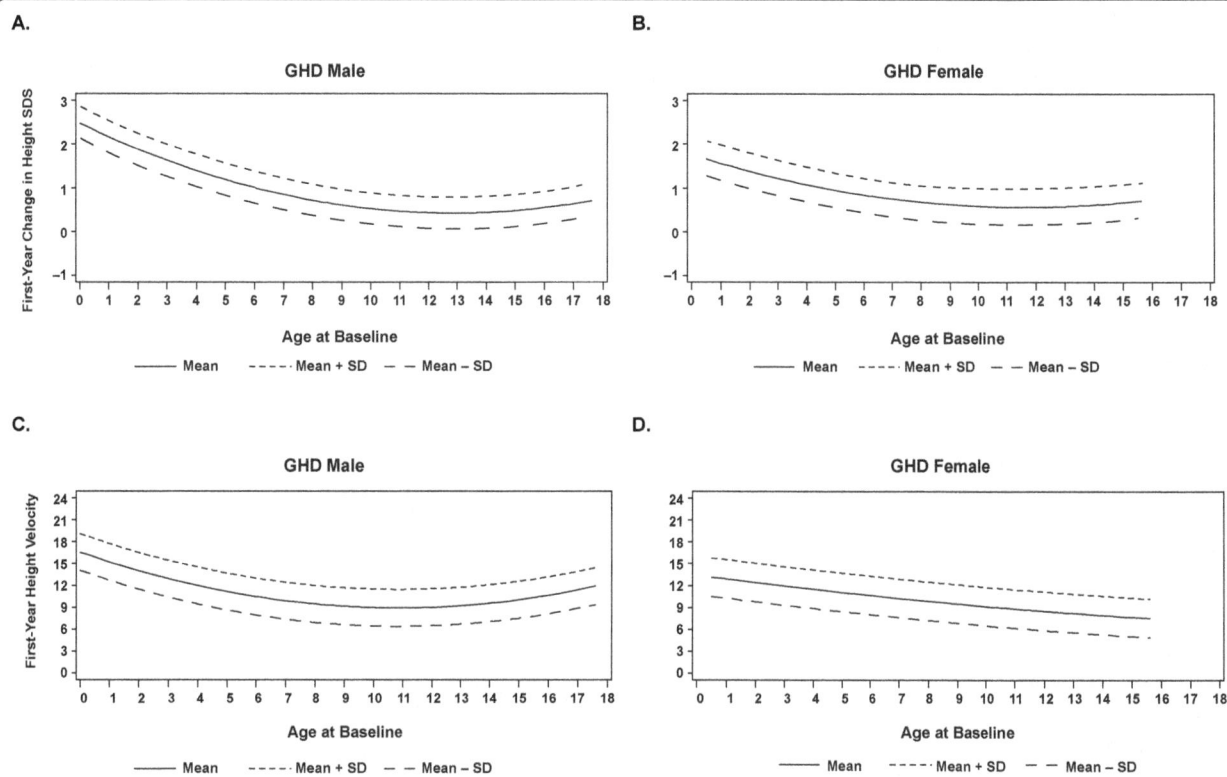

Figure 2 First-year change from baseline HSDS and height velocity vs baseline age for patients with GHD (A, Change in baseline HSDS in male patients with GHD; B, Change in baseline HSDS in female patients with GHD; C, Change in height velocity in male patients with GHD; D, Change in height velocity in female patients with GHD).

significantly influenced by weekly GH dose, chronological age, HSDS, body weight SDS, number of GH injections per week, and adjunctive oxandrolone treatment [26]. Predictors of the growth response over a longer duration of treatment (2-4 years) included HV during previous years, weekly GH dose, weight SDS, age, and oxandrolone treatment [26]. In SGA patients, results from one study found that first-year growth response to GH treatment was the most important predictor of second-year growth response [21]. Other variables that were significantly correlated with the growth response to GH included GH dose, weight and age at the start of treatment, and midparental HSDS [21]. Studies in the ISS patient population have identified additional factors as predictors of longer-term responses to GH, including baseline HSDS, GH dose, weight at the start of treatment, and first-year growth response [13,14]. It is important to recognize that this category may be the most heterogenous, with growth failure being a consequence of many different etiologies.

Specific results from other studies that are consistent with the present analysis, include the lack of gender effect on response to GH treatment. Analysis of results from the Pfizer Kabi International Growth Study database found no significant gender-related differences in

effects of GH in HV or HSDS over 2 or 3 years of treatment [34]. In 8,018 patients with ISS in the National Cooperative Growth Study there was no significant effect of gender on first-year HV or first-year change from baseline in height SDS [35]. In a recent report, a large cohort of male and female patients with GHD, MPHD, TS, SGA, NS, and ISS from the ANSWER Program registry was used to assess gender-related differences in ΔHSDS following 2 years of GH treatment. Results demonstrated increased ΔHSDS in all patients, however, clinically relevant gender differences were not observed [36]. The importance of early timing for initiation of treatment from the present analysis is also consistent with previous findings. A National Registry of Growth Hormone Treatment report in the Netherlands that included 342 patients (diagnosis of GHD or a maximal GH response during provocation tests of less than 11 ng/mL) indicated that initiation of treatment before puberty resulted in a change from baseline in HSDS of 0.71 vs 0.58 for those who initiated treatment after puberty [19]. Results from the French registry of 2,852 patients with idiopathic GHD also indicated that prepubertal initiation of GH treatment was associated with significantly greater adult height gain [37]. Although in this study it is not known what proportion of patients across the different diagnostic categories may have been in puberty, the mean baseline chronological and bone ages are consistent with the majority of patients being prepubertal, and this likely lessens the impact of puberty on the observed growth responses.

The different correlations between baseline age, HSDS, BMI SDS, and IGF-I SDS, with growth response over 2 years of treatment with GH, carry implications for clinical practice. The correlation of baseline age with ΔHSDS and HV in the patients with GHD further support the initiation of GH at as young an age as possible to promote optimal growth. This concept is supported by results from another study that demonstrated a relationship between baseline age and first-year HV for patients with GHD, MPHD, and TS [15]. Several consensus statements endorse the use of GH treatment as soon as a diagnosis is made or growth failure is demonstrated for patients from several diagnostic categories [38-41]. The inverse relationship observed between baseline IGF-I and the two-year change in HSDS is consistent with an increased sensitivity to the effects of GH in patients who have a greater degree of GHD. In this non-interventional observational study, serum IGF-I was measured at a number of commercial laboratories reflecting routine clinical practice. IGF-I SDS was calculated using one formula which provided consistency to the analysis. This is also reflected in the finding that mean baseline IGF-I SDS in both the GHD and MPHD populations was lower than that observed in non-GHD patients. The positive correlation observed between baseline BMI SDS and ΔHSDS may emphasize the importance of nutrition in patients with growth failure [33,40]. An abnormally low BMI in pediatric patients may be a sign of malnutrition, which can also be associated with growth disturbances. In the end, the role of baseline age, HSDS, BMI SDS, and IGF-I SDS in the response of individual patients to GH therapy should all be considered for optimal management of short stature or growth failure.

Conclusion
The present results from a large patient cohort enrolled in the ANSWER Program registry demonstrate gradual increases in ΔHSDS over time for all diagnostic categories. For patients with GHD, greater HV at 4 months is the most significant predictor of ΔHSDS over the first 2 years of GH treatment, while gender did not have any influence.

Acknowledgements
The authors would like to thank Bob Rhoads, PhD and Jennifer R. Kent, PhD, of MedVal Scientific Information Services, LLC, for providing writing and editorial assistance. Funding to support the preparation of this manuscript was provided by Novo Nordisk, Inc. Data from this paper were presented at the 49th Annual Meeting of the European Society for Paediatric Endocrinology (ESPE) in Prague, Czech Republic, 22-25 September 2010.

Author details
[1]Department of Pediatrics, Milton S. Hershey Medical Center, Penn State College of Medicine, Hershey, PA, USA. [2]Novo Nordisk Inc, Princeton, NJ, USA. [3]Department of Pediatrics, Thomas Jefferson University duPont Hospital for Children, Philadelphia, PA, USA.

Authors' contributions
All authors contributed equally to this work and were involved in determining the study concept and design as well as providing data analysis and interpretation. RG and JG provided access to the registry data. NK performed the regression analysis. At all stages, the authors discussed the results and implications of the data and commented on the manuscript. All authors read and approved the final manuscript."

Competing interests
PAL is a consultant for Abbott and Novo Nordisk, and has received clinical study support from Abbott, Novo Nordisk, Eli Lilly, Pfizer, and Ipsen. JR is a consultant for Novo Nordisk and Eli Lilly, and has received clinical study support from Novo Nordisk, Eli Lilly, and Pfizer. JG, RG, and NK are employees of Novo Nordisk.

References
1. Grumbach MM, Bin-Abbas BS, Kaplan SL: The growth hormone cascade: progress and long-term results of growth hormone treatment in growth hormone deficiency. Horm Res 1998, 49(suppl 2):41-57.
2. Mazzanti L, Tamburrino F, Bergamaschi R, Scarano E, Montanari F, Torella M, Ballarini E, Cicognani A: Developmental syndromes: growth hormone deficiency and treatment. Endocr Dev 2009, 14:114-134.
3. Harris M, Hofman PL, Cutfield WS: Growth hormone treatment in children: review of safety and efficacy. Paediatr Drugs 2004, 6:93-106.
4. Richmond E, Rogol AD: Current indications for growth hormone therapy for children and adolescents. Endocr Dev 2010, 18:92-108.
5. Bryant J, Baxter L, Cave CB, Milne R: Recombinant growth hormone for idiopathic short stature in children and adolescents. Cochrane Database Syst Rev 2007, CD004440.
6. Baxter L, Bryant J, Cave CB, Milne R: Recombinant growth hormone for children and adolescents with Turner syndrome. Cochrane Database Syst Rev 2007, CD003887.
7. Maiorana A, Cianfarani S: Impact of growth hormone therapy on adult height of children born small for gestational age. Pediatrics 2009, 124: e519-e531.
8. Crabbe R, von HM, Engrand P, Chatelain P: Recombinant human growth hormone for children born small for gestational age: meta-analysis confirms the consistent dose-effect relationship on catch-up growth. J Endocrinol Invest 2008, 31:346-351.
9. Pasquino AM, Passeri F, Municchi G, Segni M, Pucarelli I, Larizza D, Bossi G, Severi F, Galasso C: Final height in Turner syndrome patients treated with growth hormone. Horm Res 1996, 46:269-272.
10. Ranke MB, Lindberg A, KIGS International Board: Height at start, first-year growth response and cause of shortness at birth are major determinants of adult height outcomes of short children born small for gestational age and Silver-Russell syndrome treated with growth hormone: analysis of data from KIGS. Horm Res Paediatr 2010, 74:259-266.
11. Sas TC, de Ridder MA, Wit JM, Rotteveel J, Oostdijk W, Reeser HM, Otten BJ, de Muinck Keizer-Schrama SM: Adult height in children with growth hormone deficiency: a randomized, controlled, growth hormone dose-response trial. Horm Res Paediatr 2010, 74:172-181.
12. Hintz RL: Growth hormone treatment of idiopathic short stature: clinical studies. Growth Horm IGF Res 2005, 15(suppl A):S6-S8.
13. Zucchini S: Growth hormone use in the treatment of idiopathic short stature. Curr Opin Invest Drugs 2008, 9:396-401.
14. Ranke MB, Lindberg A, Price DA, Darendeliler F, bertsson-Wikland K, Wilton P, Reiter EO: Age at growth hormone therapy start and first-year responsiveness to growth hormone are major determinants of height outcome in idiopathic short stature. Horm Res 2007, 68:53-62.

15. Bakker B, Frane J, Anhalt H, Lippe B, Rosenfeld RG: Height velocity targets from the national cooperative growth study for first-year growth hormone responses in short children. *J Clin Endocrinol Metab* 2008, 93:352-357.

16. Lechuga-Sancho A, Lechuga-Campoy JL, del Valle-Nunez J, Rivas-Crespo F: Predicting the growth response of children with idiopathic growth hormone deficiency to one year of recombinant growth hormone treatment: derivation and validation of a useful method. *J Pediatr Endocrinol Metab* 2009, 22:501-509.

17. Land C, Blum WF, Shavrikova E, Kloeckner K, Stabrey A, Schoenau E: Predicting the growth response to growth hormone (GH) treatment in prepubertal and pubertal children with isolated GH deficiency-model validation in an observational setting (GeNeSIS). *J Pediatr Endocrinol Metab* 2007, 20:685-693.

18. Sudfeld H, Kiese K, Heinecke A, Bramswig JH: Prediction of growth response in prepubertal children treated with growth hormone for idiopathic growth hormone deficiency. *Acta Paediatr* 2000, 89:34-37.

19. de Ridder MA, Stijnen T, Hokken-Koelega AC: Prediction of adult height in growth-hormone-treated children with growth hormone deficiency. *J Clin Endocrinol Metab* 2007, 92:925-931.

20. Ranke MB, Lindberg A, Chatelain P, Wilton P, Cutfield W, bertsson-Wikland K, Price DA: Derivation and validation of a mathematical model for predicting the response to exogenous recombinant human growth hormone (GH) in prepubertal children with idiopathic GH deficiency. KIGS International Board. Kabi Pharmacia International Growth Study. *J Clin Endocrinol Metab* 1999, 84:1174-1183.

21. Ranke MB, Lindberg A, Cowell CT, Wikland KA, Reiter EO, Wilton P, Price DA: Prediction of response to growth hormone treatment in short children born small for gestational age: analysis of data from KIGS (Pharmacia International Growth Database). *J Clin Endocrinol Metab* 2003, 88:125-131.

22. de Zegher F, Albertsson-Wikland K, Wollmann HA, Chatelain P, Chaussain JL, Lofstrom A, Jonsson B, Rosenfeld RG: Growth hormone treatment of short children born small for gestational age: growth responses with continuous and discontinuous regimens over 6 years. *J Clin Endocrinol Metab* 2000, 85:2816-2821.

23. Dahlgren J, Kristrom B, Niklasson A, Nierop AF, Rosberg S, Albertsson-Wikland K: Models predicting the growth response to growth hormone treatment in short children independent of GH status, birth size and gestational age. *BMC Med Inform Decis Mak* 2007, 7:40.

24. Mehls O, Lindberg A, Nissel R, Haffner D, Hokken-Koelega A, Ranke MB: Predicting the response to growth hormone treatment in short children with chronic kidney disease. *J Clin Endocrinol Metab* 2010, 95:686-692.

25. Spagnoli A, Spadoni GL, Boscherini B: Preliminary validation of a prediction model for the short-term growth response to growth hormone therapy in children with idiopathic short stature. *Acta Paediatr Suppl* 1996, 417:66-68.

26. Ranke MB, Lindberg A, Chatelain P, Wilton P, Cutfield W, bertsson-Wikland K, Price DA: Prediction of long-term response to recombinant human growth hormone in Turner syndrome: development and validation of mathematical models. KIGS International Board. Kabi International Growth Study. *J Clin Endocrinol Metab* 2000, 85:4212-4218.

27. Ranke MB: New paradigms for growth hormone treatment in the 21st century: prediction models. *J Pediatr Endocrinol Metab* 2000, 13(suppl 6):1365-1369.

28. Ranke MB, Lindberg A: Observed and predicted growth responses in prepubertal children with growth disorders: guidance of growth hormone treatment by empirical variables. *J Clin Endocrinol Metab* 2010, 95:1229-1237.

29. Geffner ME, Dunger DB: Future directions: growth prediction models. *Horm Res* 2007, 68(suppl 5):51-56.

30. Ranke MB, Lindberg A: Predicting growth in response to growth hormone treatment. *Growth Horm IGF Res* 2009, 19:1-11.

31. Novo Nordisk: Norditropin cartridges (somatropin [rDNA origin] injection) for subcutaneous use [prescribing information]. Princeton, NJ; 2010.

32. US Centers for Disease Control and Prevention: Percentile data files with LMS values.[http://www.cdc.gov/growthcharts/percentile_data_files.htm].

33. Farber RS, Kerrigan JR: The multiple indications for growth hormone treatment of pediatric patients. *Pediatr Ann* 2006, 35:926-932.

34. Rose SR, Shulman DI, Larsson P, Wakley LR, Wills S, Bakker B: Gender does not influence prepubertal growth velocity during standard growth hormone therapy-analysis of United States KIGS data. *J Pediatr Endocrinol Metab* 2005, 18:1045-1051.

35. Kemp SF, Kuntze J, Attie KM, Maneatis T, Butler S, Frane J, Lippe B: Efficacy and safety results of long-term growth hormone treatment of idiopathic short stature. *J Clin Endocrinol Metab* 2005, 90:5247-5253.

36. Ross J, Lee PA, Gut R, Germak J: Factors influencing the one- and two-year growth response in children treated with growth hormone: analysis from an observational study. *Int J Pediatr Endocrinol* 2010, 2010:494656.

37. Carel JC, Ecosse E, Nicolino M, Tauber M, Leger J, Cabrol S, Bastie-Sigeac I, Chaussain JL, Coste J: Adult height after long term treatment with recombinant growth hormone for idiopathic isolated growth hormone deficiency: observational follow up study of the French population based registry. *BMJ* 2002, 325:70.

38. Cohen P, Rogol AD, Deal CL, Saenger P, Reiter EO, Ross JL, Chernausek SD, Savage MO, Wit JM: Consensus statement on the diagnosis and treatment of children with idiopathic short stature: a summary of the Growth Hormone Research Society, the Lawson Wilkins Pediatric Endocrine Society, and the European Society for Paediatric Endocrinology Workshop. *J Clin Endocrinol Metab* 2008, 93:4210-4217.

39. Lee PA, Chernausek SD, Hokken-Koelega AC, Czernichow P: International Small for Gestational Age Advisory Board consensus development conference statement: management of short children born small for gestational age, April 24-October 1, 2001. *Pediatrics* 2003, 111:1253-1261.

40. Growth Hormone Research Society: Consensus guidelines for the diagnosis and treatment of growth hormone (GH) deficiency in childhood and adolescence: summary statement of the GH Research Society. GH Research Society. *J Clin Endocrinol Metab* 2000, 85:3990-3993.

41. Bondy CA: Care of girls and women with Turner syndrome: A guideline of the Turner Syndrome Study Group. *J Clin Endocrinol Metab* 2007, 92:10-25.

2

Hormonal profile and androgen receptor study in prepubertal girls with hypertrichosis

Maria Isabel Hernandez[1]*, Andrea Castro[1], Ketty Bacallao[1], Alejandra Avila[1,2], Aníbal Espinoza[3], Leon Trejo[1], Germán Iñiguez[1], Ethel Codner[1] and Fernando Cassorla[1]

Abstract

Background: Prepubertal hypertrichosis is a reportedly benign condition characterized by an excessive growth of vellous hair in non-androgen dependent areas of the body compared to the amount usually present in normal subjects of the same age, race and sex. Although this condition is usually considered idiopathic and regarded as benign, it may be very disturbing cosmetically, causing significant patient and parental anxiety.

Method: We performed a hormonal and androgen receptor study in 42 prepubertal girls with hypertrichosis and 29 control girls from 2 to 8 years of age. Both groups underwent a determination of basal LH, FSH, 17OH progesterone, androstenedione, testosterone, estradiol and SHBG, abdominal ultrasound to assess ovarian morphology, and the number of androgen receptor CAG/GGC repeats in DNA obtained from peripheral leukocytes.

Results: The hypertrichosis score was higher in the cases compared to controls. Serum gonadotropins and sex steroids were similar in both groups, but SHBG was significantly lower in the girls with hypertrichosis (71.1 ± 2.9 vs 81.9 ± 3.0 nmol/L, $p < 0.02$). The distribution of shorter, larger and total alleles was not statistically different between cases and controls. The combined analysis of CAG/GGC, however, showed a significantly higher prevalence of the most androgen-sensitive haplotypes (1–2: <22CAG + 17/17GGC- < 14CAG + 17/18GGC) in girls with hypertrichosis compared to controls.

Conclusions: We conclude that girls with hypertrychosis exhibit AR(s) with enhanced sensitivity, which may facilitate the growth of their body hair.

Keywords: Hypertricosis, Prepubertal girls, Androgen receptor, Body hair, Androgen metabolism

Introduction

Prepubertal hypertrichosis is a reportedly benign condition characterized by an excessive growth of vellous hair in non-androgen dependent areas of the body compared to the amount usually present in normal subjects of the same age, race and sex [1]. Characteristically, the hair in subjects with hypertrichosis usually grows on the trunk, arms and legs. This form of hypertrichosis was described by Barth et al. in 1988 [2], and differs from universal congenital hypertrichosis [3,4] and hypertrichosis laguginosa [5]. Although this condition is usually considered idiopathic and regarded as benign, it may be very disturbing cosmetically, causing significant patient and parental anxiety. In addition, hypertrichosis may be associated with metabolic or genetic disorders, and with the use of drugs [6-11].

Studies concerning the hormonal profile of subjects with hypertrichosis are relatively few and difficult to compare, due to the various definitions of this condition. In addition, the investigation of androgen metabolism has not shown significant differences between girls with hypertrichosis and controls [12,13].

The human androgen receptor (AR) is the main regulator of androgen signaling in the cell [14] and is encoded by the AR gene encoded in the X-chromosome [15]. The transactivator domain of the AR protein contains two polymorphic trinucleotide repeats segments that encode poly -glutamine $(CAG)_n$ and –glycine $(GGN)_n$ tracts within exon 1. There are considerable data linking the length of CAG repeats to androgen sensitivity *in vivo* as well as *in vitro*, that suggests

* Correspondence: mihernandezc@gmail.com
[1]Institute of Maternal and Child Research (IDIMI), Faculty of Medicine, University of Chile, Santa Rosa 1234, 2nd floor IDIMI, Casilla, 226-3 Santiago, Chile
Full list of author information is available at the end of the article

an inverse relationship between length repeats and androgen receptor sensitivity [16]. In the case of GGC, AR with repeats number other than 17 GGC(23GGN), exhibit lower transactivation in response to androgens, suggesting a relationship between repeat lengths and AR function [16].

The aim of our study was to evaluate the clinical and hormonal characteristics of a large group of girls with hypertrichosis, and to assess the number of CAG and GGC repeats in their androgen receptor gene.

Subjects and methods

Subjects

A group of 42 prepubertal girls with hypertrichosis was recruited from our endocrine clinic, and matched by age with a group of 29 prepubertal control girls without hypertrichosis. The age of both groups of girls ranged between 2 to 8 years. Exclusion criteria were: 1) Any clinical sign of puberty according to Marshall and Tanner stages, ultrasonography or hormonal profile. 2) Chronic disease (including congenital adrenal hyperplasia) 3) Medication that could induce hypertrichosis or hyperandrogenism. 4) Low birth weight and 5) Maternal history of polycystic ovary syndrome.

Study protocol

After an overnight fast, all girls were evaluated at the Institute of Maternal and Child Research of the University of Chile. The patients and control girls underwent a careful physical examination performed by a single pediatric endocrinologist (MIH), to determine their hypertrichosis score according to Gryngarten et al. [13]. As indicated by this author, a score above 7 was considered positive for hypertrichosis.

Height was measured using a Harpenden stadiometer (Holtain, UK). Weight was measured using a manual scale with a 10-g gradation (Seca; Quickmedical, Snoqualme,WA). All the measurements were expressed as SDS for chronological age.

We obtained a hand x-ray to determine the bone age according to the method of Greulich and Pyle [17]. This determination was performed by a single observer (AE), who was blinded to the condition of the girls. A transabdominal ultrasound was performed by a single ultrasonographist (AE) with a 5-MHz transducer in Sonoace 6000C equipment (Madison Co., Seoul, Korea). Ovarian volume was calculated using the simplified formula for a prolate ellipsoid [18] and we determined the number of follicles in each ovary.

Basal levels of androstenedione, FSH, LH, estradiol, testosterone, 17 hydroxyprogesterone (17OH Prog), SHBG, antimullerian hormone (AMH) and inhibin-B were obtained and measured in a fasting sample at 8:00 AM. SHBG and testosterone were used to calculate the free androgen index (FAI), as previously reported [19].

Hormone assays

Serum testosterone, androstenedione, 17OH Prog, DHEA-S and estradiol were determined by competitive specific binding RIA, and serum LH, FSH, and SHBG were measured by immunoradiometric assays. All kits were supplied by Diagnostic System Laboratories (Webster, TX). Intra-assay coefficients of variation were 5.1% for testosterone, 3.2% for androstenedione, 4.2% for 17-OH Prog, 3.5% for DHEA-S, 4,1% for estradiol, 6.5% for LH, 3.6% for FSH, and 3.9% for SHBG. Interassay coefficients of variation were 6.4% for testosterone, 6.1% for androstenedione, 5.5% for 17-OH Prog, 5.1% for DHEA-S, 6.7% for estradiol, 7.6% for LH, 6.2% for FSH, and 6.9% for SHBG. Serum AMH was assayed using the AMH/MIS ELISA kit (Immunotech-Beckman, Marseilles, France). The AMH assay had a sensitivity of 0.7 pmol/L, and intra- and interassay coefficients of variation of 5.3% and 8.7% respectively. Serum inhibin B was measured using specific two-site ELISAs (Diagnostic Systems Labs, Webster TX). The assay sensitivity was 7 pg/mL, and intra- and inter-assay coefficients of variation were 4.8% and 7.1% respectively.

Determination of CAG and GGC repeats

Genomic DNA was extracted from peripheral blood lymphocytes using a DNA blood Wizard kit. The AR exon 1 region encoding the polyglutamine repeat was amplified using PCR. To determine the length of the CAG and GGC repeats, we amplified the corresponding regions located on exon 1 of the AR gene (Genebank accession n° AL049564) using a pair of primers whose sequence has been previously reported [20,21]. One primer from each pair was marked with fluorescent dye (FAM or NED). Amplification was performed in a 15 μL reaction volume, containing 150 ng of DNA, 200 M of each deoxynucleotide triphosphate (Invitrogen, USA), 1X Mg^{2+}-free DyNAzime EXT Buffer (FINNZYMES OY, Finland), 8% DMSO (FINNZYMES OY, Finland), 2.5 mM $MgCl_2$ (FINNZYMES OY, Finland), 1 μM of GGC or CAG primers and 0.6 U of DyNAzime EXT DNA polymerase (FINNZYMES OY, Finland). PCR conditions for CAG were: 35 cycles of 95°C for 45 sec, 60°C for 45 sec, and 72°C for 1 min. PCR conditions for CGC were: 30 cycles of 95°C for 1 min, 55°C for 2 min, and 72°C for 2 min. PCR for CAG and GGC were initiated with a denaturation step of 95°C for 5 min, and terminated with an extension step at 72°C for 10 or 5 min, respectively.

PCR fragments separation of PCR product were performed by automated capillary electrophoresis, using an ABI PRISM 310 Genetic Analyzer (Applied Biosystems), and the length was determined with Genemapper Analysis Software (version V.3.2) (Applied Biosystems). 2 μL of the PCR product was mixed with 10 μL of formamide and 0.3 μL of GeneScan ROX-500 Size Standard (Applied

Biosystems, USA CA), denatured at 98°C for 5 min. and cooled on ice.

The fragments size were compared in each capillary electrophoresis with PCR products obtained from men whose repeat lengths were known (standard automated sequencing, Macrogen Inc, Korea) in a single and pooled forms for CAG (13, 14, 17, 18, 19, 21, 22, 23, 24, 25, 28) and GGC (9, 13, 14, 17, 18). Standard automated sequencing was performed using two different amplicons that contained CAG or GGC repeats. The CAG and GGC amplicons were obtained after PCR reactions with CAG (A0 and A5) and GGC pair of primers (A3n and A10) as previously described [22]. Amplification was performed in a 25 L reaction volume, containing 150 ng of DNA, 200 M of each deoxynucleotide triphosphate (Invitrogen, USA), 1X Optimized DyNAzime EXT Buffer (FINNZYMES OY, Finland), 8% DMSO (FINNZYMES OY, Finland), 0.3 µM of each one sense or antisense primer and 1 U of DyNAzime EXT DNA polymerase (FINNZYMES OY, Finland). Both PCR reactions were performed under the same conditions: 37 cycles of 94°C for 1 min, 58°C for 1 min and 72°C for 1 min; initiated with a denaturation step of 94°C for 3 min, and terminated with an extension step at 72°C for 10 min.

The protocol was approved by the Institutional Review Boards of the Hospital San Borja Arriaran and the Faculty of Medicine, University of Chile. All parents signed an informed consent at the beginning of the study.

Statistical analysis

Results are expressed as mean ± SD. Statistical analysis was performed using SPSS 10.0 for Windows (SPSS Inc., Chicago, IL). Normality of variables was assessed using the Kolmogorov-Smirnov test. Differences between girls with hypertrichosis and control girls were assessed by the Kruskall-Wallis or the Mann–Whitney test for nonparametric variables. To compare the number of CAG and GGC repeats in short, large and total alleles between girls with hipertrichosis and control girls we used the chisquare test. $P < 0.05$ was considered statistically significant.

Results

Hypertrichosis score and general assessment

The mean hypertrichosis score in the control group was 3 ± 2 and, as expected, none of these girls expressed concern about their body hair. The mean score observed in the girls with hypertrichosis was 16 ± 7, which was significantly higher compared to the control group (Table 1). The girls with hypertrichosis had long and dense vellous hair covering mainly the trunk, sacrum, upper and lower limbs, exceeding what is commonly observed in our population of prepubertal girls.

The mean chronological and bone age was similar in the girls with hypertrichosis and the control group, as

Table 1 Baseline characteristics of cases and controls

	Cases	Controls
Age (yrs)	6 ± 2	6 ± 2
Bone Age (yrs)	5.5 ± 0.3	6.7 ± 0.4
Hypertrichosis score	**16 ± 4**	**3 ± 2****
BMI (k/m²) SDS	1 ± 0.1	0.9 ± 0.3
Follicle number per ovary	4.8 ± 2.4	3.7 ± 1.3

mean ± SD; Kruskall-Wallis test **P < 0.01 cases vs controls.

shown in Table 1. Their weight and BMI were also comparable (Table 1).

Ultrasound study

We did not find any differences in uterine or ovarian size between both groups of girls. The number of follicles per ovary, however, was higher in girls with hypertrichosis compared with controls (4.8 ± 0.5 vs 3.7 ± 0.3, p < 0.05) (Table 1).

Hormone assays

Basal serum levels of LH, FSH and estradiol levels were similar in both groups of girls, and in the range usually observed in prepubertal girls. Basal DHEA-S, 17OH progesterone, androstenedione, inhibin-B and AMH were similar in both groups, and 17 OH progesterone and androstenedione. Interestingly, girls with hypertrichosis had significantly lower levels of SHBG than control girls (71.16 ± 16 vs 82 ± 15, p < 0.05). We did not observe statistically significant differences in the free androgen index between both groups of girls (0.83 ± 0.67 vs 0.62 ± 0.36 in hypertrichosis vs controls, p = NS) (Table 2).

CAG repeats analysis

The mean number of CAG repeats was 17.5 ± 3.1 vs 17.4 ± 3.0 in girls with hypertrichosis and control girls respectively, which was within the normal range observed in the general population [23,24]. Allele distribution for CAG repeats length was homozygous in 5 and

Table 2 Hormonal profile of cases and controls

	Cases	Controls
Testosterone (ng/mL)	0.14 ± 0.06	0.14 ± 0.06
Androstenedione (ng/mL)	0.3 ± 0.4	0.2 ± 0.2
DHEAS (ng/mL)	116 ± 162	96 ± 84
SHBG (nmol/L)	**71 ± 16**	**82 ± 15***
Free androgen index	0.83 ± 0.67	0.62 ± 0.36
Estradiol (pg/mL)	7.85 ± 5.0	8.2 ± 4.5
Inhibin (pg/mL)	16 ± 14	11 ± 4
AMH(pM)	23.4 ± 2.0	29.6 ± 4.2
Insulin (uUI/ml)	5.9 ± 0.6	5.6 ± 0.1

mean ± SD; Kruskall-Wallis test *P < 0.05 cases vs controls.

7% of cases and control girls respectively, and heterozygous in 95% and 93% of cases and control girls respectively, not showing any differences between cases and controls.

GGC repeat analysis

The mean number of GGC repeats was not statistically significantly different between both groups (17.4 ± 1.1 vs 17.4 ± 0.61 in cases and controls respectively), and remained within the normal range for the general population [23,24]. Examination of the allele distribution did not reveal any difference in alleles with 17 or less repeats in the girls with hypertrichosis compared with controls. The GGC repeats length was homozygous in 70% and 69% of cases and controls, respectively, and heterozygous in 30% and 31% of cases and controls, respectively.

The combined analysis of CAG/GGC, however, showed a significantly higher prevalence of the most androgen-sensitive haplotypes (1–2: <22CAG + 17/17GGC - <14CAG + 17/18GGC) in the girls with hypertrichosis compared with controls (36% vs 14%, p < 0.05). Distribution of combination CAG/GGC haplotypes is shown in Table 3. In girls with the most androgen-sensitive haplotypes testosterone, DHEAS and androstenedione levels were significantly lower than in the girls with less sensitive haplotypes (p < 0.03).

The hormonal levels according to CAG/GGC haplotypes are shown in Table 4. We observed that girls with hypertrichosis who harbor haplotypes 3–5 have lower SHBG concentrations compared to controls with the same haplotype.

In contrast, we observed that cases with the haplotypes 1–2 have normal androgen levels.

Discussion

Prepubertal hypertrichosis is a poorly understood clinical entity which may cause significant patient and parental anxiety. In this study, we performed an assessment of ovarian function and androgen receptor repeat polymorphisms in a large group of carefully selected prepubertal

girls with this condition, which were compared with a group of control girls.

The limited data available regarding the androgen profile of girls with prepubertal hypertrichosis are somewhat controversial. Balducci and Toscano demonstrated elevated concentrations of serum dihydrotestosterone (DHT) in a small group of prepubertal girls with hypertrichosis compared with age-matched controls. These authors, however, did not observe a concomitant increase in the levels of the DHT metabolite 3α-androstanediol glucuronide [12]. Gryngarten et al. observed increased serum testosterone levels and FAI in a group of prepubertal girls with hypertricosis compared to controls. In addition, they observed a slight increase in 3α-androstanediol glucuronide concentrations in approximately half of their girls with hypertrichosis [13].

We evaluated 42 prepubertal girls with hypertrichosis that were matched with 29 control prepubertal girls. We did not observe any differences in the androgen profile of both groups, except for lower levels of SHBG in the girls with hypertrichosis, although FAI was not different. In addition, serum AMH levels and pelvic ultrasound were similar in both groups. We also performed an hormonal study in both groups of girls, but we did not observe any differences in the basal concentrations of gonadotropins or sex steroid concentrations.

The investigation of the androgen receptor repeat polymorphisms provided the most interesting results of this study. Androgen receptor CAG repeats usually range between 11 and 35, and a decreased CAG repeat number has been linked to an increased transcriptional response to androgens [25]. Van Nieuwerburgh et al. studied 97 oligo-anovulatory women with ultrasound features of PCOS, and observed that patients with a bi-allelic mean lower than 21 repeats had lower androgen levels, but more florid clinical evidence of acne and/or hirsutism [26]. Ibañez et al. observed that girls with precocious pubarche had shorter mean CAG repeats and a greater proportion of short alleles (20 repeats or less) compared to controls. They concluded that shorter androgen receptor CAG number is indicative of increased

Table 3 Distribution of combination CAG/GGC haplotypes

Hap N°	CAG/GGC haplotypes definition	Girls		Total
		Hypertrichosis	Controls	(n)
1	<22CAG + 17/17GGC	12 (28.6%)	4 (13.8%)	16
2	<14CAG + 17/18GGC	3 (7.1%)	0 (0%)	3
3	(≥18 and < 22)CAG + 17/18GGC	3 (7.1%)	6 (20.7%)	9
4	<22CAG + (<17 and/or >17)GGC	5 (11.9%)	6 (20.7%)	11
5	≥22/22CAG + (17 and/or 18)GGC	18 (42.9%)	13 (44.8%)	31
	Total (n)	41	29	70

One girl with hypertrichosis had a genotype: 20/27 CAG and 14/17 GGC and therefore did not classify in any of this haplotypes.
The prevalence of the most sensitive combinations (1 and 2) was significantly higher in girls with hypertrichosis than in controls (37.5% vs 13.8% P = 0.04 Chi^2 test).

Table 4 Hormonal levels according to CAG/GGC haplotypes

	Cases (n)		Controls (n)	
	Hap 1-2	Hap 3-5	Hap 1-2	Hap 3-6
Age (years)	5.9 ± 2.2 (13)	59 ± 1.(23)	7.0 ± 1 8 (4)	6.0 ± 1.5 (25)
Hypertrichosis score	16.0 ± 3.3 (13)&	17.1 ± 3.2 (23)&	1.8 ± 1.0 (4)	3.5 ± 2.0 (25)
Follicle number per ovary	4.9 ± 1.5 (9)	5.0 ± 3.0 (17)	3.3 ± 1.0 (3)	3.8 ± 1.4 (15)
LH (mUI/mL)	0.5 ± 0.4 (11)	0.4 ± 0.1 (19)&	0.5 ± 0.1 (4)	0.5 ± 0.2 (22)
FSH	2,0 ± 1.0 (11)	2.0 ± 1.1 (19)	2.4 ± 0.8 (4)	2.9 ± 3.2 (22)
Testosterone (ng/mL)	0.1 ± 0.06 (11)*	0.2 ± 0.06 (23)	02 ± 0.08 (4)	0.1 ± 0.06 (23)
Androstenedione (ng/mL)	0.2 ± 0.6 (11)*	0.4 ± 0.49 (20)	0.2 ± 0.08 (4)	0.2 ± 0.16 (22)
DHEAS (ng/mL)	38 ± 39 (11)*	161 ± 190 (22)	81 ± 82 (4)	98 ± 86 (23)
17OH progesterone (ng/mL)	0.5 ± 0.2 (12)	0.7 ±0.4 (20)	04 ± 0.15 (4)*	0.8 ± 0.5 (22)
Estradiol	8.74 ± 6.5 (11)	749 ± 4.2 (19)	7.45 ± 3.7 (4)	8.38 ± 4.7 (22)
SHBG (nmoL/L)	77.2 ± 16.7 (12)	68.2 ± 15.6 (19)&	79.3 ± 18 (4)	82.4 ± 15 (22)
FAI	0.54 ± 0.36 (11)	0.98 ± 0.77 (22)&	0.64 ± 0.18 (41)	0.62 ± 0.39 (23)
AMH (pmol/L)	41.6 ± 24.7 (12)*	23.8 ± 17.9 (20)	30.1 ± 5.9 (4)	22.4 ± 10.2 (22)
Inhibin B (pg/mL)	18.9±18 (12)&	14 ± 11 (20)	8.3 ± 3.3 (4)	12 ± 4.1 (22)

Values are mean ± DS. *P<0.03 hap 1–2 versus hap 3–6 in cases or controls; &P<0.05 cases vs controls. Krustal Wallis Test.

androgen sensitivity, and subsequent ovarian hyperandrogenism [27]. In addition, Vottero et al. reported a reduced androgen receptor gene methylation pattern, which was associated with the presence of shorter CAG repeats, in girls with precocious pubarche. This constellation of findings might lead to hypersensitivity of the hair follicles to androgens, and therefore to the premature development of pubic hair [28].

On the other hand, *in vitro* characterization has showed a higher transactivating capacity for GGN 23 allele (GGC 17), and GGN 27 or GGN 10, compared to GGN 24 with a constant CAG repeat number of CAG 22, in response to testosterone analogs (R1881) and 5-α dihydrotestosterone. In accordance with several reports, our GGC distribution showed that GGC 17 and GGC 18 were the most frequent alleles in our population.

In the present study we did not find differences in the mean number of CAG or GGC repeats. In order to investigate the combined contribution of the CAG and GGC alleles to androgen sensitivity, we performed a study of the joint distribution of these alleles. The combined analysis of CAG/GGC showed a significantly higher prevalence of the most androgen-sensitive combinations (<18 CAG + 17/17 GGC and <14 CAG + 17/18 GGC) in the girls with hypertrychosis. The normal androgen levels in haplotypes 1 and 2 indicates that they may develop hypertrichosis due to enhanced androgen receptor sensitivity. The higher AMH and inhibin B levels observed in these patients, suggests that they appear to have a higher number of small antral follicles, as observed in patients with PCO. In addition, the girls who harbored combinations 3 – 5 had lower SHBG

concentrations compared to controls. This hormonal pattern may lead to the development of hypertrichosis due to a higher free androgen index. The lower LH levels observed in these patients may be consequence of the central negative feedback by androgens.

Although it is known that analyzing blood DNA may not reflect target tissue AR sensitivity, we did not perform skin biopsies to study AR sensitivity due to ethical considerations.

Conclusions

In conclusion, we have studied the hormonal profile and androgen receptor polymorphisms in a group of prepubertal girls with hypertrichosis. Girls with hypertrichosis exhibited lower levels of SHBG, but had otherwise normal androgen levels. The association of GGC 17 + CAG < 18 repeats suggests that some girls with hypertrichosis may have androgen receptors with enhanced sensitivity, which may facilitate the growth of their body hair. In order to clarify the contribution of each androgen receptor repeat, it will be important to study the methylation of the androgen receptor in these patients.

Competing interests
The authors declare that they have no competing interests.

Authors' contributions
MIH: Conceived the study, participated in the design of the study, recruited the patients and controls, performed the physical examination, performed the statistical analysis and drafted the manuscript. AC: Participated in the determination of CAG and GGC repeats, molecular analysis and statistical analysis. KB: Participated in the determination of CAG and GGC repeats and molecular analysis. AA: Nurse who drew the blood samples. AE: Participated evaluating the bone age. LT: Participated performing the Ultrasound.

GI: Participated carried out the immunoassays and statistical analysis. EC: Participated in the design of the study. FC: Participated in the design of the study and helped to draft the manuscript. All the authors read an approved the final manuscript.

Acknowledgments
We want to thanks Drs Maria Eugenia Willshaw, Alex Passeron, Marta Arriaza and Vinka Giadrosich for referring patients for this study.
Supported in part by Fondecyt project n° 11121427.

Author details
[1]Institute of Maternal and Child Research (IDIMI), Faculty of Medicine, University of Chile, Santa Rosa 1234, 2nd floor IDIMI, Casilla, 226-3 Santiago, Chile. [2]Departments of Pediatrics, Hospital Clínico San Borja Arriarán, Santiago, Chile. [3]Department of Radiology, Hospital Clínico San Borja Arriarán, Santiago, Chile.

References
1. Beighton P: **Familial hypertrichosis cubiti: hairy elbows syndrome.** *J Med Genet* 1970, **7:**158–160.
2. Barth JH, Wilkinson JD, Dawber RP: **Prepubertal hypertrichosis: normal or abnormal?** *Arch Dis Child* 1988, **63:**666–668.
3. Baumeister FA, Egger J, Schildhauer MT, Stengel-Rutkowski S: **Ambras syndrome: delineation of a unique hypertrichosis universalis congenita and association with a balanced pericentric inversion(8)(p11.2; q22).** *Clin Genet* 1993, **44:**121–128.
4. Baumeister FA: **Differentiation of Ambras syndrome from Hypertrichosis Universalis.** *Clin Genet* 2000, **57:**157–158.
5. Beighton P: **Congenital hypertrichosis lanuginosa.** *Arch Dermatol* 1970, **101:**669–672.
6. Trüeb RM: **Causes and management of hypertrichosis.** *Am J Clin Dermatol* 2002, **3:**617–627.
7. Hassan G, Khalaf H, Mourad W: **Dermatologic complications after liver transplantation: a single-center experience.** *Transplant Proc* 2007, **39:**1190–4194.
8. Hengge UR, Ruzicka T, Schwartz RA, Cork MJ: **Adverse effects of topical glucocorticosteroids.** *J Am Acad Dermatol* 2006, **54:**1–15.
9. Mihatsch MJ, Kyo M, Morozumi K, Yamaguchi Y, Nickeleit V, Ryffel B: **The side-effects of ciclosporine-A and tacrolimus.** *Clin Nephrol* 1998, **49:**356–363.
10. Tosi A, Misciali C, Piraccini BM, Peluso AM, Bardazzi F: **Drug-induced hair loss and hair growth. Incidence, management and avoidance.** *Drug Saf* 1994, **10:**310–317.
11. Vanderveen EE, Ellis CN, Kang S, Case P, Headington JT, Voorhees JJ, Swanson NA: **Topical minoxidil for hair regrowth.** *J Am Acad Dermatol* 1984, **11:**416–421.
12. Balducci R, Toscano V: **Bioactive and peripheral androgens in prepubertal simple hypertrichosis.** *Clin Endocrinol (Oxf)* 1990, **33:**407–414.
13. Gryngarten M, Bedecarràs P, Ayuso S, Bergadà C, Campo S, Escobar ME: **Clinical assessment and serum hormonal profile in prepubertal hypertrichosis.** *Horm Res* 2000, **54:**20–25.
14. Eder IE, Culig Z, Putz T, Nessler-Menardi C, Bartsch G, Klocker H: **Molecular biology of the androgen receptor: from molecular understanding to the clinic.** *Eur Urol* 2001, **40:**241–251.
15. Mangelsdorf DJ, Thummel C, Beato M, Herrlich P, Schütz G, Umesono K, Blumberg B, Kastner P, Mark M, Chambon P, Evans RM: **The nuclear receptor superfamily: the second decade.** *Cell* 1995, **83:**835–839.
16. Lundin KB, Giwercman A, Dizeyi N, Giwercman YL: **Functional in vitro characterisation of the androgen receptor GGN polymorphism.** *Mol Cell Endocrinol* 2007, **264:**184–187.
17. Greulich WW, Pyle SI: *Radiographics atlas of skeletal development of the hand and wrist.* 2nd edition. Standford (CA): Standford Universtity Press; 1959.
18. Swanson M, Sauerbrei EE, Cooperberg PL: **Medical implications of ultrasonically detected polycystic ovaries.** *J Clin Ultrasound* 1981, **9:**219–222.
19. Vermeulen A, Verdonck L, Kaufman JM: **A critical evaluation of simple methods for the estimation of free testosterone in serum.** *J Clin Endocrinol Metab* 1999, **84:**3666–3672.
20. Edwards SM, Badzioch MD, Minter R, Hamoudi R, Collins N, Ardern-Jones A, Dowe A, Osborne S, Kelly J, Shearer R, Easton DF, Saunders GF, Dearnaley DP, Eeles RA: **Androgen receptor polymorphisms: association with prostate cancer risk, relapse and overall survival.** *Int J Cancer* 1999, **84:**458–465.
21. Vottero A, Stratakis CA, Ghizzoni L, Longui CA, Karl M, Chrousos GP: **Androgen receptor-mediated hypersensitivity to androgens in women with nonhyperandrogenic hirsutism: skewing of X-chromosome inactivation.** *J Clin Endocrinol Metab* 1999, **84:**1091–1095.
22. Ferlin A, Garolla A, Bettella A, Bartoloni L, Vinanzi C, Roverato A, Foresta C: **Androgen receptor gene CAG and GGC repeat lengths in cryptorchidism.** *Eur J Endocrinol* 2005, **152:**419–425.
23. Esteban E, Rodon N, Via M, Gonzalez-Perez E, Santamaria J, Dugoujon JM, Chennawi FE, Melhaoui M, Cherkaoui M, Vona G, Harich N, Moral P: **Androgen receptor CAG and GGC polymorphisms in Mediterraneans: repeat dynamics and population relationships.** *J Hum Genet* 2006, **51:**129–136.
24. Kittles RA, Young D, Weinrich S, Hudson J, Argyropoulos G, Ukoli F, Adams-Campbell L, Dunston GM: **Extent of linkage disequilibrium between the androgen receptor gene CAG and GGC repeats in human populations: implications for prostate cancer risk.** *Hum Genet* 2001, **109:**253–261.
25. Chamberlain NL, Driver ED, Miesfeld RL: **The length and location of CAG trinucleotide repeats in the androgen receptor N-terminal domain affect transactivation function.** *Nucleic Acids Res* 1994, **22:**3181–3186.
26. Van Nieuwerburgh F, Stoop D, Cabri P, Dhont M, Deforce D, De Sutter P: **Shorter CAG repeats in the androgen receptor gene may enhance hyperandrogenicity in polycystic ovary syndrome.** *Gynecol Endocrinol* 2008, **24:**669–673.
27. Ibáñez L, Ong KK, Mongan N, Jääskeläinen J, Marcos MV, Hughes IA, De Zegher F, Dunger DB: **Androgen receptor gene CAG repeat polymorphism in the development of ovarian hyperandrogenism.** *J Clin Endocrinol Metab* 2003, **88:**3333–3338.
28. Vottero A, Capelletti M, Giuliodori S, Viani I, Ziveri M, Neri TM, Bernasconi S, Ghizzoni L: **Decreased androgen receptor gene methylation in premature pubarche: a novel pathogenetic mechanism?** *J Clin Endocrinol Metab* 2006, **91:**968–972.

3

Presenting features and long-term effects of growth hormone treatment of children with optic nerve hypoplasia/septo-optic dysplasia

Amy M Vedin[1*], Hanna Karlsson[2], Cassandra Fink[3], Mark Borchert[3,4] and Mitchell E Geffner[1,4]

Abstract

Background: Optic nerve hypoplasia (ONH) with/or without septo-optic dysplasia (SOD) is a known concomitant of congenital growth hormone deficiency (CGHD).

Methods: Demographic and longitudinal data from KIGS, the Pfizer International Growth Database, were compared between 395 subjects with ONH/SOD and CGHD and 158 controls with CGHD without midline pathology.

Results: ONH/SOD subjects had higher birth length/weight, and mid-parental height SDS. At GH start, height, weight, and BMI SDS were higher in the ONH/SOD group. After 1 year of GH, both groups showed similar changes in height SDS, while weight and BMI SDS remained higher in the ONH/SOD group. The initial height responses of the two groups were similar to those predicted using the KIGS-derived prediction model for children with idiopathic GHD. At near-adult height, ONH/SOD and controls had similar height, weight, and BMI SDS.

Conclusions: Compared to children with CGHD without midline defects, those with ONH/SOD presented with greater height, weight, and BMI SDS. These differences persisted at 1 year of GH therapy, but appeared to be overcome by long-term GH treatment.

Background

Optic nerve hypoplasia (ONH) is a congenital anomaly often associated with hypopituitarism and brain malformations. It is relatively rare, with an incidence of 1 in 10,000 live births, and it equally affects boys and girls [1]. The term septo-optic dysplasia (SOD), historically and even today, is widely used interchangeably with that of ONH. However, it is now known that absence of the septum pellucidum *per se* does not confer increased risk for growth hormone (GH) deficiency alone or as a component of hypopituitarism in children with ONH [2,3].

In a study of 47 subjects [age (mean ± SD) 15.2 ± 10.6 months] with ONH followed until 59.0 ± 6.2 months of age, Ahmad, *et al* reported a prevalence of endocrinopathies of 71.7% (including 64.1% with GH-IGF-I axis abnormalities); these were not associated with ONH laterality, absence of septum pellucidum, or pituitary abnormalities on neuro-imaging [2]. The only prior large,

long-term study looking at growth outcomes in children described as having SOD treated with GH included 582 children enrolled in the National Cooperative Growth Study (NCGS) (Genentech, S. San Francisco CA). Among this cohort, 71 reached near-adult height (NAH) (mean -1.57 ± 1.27 SD), representing a mean gain of 1.17 ± 1.49 SD after 6-7 years of GH treatment [4].

More recently, it has been suggested that obesity is a frequent occurrence in children with ONH perhaps on a hypothalamic basis [5,6]. In his cohort of 47 subjects with ONH, Ahmad found that 44% had a body mass index (BMI) > 85th percentile at 5 years of age [2]. In the large NCGS study, no weight or BMI data were reported [4].

The purpose of the current analyses is to compare presenting features and short- and long-term auxological outcomes of GH treatment in children with ONH to those of patients with congenital growth hormone deficiency (CGHD) without non-pituitary midline defects or ONH using data from KIGS (the Pfizer International Growth Database).

* Correspondence: avedin@chla.usc.edu
[1]Center for Endocrinology, Diabetes, and Metabolism, Children's Hospital Los Angeles, 4650 Sunset Boulevard, Mailstop #61, Los Angeles, CA 90027, USA
Full list of author information is available at the end of the article

Methods

The KIGS database, established in 1987 and containing data from over 70,000 patients in 51 different countries, is an international registry developed with the main objective of documenting the long-term outcomes and safety of Somatonorm® and Genotropin® GH products (Pfizer, Inc). The KIGS survey is performed in accordance with the recommendations adopted by the 18th World Medical Assembly (held in Helsinki, Finland in 1964) and any subsequent revisions which exist to guide physicians carrying out biomedical research involving human individuals. Each subject and/or his/her legal representative receive adequate information, has the right to withdraw from the survey at any time, and consents his/her participation, although, during the first decade of its existence, this kind of registry or non-interventional trial that KIGS represents did not require informed consent from the subjects or legally acceptable representatives in many countries.

To capture subject data from KIGS for the current investigation, we included the diagnoses, ONH *and/or* SOD, since the latter is still widely used to describe patients with ONH whether or not the presence of the septum pellucidum is documented. Hereafter, for simplicity, we refer to the study condition as ONH/SOD. As of January 2009, there were 565 subjects identified as having CGHD secondary to ONH/SOD and 244 control subjects with CGHD unrelated to ONH/SOD and without extra-pituitary midline pathology. A list of the diagnostic codes included in the non-ONH/SOD CGHD group is included in Table 1. Subjects that were prepubertal and had at least one year of longitudinal data while receiving GH were included in the data analysis (ONH/SOD group n = 395 and CGHD group n = 158).

Background demographic characteristics, birth measurements, GH stimulation test results, and prevalence of associated hypothalamic-pituitary deficiencies affecting thyroid function, glucocorticoid production, and water metabolism (diabetes insipidus) were collected from KIGS. The prevalence of hypogonadism could only be obtained in older subjects who reached NAH. The

subjects' additional hormonal deficiencies were also managed by their treating physicians. Auxological data at the time of initiation of GH therapy and after one year of treatment were also collected. Similar data of the subsets of the two groups who attained NAH were compared. NAH was defined by height velocity (< 2 cm/year), bone age (≥ 14 years in females or ≥ 16 years in males), and/or chronological age (> 15 years in females and > 17 years in males).

Growth parameters are reported as standard deviation scores (SDS) which were calculated based on standards from Prader *et al* [7] and, for weight data, from Freeman *et al* [8]. Birth weight and length SDS were calculated using the reference of Niklasson *et al* [9]. Bone age readings were taken as reported by physicians and were based on the methods of Greulich and Pyle [10] or Tanner *et al* [11,12]. Data were not normally distributed and, therefore, are presented as median and 10th and 90th percentiles. Wilcoxon rank-sum test was used to detect differences between the two groups.

The heights of subjects in both groups were analyzed using the previously published KIGS prediction model for idiopathic GHD excluding GH maximum peak [13]. Differences between observed and predicted height velocities are expressed in terms of Studentized residuals. The residual is calculated as the observed height velocity minus the predicted height velocity for each observation, and the Studentized residual is the residual divided by its standard error.

Results

Background characteristics were compared between the two groups (Table 2). The birth length and weight SDS were significantly greater in the ONH/SOD group compared to the non-ONH/SOD CGHD group [birth length SDS median (0.27); 10th and 90th percentiles (-1.3, 2.0) vs. median (-0.62); 10th and 90th percentiles (-2.5, 1.2); p < 0.001) and birth weight SDS (-0.31; -1.7, 1.1) vs. (-0.58; -2.0, 1.0); p = 0.021]. Mid-parental height SDS was also significantly greater in the ONH/SOD group (-0.23; -1.8, 1.3) compared to the non-ONH/SOD CGHD group [(-1.04; -3.0, 0.5); p < 0.001]. Peak GH levels on stimulation testing were similar between the two groups. The ONH/SOD group had significantly more subjects with other hypothalamic-pituitary hormone deficiencies compared to the non-ONH/SOD CGHD group (72.7% vs. 51.9%; p < 0.001), with involvement of the thyroid and adrenal axes being the most common.

At the start of GH therapy, both groups had similar chronological ages and bone ages. However, the ONH/SOD group had significantly greater height SDS [(-3.00; -4.8, -0.9) vs. (-3.68; -6.7, -1.9); p < 0.001], weight SDS [(-1.56; -4.2, 0.5) vs. (-2.56; -5.7, -0.6); p < 0.001], and

Table 1 KIGS diagnostic codes included in non-ONH/SOD CGHD (cross-sectional numbers)

KIGS Diagnostic Codes	n	Description
2.1.1.1	23	*GH gene-defect (Type 1A dominant or recessive)*
2.1.1.2	25	*GH gene-defect*
2.1.1.3	4	*GHRH gene-defect*
2.1.1.9	192	Other genetic cause of GHD
Total	**244**	

GH, growth hormone; GHRH, growth hormone releasing hormone; GHD, growth hormone deficiency

Table 2 Characteristics at background, GH start, and 1st year on GH

	N	Median	10th, 90th percentiles	N	Median	10th, 90th percentiles	P-value
		ONH/SOD			Non-ONH/SOD		
		Background					
Gender, males	395	227 (57.5%)		158	101 (63.9%)		
Birth Length SDS	206	0.27	-1.3, 2.0	104	-0.62	-2.5, 1.2	< 0.001
Birth Weight SDS	349	-0.31	-1.7, 1.1	133	-0.58	-2.0, 1.0	0.021
Mid-Parental Height SDS	324	-0.23	-1.8, 1.3	140	-1.04	-3.0, 0.5	< 0.001
Peak GH (μg/L)	307	2.60	0.8, 7.2	131	3.30	0.5, 10.8	0.053
Other Pituitary Hormone Deficiencies	395	287 (72.7%)		158	82 (51.9%)		< 0.001
Hypothyroidism	395	250 (63.3%)		158	74 (46.8%)		< 0.001
Glucocorticoid deficiency	395	206 (52.2%)		158	46 (29.1%)		< 0.001
Diabetes insipidus	395	51 (12.9%)		158	6 (3.8%)		< 0.001
		At GH Start					
Age (years)	395	3.99	0.9, 9.8	158	4.47	0.7, 10.7	0.498
Bone Age (years)	77	3.50	1.4, 8.7	41	4.00	1.2, 10.0	0.784
Height SDS	395	-3.00	-4.8, -0.9	158	-3.68	-6.7, -1.9	< 0.001
Height - Mid-Parental Height SDS	324	-2.74	-4.67, -0.62	140	-2.42	-4.94, -0.72	0.305
Height Velocity (cm/year)	147	5.46	2.35, 12.07	45	5.23	3.19, 9.76	0.904
Weight SDS	395	-1.56	-4.2, 0.5	158	-2.56	-5.7, -0.6	< 0.001
BMI SDS	395	0.22	-1.8, 2.1	158	-0.18	-2.1, 1.6	0.001
GH Dose (mg/kg/week)	395	0.24	0.16, 0.33	158	0.22	0.16, 0.39	0.395
		1st yr on GH					
Age (years)	395	5.01	1.87, 10.74	158	5.46	1.64, 11.75	0.500
Bone Age (years)	96	4.40	2.00, 9.00	53	4.17	2.00, 11.5	0.429
Height SDS	395	-1.95	-4.0, 0.0	158	-2.37	-4.7, -0.9	< 0.001
Δ Height SDS	395	1.02	0.0, 2.0	158	1.10	0.3, 2.7	0.066
Height - Mid-Parental Height SDS	324	-1.70	-3.78, 0.29	140	-1.29	-3.15, 0.23	0.010
Height Velocity (cm/year)	395	11.25	6.74, 16.18	158	10.54	6.98, 18.97	0.863
Weight SDS	393	-0.91	-3.3, 1.3	158	-1.81	-3.9, -0.0	< 0.001
BMI SDS	393	0.05	-1.8, 2.3	158	-0.43	-2.1, 1.2	< 0.001
GH Dose (mg/kg/week)	388	0.23	0.14, 0.33	156	0.21	0.13, 0.33	0.068
		IGHD Prediction Model (Without GH Peak) at 1 year					
Predicted Height Velocity	186	10.69	9.03, 12.51	73	9.99	8.28, 11.86	< 0.001
Actual Height Velocity (cm/year)	186	10.72	6.66, 14.37	73	9.49	7.16, 13.77	0.305
Studentized Residual	186	-0.11	-2.53, 1.98	73	-0.04	-1.61, 1.95	0.565

SDS, standard deviation score; GH, growth hormone

BMI SDS [(0.22; -1.8, 2.1) vs. (-0.18; -2.1, 1.6); p = 0.001] (Table 2).

After one year on GH therapy, the two groups had similar changes in height SDS (p = 0.066). The ONH/SOD group continued to have a significantly higher height SDS, weight SDS, and BMI SDS after one year of GH therapy (all p < 0.001). However, height SDS corrected for family height genetics was significantly greater in the comparator group after the first year of GH treatment (Figure 1). Use of the prediction model for first-year growth response in children with idiopathic GHD showed that, although there was a slightly greater than predicted response in the ONH/SOD group versus the non-ONH/SOD CGHD group, there was no difference in actual height response between both groups, with Studentized residuals equivalent in both groups (Figure 2).

NAH data were available for 59 subjects in the ONH/SOD group and 23 subjects in the non-ONH/SOD CGHD group (Table 3). The two groups had similar NAH at approximately -1 SDS (p = 0.430). The non-ONH/SOD CGHD attained a NAH that was closer to their mid-parental height (p < 0.05). The two groups had similar weight SDS and BMI SDS at time of NAH (Figure 3). At NAH, the two groups had the same prevalence of hypogonadism.

Discussion

Although over half of the patients with ONH/SOD will develop an abnormality in their GH-IGF-I axis [2],

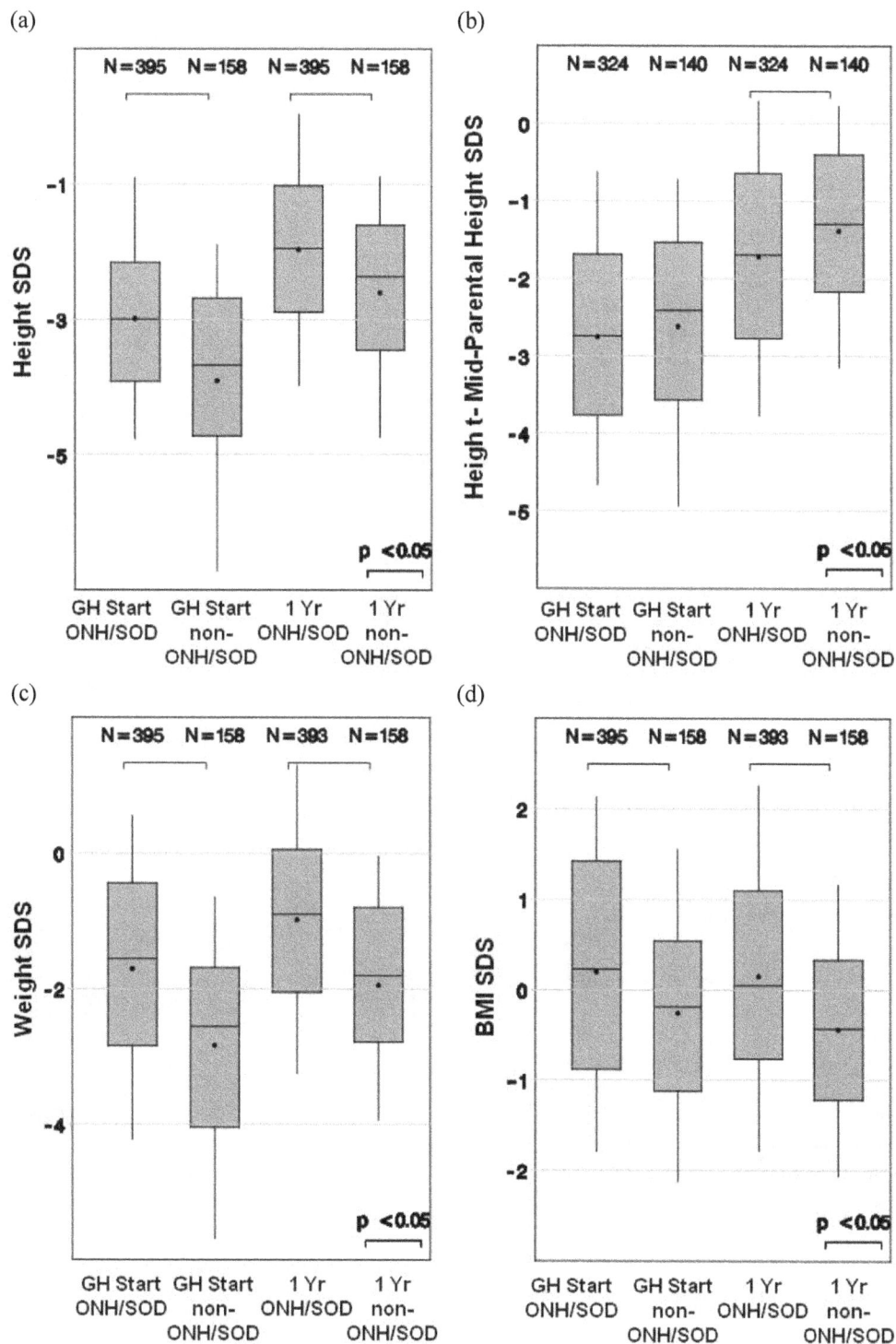

Figure 1 Comparison between groups. Comparison between groups with ONH/SOD vs. non-ONH/SOD CGHD of (a) height SDS, (b) height - MPH SDS, (c) weight SDS, and (d) BMI SDS at start and after 1 year of GH therapy.

little is known about their clinical presentations and auxological responses to GH, especially in comparison to those of similar patients with non-ONH/SOD CGHD.

In our study, the birth length and weight were significantly greater in the ONH/SOD group. It is unclear whether these differences can be fully explained by the increased mid-parental height seen in

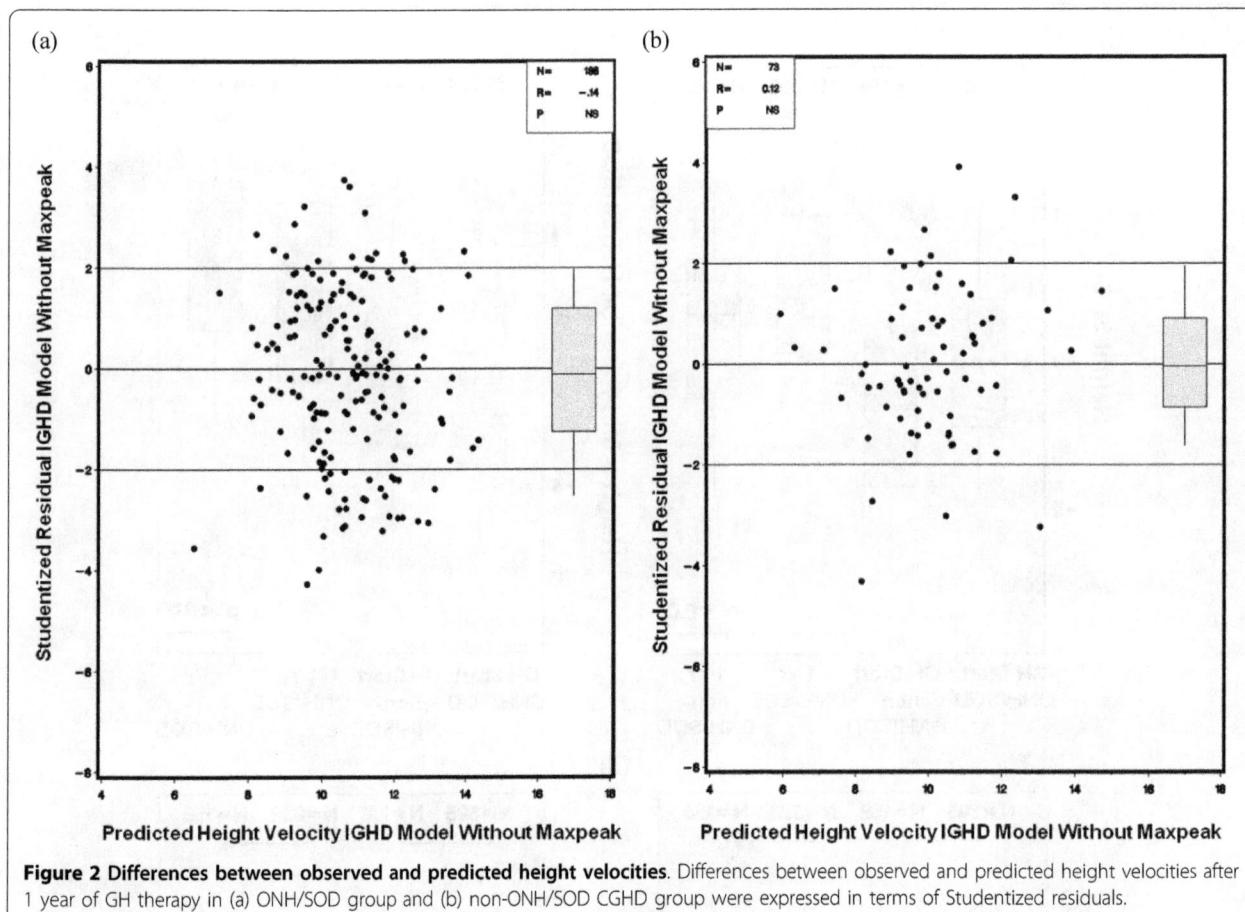

Figure 2 Differences between observed and predicted height velocities. Differences between observed and predicted height velocities after 1 year of GH therapy in (a) ONH/SOD group and (b) non-ONH/SOD CGHD group were expressed in terms of Studentized residuals.

Table 3 Characteristics at Near-Adult Height

	N	ONH/SOD Median	10th, 90th percentiles	N	Non-ONH/SOD Median	10th, 90th percentiles	P-value
		At GH Start					
Gender, males	59	26 (44.1%)		23	10 (43.5%)		
Age (years)	59	5.64	2.14, 11.76	23	5.12	2.09, 12.04	0.546
Height SDS	59	-3.77	-5.51, -1.96	23	-4.97	-7.73, -2.98	< 0.001
Height - Mid-Parental Height SDS	48	-3.41	-5.85, -1.78	22	-3.30	-5.81, -0.91	0.658
Weight SDS	59	-2.23	-4.44, -0.72	23	-3.49	-5.92, -0.80	0.013
BMI SDS	59	-0.13	-2.02, 1.86	23	0.09	-1.64, 1.56	0.955
GH Dose (mg/kg/week)	59	0.21	0.14, 0.31	23	0.21	0.14, 0.43	0.996
		At NAH					
Age (years)	59	17.73	15.5, 20.5	23	17.30	15.3, 19.4	0.369
Height SDS	59	-0.87	-2.8, 0.6	23	-1.37	-2.7, 0.2	0.430
Δ Height SDS (Latest minus Start)	59	2.75	1.1, 4.4	23	3.37	1.6, 6.1	0.025
Height - Mid-Parental Height SDS	48	-0.63	-2.35, 0.87	22	0.37	-1.59, 1.43	0.004
Weight SDS	59	-0.53	-2.6, 2.7	23	-0.22	-2.1, 1.9	0.988
BMI SDS	59	0.32	-1.90, 2.50	23	0.59	-0.90, 2.50	0.581
Mean Total GH Dose (mg/kg/week)	59	0.19	0.13, 0.28	23	0.19	0.14, 0.25	0.722
Years on GH Treatment	59	11.15	6.69, 16.37	23	11.51	6.71, 14.69	0.996
Hypogonadism	59	23 (39.0%)		23	9 (39.1%)		

SDS, standard deviation score; GH, growth hormone

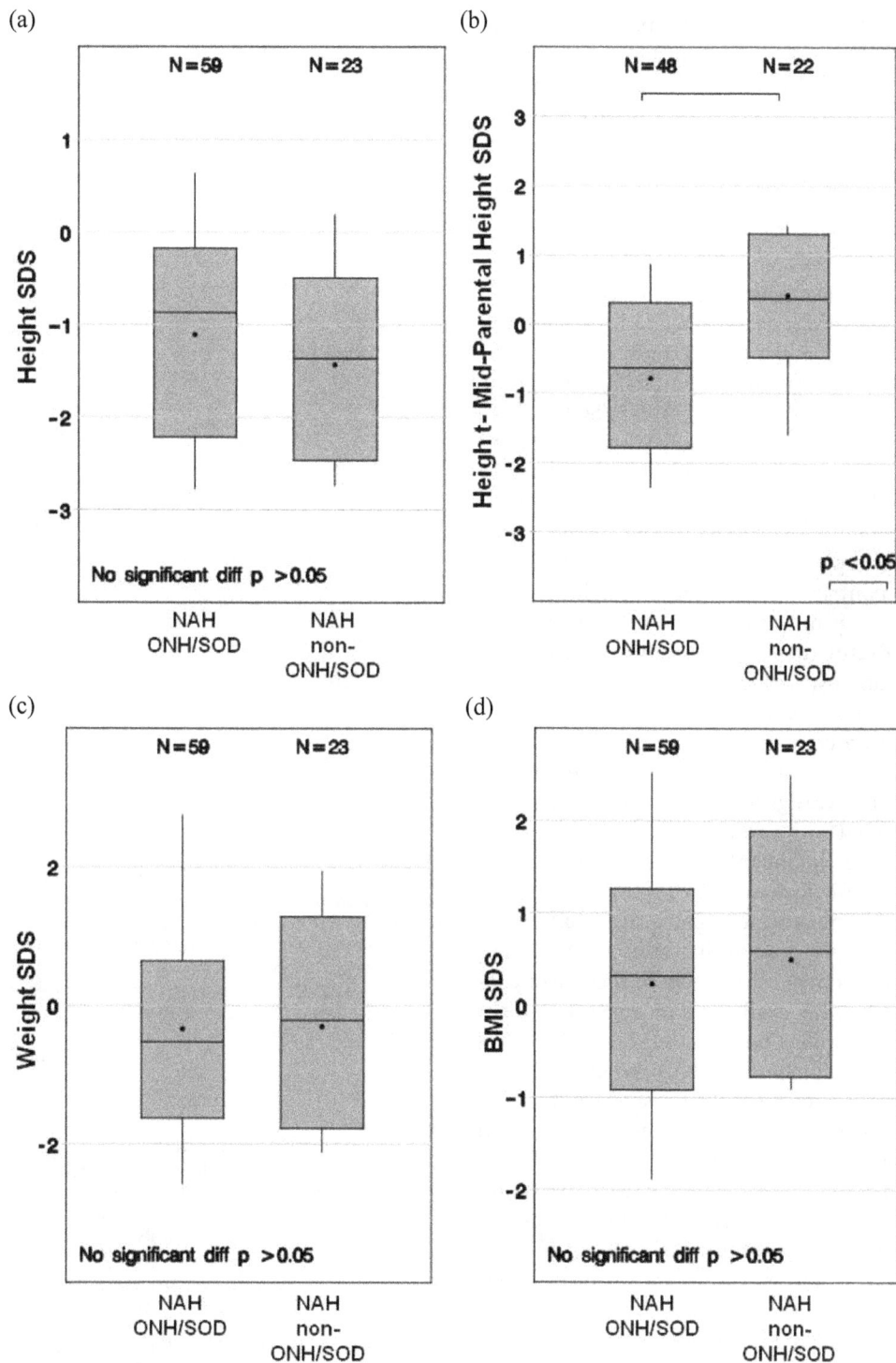

Figure 3 Comparison between groups with ONH/SOD vs. non-ONH/SOD CGHD. Comparison between groups with ONH/SOD vs. non-ONH/SOD CGHD of (a) height SDS, (b) height - MPH SDS, (c) weight SDS, and (d) BMI SDS at near-adult height.

the ONH/SOD group or if there might be other disease-specific explanations. Some of this difference in mid-parental height may be due to the parents of those children with non-ONH/SOD CGHD also having the same gene defect causing short stature. At the time of diagnosis, the two groups had similar stimulated peak GH levels suggesting a comparable degree of GH deficiency.

The higher prevalence of pituitary hormone deficiencies seen in the ONH/SOD group compared to the non-ONH/SOD CGHD group is not surprising given the known association of ONH/SOD with hypopituitarism. However, our study found, at the time of GH initiation, for no obvious reason, a much higher prevalence of associated hormone deficiencies in the ONH/SOD group compared to the data reported in the NCGS study (hypothyroidism: 63.2% vs 27%, glucocorticoid deficiency: 52.2% vs 24%, and diabetes insipidus: 12.9% vs 5%) [4]. In a smaller subset who reached NAH, 39% of subjects in our cohort had hypogonadism while this data was not reported in the NCGS study.

At the time of GH initiation, the ONH/SOD group was significantly larger than the non-ONH/SOD CGHD group in all measures (height, weight, and BMI). The taller heights at diagnosis in the ONH/SOD group might relate to the associated ophthalmological manifestations of the condition leading to nystagmus and earlier referral. This group's greater genetic height potential might also be contributory. As for the higher weight and BMI, this may be associated with the intrinsic hypothalamic dysfunction seen in some patients with ONH/SOD causing hyperphagia.

The two groups responded similarly to one year of GH therapy with a comparable increase in height and similar to that predicted using the KIGS-derived prediction model for first-year growth in GH-treated children with idiopathic GHD. As a result, the ONH/SOD group continued to have significantly greater height, along with weight and BMI, than did the non-ONH/SOD CGHD group. Although we recognize the small size of the subsets from both groups that attained NAH and the inherent uncertainty of being able to draw firm conclusions as a result, the available data suggest that the two groups have similar height, weight, and BMI at NAH. With height outcomes in both groups within 1 SD of the mean (corrected for their respective mid-parental heights), this suggests that there is excellent adult height potential in children with congenital GH deficiency. Furthermore, these results suggest that long-term GH therapy can possibly prevent, minimize, and/or reverse the obesity that has been described in patients with ONH/SOD. Additional randomized prospective studies of GH therapy in patients with ONH/SOD are needed to investigate the effects of GH therapy specifically on obesity and body composition.

In summary, children with ONH/SOD have different presenting characteristics, but similar and normal final height responses to GH therapy compared to children with non-ONH/SOD CGHD. Because ONH/SOD is a major risk factor for CGHD and these patients may not be as short as those with non-ONH/SOD CGHD, it is important for clinicians to have a high index of suspicion and begin screening these patients for CGHD as early as possible. GH therapy may have additional benefits in this patient population as well with regard to body composition thus making early diagnosis and treatment even more important.

Abbreviations
ONH: Optic nerve hypoplasia; SOD: septo-optic dysplasia; GH: growth hormone; NCGS: National Cooperative Growth Study; NAH: near-adult height; CGHD: congenital growth hormone deficiency; SDS: standard deviation score

Acknowledgements
The authors express their thanks to the clinicians who provided the data on their patients. KIGS is supported by Pfizer, Inc. No authors were paid for their contributions to this manuscript.

Author details
[1]Center for Endocrinology, Diabetes, and Metabolism, Children's Hospital Los Angeles, 4650 Sunset Boulevard, Mailstop #61, Los Angeles, CA 90027, USA. [2]Pfizer Inc., Pfizer Endocrine Care, KIGS/KIMS/ACROSTUDY, SE-191 90 Sollentuna, Sweden. [3]The Vision Center, Children's Hospital Los Angeles, 4650 Sunset Boulevard, Mailstop #88, Los Angeles, CA 90027, USA. [4]Saban Research Institute of Children's Hospital Los Angeles, 4650 Sunset Boulevard, Los Angeles, CA 90027, USA.

Authors' contributions
AV participated in the design of the study and drafted the manuscript. HK participated in the design of the study and performed the statistical analyses. CF and MB participated in the study's design and coordination. MG conceived of the study, and participated in its design and coordination. All authors read and approved the final manuscript.

Competing interests
HK is a full-time employee of Pfizer Endocrine Care, KIGS/KIMS/ACROSTUDY, Sollentuna, Sweden. MG receives funding from Pfizer for institutional participation in KIGS (Pfizer International Growth Database); for research subject participation in the multi-center clinical trial: "A Four-Year Open-Label Multi-Center Randomized Two-Arm Study of Genotropin in Idiopathic Short Stature Patients: Comparing an Individualized, Target-Driven Treatment Regimen to Standard Dosing of Genotropin," and for serving as a member of national and international KIGS advisory boards.

References
1. Patel L, McNally RJ, Harrison E, Lloyd IC, Clayton PE: **Geographical distribution of optic nerve hypoplasia and septo-optic dysplasia in Northwest England.** *J Pediatr* 2006, 148(1):85-88.
2. Ahmad T, Garcia-Filion P, Borchert M, Kaufman F, Burkett L, Geffner M: **Endocrinological and auxological abnormalities in young children with optic nerve hypoplasia.** *J Pediatr* 2006, 148(1):78-84.
3. Brodsky MC, Glasier CM: **Optic nerve hypoplasia. Clinical significance of associated central nervous system abnormalities on magnetic resonance imaging.** *Arch Ophthalmol* 1993, 111:66-74.
4. Parker KL, Hunold JJ, Blethen SL: **Septo-optic dysplasia/optic nerve hypoplasia: data from the National Cooperative Growth Study (NCGS).** *J Pediatr Endocrinol Metab* 2002, 15(suppl 2):697-700.
5. Borchert M, Garcia-Filion P: **The syndrome of optic nerve hypoplasia.** *Curr Neurol Neurosci Rep* 2008, 8(5):395-403.
6. Webb EA, Dattani MT: **Septo-optic dysplasia.** *Eur J Hum Genet* 2010, 18(4):393-397.
7. Prader A, Largo RH, Molinari L, Issler C: **Physical growth of Swiss children from birth to 20 years of age; first Zurich longitudinal study of growth and development.** *Helv Paediatr Acta* 1989, 52(suppl):1-125.

8. Freeman JV, Cole TJ, Chinn S, Jones PR, White EM, Preece MA: **Cross sectional stature and weight references for the UK, 1990.** *Arch Dis Child* 1995, **73**:17-24.

9. Niklasson A, Ericson A, Fryer JG, Karlberg J, Lawrence C, Karlberg P: **An update of the Swedish reference standards for weight, length and head circumference at birth for given gestational age (1977-1981).** *Acta Paediatr Scand* 1991, **80**:756-762.

10. Greulich WW, Pyle SI: **Radiographic Atlas of Skeletal Development of Hand and Wrist.** Stanford, Stanford University Press;, 2 1959.

11. Tanner JM, Landt KW, Cameron N, Carter BS, Patel J: **Prediction of adult height and bone age in children. A new system of equations (TW mark II) based on sample including very tall and very short children.** *Arch Dis Child* 1983, **58**:767-776.

12. Tanner JM, Healy MJR, Goldstein H, Cameron N: **Assessment of Skeletal Maturity and Prediction of Adult Height (TW3) Method.** Singapore, WB Saunders;, 3 2001.

13. Ranke MB, Lindberg A, Chatelain P, Wilton P, Cutfield W, Albertsson-Wikland K, Price DA: **Derivation and validation of a mathematical model for predicting the response to exogenous recombinant human growth hormone (GH) in prepubertal children with idiopathic GH deficiency.** *J Clin Endocrinol Metab* 1999, **84**:1174-1183.

4

Impaired endothelial function in pediatric patients with Turner Syndrome and healthy controls: a case-control study

Clodagh S O'Gorman[1,3,4,5*], Catriona Syme[4], Tim Bradley[2,3], Jill Hamilton[1,3,4] and Farid H Mahmud[1,3,4]

Abstract

Background: Turner Syndrome women are at high risk of vascular disease and the assessment of early risk factors in Turner Syndrome girls is an emerging focus of research. Our objective was to evaluate endothelial function (EF), a preclinical measure of atherosclerosis, in Turner Syndrome girls compared with controls.

Methods: A cross-sectional case-control study of Turner Syndrome girls and healthy controls. Subjects underwent fasting insulin and glucose with calculation of HOMA-IR, fasting lipid profile, anthropometrics, and EF testing using peripheral arterial tonometry (PAT). Subjects, aged 10-18 years, had karyotype-confirmed Turner Syndrome; growth hormone (GH), thyroxine and estrogen use were not exclusion criteria. Controls were age- and BMI-matched healthy girls. Fifteen Turner Syndrome and 15 controls were recruited.

Results: Turner Syndrome girls had lower height, higher HDL and higher waist:height ratio than controls. PAT-hyperemia ratio (RH-PAT) scores were lower in Turner Syndrome (1.64 ± 0.34 vs. 2.08 ± 0.32, $p = 0.002$) indicating impaired EF. Among Turner Syndrome, RH-PAT did not vary with estrogen therapy or with karyotype 45,XO compared with other karyotypes. However, endothelial function was better in GH-treated compared with GH-untreated Turner Syndrome (1.80 ± 0.36 vs. $1.4 + 0.22$, $p = 0.02$) although there were no differences in HOMA-IR, adiponectin or IGF-1.

Conclusion: Girls with Turner Syndrome exhibit impaired endothelial function compared with controls, which may explain higher risk for vascular disease. GH may protect endothelial function in Turner Syndrome.

Keywords: Turner syndrome, Endothelial function, Adolescents, Pediatrics

Introduction

Turner Syndrome, a common genetic disorder affecting 1 in 2500 live-born females, is caused by complete or partial loss of × chromosome [1]. Despite significant advances in diagnosis and treatment in pediatric settings, Turner Syndrome patients experience high rates of cardiovascular disease such that adult females with Turner Syndrome have 3.47 and 2.21 standardized mortality ratios of coronary and cerebrovascular death respectively [2]. The majority of this excess mortality risk encompasses non-congenital circulatory disease [3]. However, this relates to underlying congenital structural and functional arterial abnormalities, which predispose these patients to aortic dilatation and aneurysm [4]. Additionally, Turner Syndrome patients exhibit a clustering of acquired cardiovascular disease risk factors, including increased rates of hypertension, glucose intolerance, obesity and dyslipidemia, which are also impacted by treatment regimens including growth hormone (GH) and estrogen [1].

Adolescents and young adults rarely experience cardiovascular events, and surrogate markers of cardiovascular disease are needed to evaluate asymptomatic patients. Impaired endothelial function is an initial step in the development of atherosclerosis, and represents an early and reversible step in the vascular disease process [5,6]. The measurement of endothelial function can be used as a surrogate marker to assess cardiovascular risk [7-10].

* Correspondence: clodagh.ogorman@ul.ie
[1]Divisions of Endocrinology, The Hospital for Sick Children Research Institute, University of Toronto, Toronto, Canada
Full list of author information is available at the end of the article

In prior clinical studies, peripheral arterial tonometry (PAT) testing has been used to measure endothelial function in both high risk adult [11] and pediatric populations [12,13]. Assessment of endothelial function has not previously been reported in pediatric Turner Syndrome populations and it is unclear whether Turner Syndrome is an independent risk factor for endothelial damage or if acquired cardiovascular risk factors impact endothelial function in this high risk patient group [14,15].

The objectives of this study were to evaluate endothelial function, as a marker of early vascular disease, in a group of pediatric Turner Syndrome girls in relation to an age-, sex- and body mass index (BMI)-matched healthy control population, and to assess the impact of disease-related treatment factors and acquired cardiovascular risk factors on endothelial function in the Turner Syndrome study group.

Materials and methods

Institutional ethical approval was obtained for this case-controlled cross-sectional study. Inclusion criteria for Turner Syndrome subjects included: karyotype-confirmed diagnosis of Turner Syndrome; patients followed in our endocrinology clinic; and aged 10-18 years. Individuals receiving human growth hormone (GH), L-thyroxine or estrogen, or with a history of congenital heart disease, were eligible for inclusion. All patients taking L-thyroxine were on stable therapy with thyroid function within the normal range. Subjects took their medications as usual on the day of the study. Controls were healthy girls, age- and BMI-matched to TS subjects and recruited as part of previous studies using the same testing protocol. Exclusion criteria included: inability of the family and/or patient to comply with study protocol; previous diagnosis of Type 1 or Type 2 Diabetes Mellitus; taking medications for the treatment of disorders of glucose, insulin or lipid metabolism.

Each subject attended the Hospital for Sick Children for full evaluation on two separate days. On one day, subjects had fasting bloodwork including cholesterol profile (triglycerides, total cholesterol, high and low density lipoprotein cholesterol [HDL and LDL]), adiponectin, insulin and glucose. Homeostatic model assessment of insulin resistance (HOMA-IR) was calculated based on fasting insulin and glucose values: [16].

$$HOMA \text{-} IR = [Glucose \; (mmol/L) \times Insulin \; (mU/L)] / 22.5$$

Brachial arterial blood pressure (BP) (systolic, diastolic, and mean) and heart rate were recorded in the left arm using an automated Dinamap sphygmomanometer (Critikon Dinamap, Minneapolis, MN, USA). Each subject underwent history, examination and anthropometrics by a single examiner. Height, in metres (m), was measured using a wall-mounted stadiometer; and weight, in kilograms (kg), was assessed using calibrated electronic scales. BMI was calculated as kg/m^2. Pubertal status was assessed by a single examiner according to the methods of Tanner [17].

On a different day, subjects returned fasting for endothelial function testing. PAT (Itamar Medical, Caesarea, Israel) is a non-invasive test which uses pneumatic probes, similar in shape to a thimble, which cover the fingertip and apply a uniform pressure field which allows for the measurement of the pulsatile oscillations of the digital vascular bed microcirculation. The PAT-hyperemia ratio (RH-PAT) shows a strong sensitivity and specificity for the detection of coronary endothelial function, which has been shown to predict cardiovascular events in adult patients [7,10]. PAT has been used previously as a surrogate marker of early endothelial function in paediatric populations [13,18] and, in adolescents it has been validated in a repeated measures study [19]. PAT probes are placed on finger II or III of each hand. After a 5 minute equilibration period, a BP cuff is inflated on the study arm 40 mmHg above systolic BP for 5 minutes. The cuff is then deflated and tonometric recording is completed for an additional 5 minutes. The RH-PAT was determined for each patient and each recording was analyzed individually. Lower RH-PAT index scores indicate worse endothelial function and increased risk for atherosclerosis.

Fifteen Turner Syndrome subjects were recruited, and matched for age and BMI with 15 healthy control girls (Table 1). All girls and their parents consented to participate. All subjects completed the protocol. For the girls with TS, karyotypes were as follows: 45,XO N = 6; 45, XO/46,XX mosaicism N = 1; 45,XO/47,XXX mosaicism N = 1; complex translocations N = 3; isochrome q material N = 2; 45,XO/46,XY mosaicism N = 2. Two subjects had aortic stenosis, including one with coarctaction repair several years previously. One additional subject had a bicuspid aortic valve. No other TS subjects had any known cardiovascular disease. Fourteen TS subjects were taking medications, including: N = 6 estrogen supplementation (N = 1 estrogen only; n = 1 estrogen and progesterone; N = 1 estrogen, progesterone and GH*; N = 3 oral contraceptive pill) and N = 7 GH supplementation (N = 4 GH only; N = 1 GH, estrogen and progesterone*; N = 1 GH and migraine prophylaxis; N = 1 GH with Ritalin and concerta) and N = 1 calcium supplementation (* denotes same patient).

Biochemical analyses

Insulin was measured by chemiluminsecence using the Siemens Immulite 2500 (range of assay 15-2165 pmol/L, intra-and inter-assay coefficient of variation [CV] <7.6%). Adiponectin was measured by ELISA (Linco Research Inc., Range: 1-100 ng/mL; inter-assay CV 2.4 - 8.4%).

Table 1 Baseline Demographics and results of investigations and PAT compared between girls with Turner Syndrome and Control girls

	Turner Syndrome N = 15	Control Subjects N = 15	p
Age	13.5 (2.4)	14.3 (1.7)	0.38
Systolic BP (mm Hg)	113.8 (12.2)	106.6 (5.5)	0.06
Diastolic BP (mm Hg)	65.8 (11.5)	70.18 (3.12)	0.21
Height (m)	1.42 (0.11)	1.64 (0.15)	**0.0019**
Weight (kg)	44.2 (13.0)	54.5 (15.5)	0.07
BMI (kg/m^2)	21.5 (4.5)	20.8 (3.4)	0.64
Waist Circumference (cm)	73.1 (10.9)	71.4 (12.8)	0.71
Waist:Height Ratio	0.51 (0.06)	0.44 (0.08)	**0.0054**
Fasting glucose (mmol/L)	4.55 (0.91)	4.65 (0.47)	0.74
LDL cholesterol (mmol/L)	2.29 (0.58)	2.56 (0.73)	0.29
HDL cholesterol (mmol/L)	1.53 (0.51)	1.00 (0.32)	**0.003**
Total cholesterol (mmol/L)	4.27 (0.57)	4.08 (0.77)	0.46
Triglycerides (mmol/L)	1.01 (0.48)	0.95 (0.34)	0.71
HDLc:Triglycerides ratio	2.17(1.82)	1.26(0.70)	0.10
RH-PAT	1.64 (0.34)	2.08 (0.32)	**0.002**

Data are expressed as mean (SD)

Data analyses

All measures are expressed as mean value ± standard deviation (SD). Baseline characteristics were compared with paired t-tests (due to age- and BMI-matching of patients) and McNemar test. Associations between baseline characteristics and RH-PAT were quantified with Pearson Correlation Coefficients. Linear regression was used to determine whether baseline factors were correlated with outcome measures. All analyses were conducted with SAS, version 9.1 (SAS Institute Inc., Cary, NC).

Results

There were no statistically significant differences between the Turner Syndrome and control groups for age, BP, weight or BMI. Control subjects were significantly taller than Turner Syndrome subjects. There was no difference in waist circumference between the groups; but, the waist:height ratio was higher in Turner Syndrome than in controls (Table 1). There were no differences between the groups for fasting glucose, LDL, total cholesterol, or triglycerides. HDL was higher in TS subjects.

The ages of GH-treated [N = 7] and GH-untreated [N = 8] Turner Syndrome girls were not different (12.7 ± 2.0 years versus 14.3 ± 2.4 years, t = -0.79, p = 0.22) and IGF-1 levels were not different between GH-treated and GH-untreated girls (423.8 ± 122.8 versus 336.7 ± 103.6 mcg/L respectively, p = 0.23). Among the GH-treated Turner Syndrome girls, GH treatment duration was 4.6 ± 1.1 years, with prescribed GH doses 0.35 mg/kg/week. There were no statistical differences in HOMA-IR, adiponectin, lipid measurements or blood glucose between GH-treated and GH-untreated Turner Syndrome girls (see Table 2).

RH-PAT scores were significantly lower in Turner Syndrome than in control subjects (1.64 ± 0.34 versus 2.08 ± 0.32, p = 0.002). Among girls with Turner Syndrome, RH-PAT scores did not vary with estrogen replacement therapy (1.56 ± 0.30 with estrogen replacement [N = 6] versus 1.69 ± 0.37 without estrogen replacement [N = 9], p = 0.64) or between those with 45,XO karyotype [N = 6] and other karyotypes [N = 9] (1.60 ± 0.46 versus 1.67 ± 0.26 respectively, p = 0.56). However, RH-PAT scores were higher in girls receiving GH therapy than in those not receiving GH therapy (1.86 ± 0.28 versus 1.44 + 0.26 respectively, p = 0.045) and in Turner Syndrome girls receiving GH therapy, PAT scores were similar to control girls (1.86 ± 0.28 versus 2.08 ± 0.32 respectively, p = 0.14).

In Turner Syndrome subjects, RH-PAT score did not correlate with any measures of glucose, adiposity or anthropometrics. In control subjects, RH-PAT correlated positively with age and systolic BP, and negatively with LDL and HDL.

Discussion

This study demonstrates that Turner Syndrome girls, compared with healthy age-, sex- and BMI-matched controls, have impaired endothelial function, an early, pre-clinical marker of vascular disease. We did not observe any significant correlations with acquired CVD risk factors present in our TS cohort, including lipid profile, BP or markers of insulin resistance.

The increased risk of cardiovascular complications in Turner Syndrome patients is complex and encompasses both congenital and acquired lesions. Recent data from the UK observed that non-congenital circulatory disease accounted for 41% of absolute excess mortality in

Table 2 Comparison of metabolic parameters between TS subjects GH-treated versus GH-untreated

	GH-untreated N = 8	GH-treated N = 7	p-value
Age (years)	14.31(2.38)	12.66(2.00)	0.22
Height (m)	1.43(0.13)	1.40(0.10)	0.95
Weight (kg)	48.01(13.75)	39.79(11.53)	0.17
BMI (kg/m^2)	23.02(4.72)	19.82(3.78)	0.24
RH-PAT	1.44(0.26)	1.86(0.28)	**0.045**
Systolic BP (mm Hg)	113.0(11.56)	114.71(13.70)	0.69
Diastolic BP (mm Hg)	64.88(6.49)	66.86(16.04)	0.65
Waist Circumference (cm)	76.19(11.90)	69.50(9.05)	0.29
Waist:Height Ratio	0.53(0.07)	0.49(0.04)	0.34
HOMA IR	1.90(1.64)	0.68(0.71)	0.06
Adiponectin (ng/mL)	16466(9186)	12995(4466)	0.53
IGF-1 (mcg/L)	423.8(122.8)	336.7(103.6)	0.43
Glucose (mmol/L)	4.79(1.20)	4.29(0.31)	0.95
Insulin (pmol/L)	61.25(44.38)	34.60(20.33)	0.24
HDL (mmol/L)	1.30(0.32)	1.80(0.57)	0.09
LDL (mmol/L)	2.49(0.66)	2.07(0.41)	0.24
Total Cholesterol (mmol/L)	4.27(0.66)	4.27(0.30)	0.78
Triglycerides (mmol/L)	1.14(0.58)	0.89(0.36)	0.33
HDL:Triglycerides Ratio	1.78(1.69)	2.56(2.00)	0.22

Data are expressed as mean(SD)

Turner Syndrome women compared with only 8% for congenital anomalies [3]. Our study describes a young cohort of reasonably healthy Turner Syndrome patients with inherent impaired vascular function, of whom only 3/15 have evidence of some cardiac lesion. The Turner Syndrome patients are compared to BMI-matched healthy controls, because obesity measures do impair endothelial function, as we have previously described in adolescents using the same measure [13]. Previous reports evaluating vascular function in Turner Syndrome have shown carotid intima media thickening present in two adult studies, without evidence of abnormal endothelial function (brachial artery reactivity or pulse wave velocity) [20,21]. However, these studies were conducted in older Turner Syndrome patients with significant differences in BP and BMI compared with healthy controls.

We identified higher HDL concentrations in Turner Syndrome subjects compared with controls, and no effect of GH treatment on any measured cholesterol parameter was observed. These results are different with respect to previous studies that have shown higher total cholesterol in TS subjects independent of age, BMI and karyotype [22] and higher total cholesterol but lower HDL in older Turner Syndrome girls compared with controls [23].

Additionally, we identified a tendency towards a decrease in fasting insulin and HOMA-IR with GH therapy. Previous reports have been mixed. One study identified increased fasting insulin and glucose in TS girls on GH therapy [24] and another found no difference in

fasting insulin prior to GH therapy in TS girls compared with controls, but found increased fasting insulin following 6-12 months of GH therapy [25]. Compared with controls, in two studies, TS girls on GH therapy had an exaggerated hyperinsulinaemic response to glucose load [24,26]. The suggestion of a protective effect of GH on insulin dynamics and endothelial function in TS girls in this report indicates that confirmatory studies are required, using various modalities to assess endothelial function and glucose-insulin dynamics in TS girls at various ages and stages of puberty.

We did observe that girls with Turner Syndrome who were receiving GH therapy had higher RH-PAT scores than girls with Turner Syndrome who were not receiving GH therapy, suggesting that GH may offer some endothelial protection in girls with Turner Syndrome. This was seen in a small number of patients, yet differences in endothelial function were not noted with estrogen replacement. Using other measures of endothelial or vascular function, previous studies have identified a protective effect of GH therapy. Flow-mediated dilatation improves in GH deficient adults following 3-18 months of GH therapy [27]. GH deficient adolescents had impaired flow-mediated dilatation, and GH induced a larger increase in blood flow in GH treated adolescents than in untreated or healthy controls [28]. Some studies have failed to identify improvements in vascular function following GH therapy, including a recent study of endothelial dysfunction in GH deficient children [29]. Both GH and sex steroids influence vascular function; GH improves cardiac contractility and vasculature tone [30] while estrogen promotes the release of nitric oxide thus resulting in vasodilation [31]. There are various mechanisms by which GH may improve endothelial function in girls with Turner Syndrome. Firstly, clinical studies suggest that GH may be beneficial in non-GH-deficient (non-Turner Syndrome) individuals with visceral obesity, by reducing abdominal fat and improving insulin sensitivity [32]. Secondly, studies suggest that the GH-IGF axis is profoundly altered in Turner Syndrome, specific alterations include a reduction in bioactive IGF-1 [33]. Finally, in studies of animal models of GH deficiency, GH treatment has resulted in increased anti-oxidant capacity and increased resistance to oxidative stressors [34,35].

Physiologically, inherent differences have been described as part of the vasculopathy associated with Turner Syndrome. The precise mechanisms underlying this are likely multi-factorial and related to endothelial injury; alterations in Turner Syndrome patients include abnormities of collagen [36] and impaired release of nitric oxide [37]. Imbalances in matrix metalloproteinases (MMP) activity necessary to maintain normal vessel structure has also been postulated to be present in TS patients [4]. These changes are important in promoting aortic dilation and aneurysm formation; they also likely act in synergy with acquired cardiovascular disease risk factors to promote accelerated atherogenesis in Turner Syndrome.

Several features of this study warrant further comment. This report is limited by the small number of patients studied and by the absence of significant correlations between RH-PAT and known traditional cardiovascular risk factors in the Turner Syndrome cohort. We did not observe any significant correlations with acquired CVD risk factors present in our cohort, including abnormal lipid profile, hypertension or insulin resistance. However, our relatively small study size and the lack of wide variation in these variables may account for this finding. We also used historical healthy controls who had undergone previous endothelial function testing using the same measure and protocol. While this did allow for matching on the basis of several confounding variables including age, sex and BMI, data relating to pubertal status or markers of insulin resistance were not available for comparison in the healthy control group. Nonetheless, given the nature of Turner Syndrome, with requirements for pubertal induction, it is unlikely that groups could be matched simultaneously for age and pubertal status [38]. Finally, we included 1 Turner Syndrome girl with a history of CoArctation repair. But this group of Turner Syndrome girls has not had cardiac MRI performed and, similar to previous studies [39], it is therefore possible that MRI would identify additional girls with structural heart defects. This study confirms that assessment of endothelial function using the PAT technique is well-tolerated and suitable for use in high risk,

adolescent pediatric cohorts. However, like other tests of endothelial functionthat serve as surrogate markers of atherosclerosis, additional longitudinal data are required to evaluate any predictive value of these measures for cardiovascular events in adulthood.

Our findings suggest that that Turner Syndrome is an independent risk factor for impaired endothelial function at a young age, but GH therapy may be protective in the Turner Syndrome population. Considering this inherent vasculopathy, it is important to monitor and intervene in these patients to reduce the additional burden of acquired cardiovascular disease risk factors (hypertension, glucose intolerance, obesity and dyslipidemia), which are commonly observed in adolescent and adult Turner Syndrome patients. Regular screening is essential so that sub-clinical treatable conditions can be identified, with the ultimate goal of improving morbidity and mortality.

Conclusions
We identified evidence of impaired endothelial function in pediatric Turner Syndrome subjects, compared with age- and BMI-matched female controls. We suggest that pediatricians need to be aware of increased risk of early atherosclerosis in pediatric age range Turner Syndrome patients, and to intervene with diet and lifestyle modifications and medications as needed. We also suggest that longitudinal studies are required to follow Turner Syndrome girls throughout the age spectrum into adulthood to identify and follow evidence of atherosclerosis.

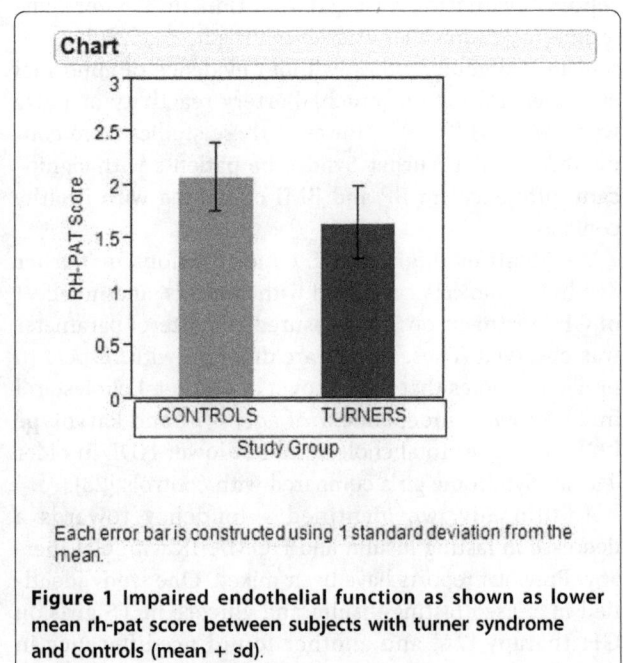

Each error bar is constructed using 1 standard deviation from the mean.

Figure 1 Impaired endothelial function as shown as lower mean rh-pat score between subjects with turner syndrome and controls (mean + sd).

Abbreviations

PAT: Peripheral Arterial Tonometry; BMI: Body Mass Index; HOMA-IR: Homeostasis Model Assessment - Insulin Resistance; RH-PAT: PAT-hyperemia ratio; HDL: High Density Lipoprotein cholesterol; GH: Growth Hormone; IGF1: Insulin-Like Growth Factor 1; LDL: Low Density Lipoprotein; BP: Blood Pressure; Kg: kilograms; M: metres; CV: coefficient of variation; SD: Standard deviation.

Acknowledgements

This study was supported by a grant from the Adrian and Rita Hudson Foundation. COG was supported by a fellowship from the SickKids Research Institute and by a research award from the Faculty of Medicine, University of Toronto. CS was supported by a fellowship from Heart and Stroke Foundation of Canada. We acknowledge the contribution of our patients and their families in supporting this research.
Disclosures
COG wrote the first draft of this manuscript, and COG was/is not in receipt of payment for writing. This study was supported by a grant from the Adrian and Rita Hudson Foundation. COG was supported by a fellowship from the SickKids Research Institute and by a research award from the Faculty of Medicine, University of Toronto. CS was supported by a fellowship from Heart and Stroke Foundation of Canada.

Author details

[1]Divisions of Endocrinology, The Hospital for Sick Children Research Institute, University of Toronto, Toronto, Canada. [2]Divisions of Cardiology, The Hospital for Sick Children Research Institute, University of Toronto, Toronto, Canada. [3]Department of Pediatrics, The Hospital for Sick Children Research Institute, University of Toronto, Toronto, Canada. [4]Physiology and Experimental Medicine Program, The Hospital for Sick Children Research Institute, University of Toronto, Toronto, Canada. [5]Department of Paediatrics, Graduate Entry Medical School, University of Limerick, Limerick, Ireland.

Authors' contributions

CSOG designed the study, collected the data, analysed the data, wrote the manuscript. CS co- collected data and co-analysed data. TB co-designed the study and co-analysed the data. JH participated in study design, data analysis and preparation of the manuscript. FHM conceived the study, designed the study, analysed the data and co-wrote the final manuscript. All authors read and approved the final manuscript.

Competing interests

The authors declare that they have no competing interests.

References

1. Hall JG, Gilchrist DM: Turner syndrome and its variants. Pediatr Clin North Am 1990, 37:1421-1440.
2. Gravholt CH, Juul S, Naeraa RW, Hansen J: Morbidity in turner syndrome. J Clin Epidemiol 1998, 51:147-158.
3. Schoemaker MJ, Swerdlow AJ, Higgins CD, Wright AF, Jacobs PA: Mortality in women with turner syndrome in Great Britain: a national cohort study. J Clin Endocrinol Metab 2008, 93:4735-4742.
4. Bondy CA: Aortic dissection in Turner syndrome. Curr Opin Cardiol 2008, 23:519-526.
5. Brunner H, Cockcroft JR, Deanfield J, Donald A, Ferrannini E, Halcox J, Kiowski W, Luscher TF, Mancia G, Natali A, et al: Endothelial function and dysfunction. part II: association with cardiovascular risk factors and diseases. a statement by the working group on endothelins and endothelial factors of the european society of hypertension. J Hypertens 2005, 23:233-246.
6. Anderson TJ, Uehata A, Gerhard MD, Meredith IT, Knab S, Delagrange D, Lieberman EH, Ganz P, Creager MA, Yeung AC, et al: Close relation of endothelial function in the human coronary and peripheral circulations. J Am Coll Cardiol 1995, 26:1235-1241.
7. Bonetti PO, Pumper GM, Higano ST, Holmes DR Jr, Kuvin JT, Lerman A: Noninvasive identification of patients with early coronary atherosclerosis by assessment of digital reactive hyperemia. J Am Coll Cardiol 2004, 44:2137-2141.
8. Bonetti PO, Barsness GW, Keelan PC, Schnell TI, Pumper GM, Kuvin JT, Schnall RP, Holmes DR, Higano ST, Lerman A: Enhanced external counterpulsation improves endothelial function in patients with symptomatic coronary artery disease. J Am Coll Cardiol 2003, 41:1761-1768.
9. Kuvin JT, Patel AR, Sliney KA, Pandian NG, Rand WM, Udelson JE, Karas RH: Peripheral vascular endothelial function testing as a noninvasive indicator of coronary artery disease. J Am Coll Cardiol 2001, 38:1843-1849.
10. Kuvin JT, Patel AR, Sliney KA, Pandian NG, Sheffy J, Schnall RP, Karas RH, Udelson JE: Assessment of peripheral vascular endothelial function with finger arterial pulse wave amplitude. Am Heart J 2003, 146:168-174.
11. Hamburg NM, Keyes MJ, Larson MG, Vasan RS, Schnabel R, Pryde MM, Mitchell GF, Sheffy J, Vita JA, Benjamin EJ: Cross-sectional relations of digital vascular function to cardiovascular risk factors in the Framingham Heart Study. Circulation 2008, 117:2467-2474.
12. Mahmud FH, Hill DJ, Cuerden MS, Clarson CL: Impaired vascular function in obese adolescents with insulin resistance. J Pediatr 2009, 155:678-682.
13. Mahmud FH, Van Uum S, Kanji N, Thiessen-Philbrook H, Clarson CL: Impaired endothelial function in adolescents with type 1 diabetes mellitus. J Pediatr 2008, 152:557-562.
14. Jarvisalo MJ, Putto-Laurila A, Jartti L, Lehtimaki T, Solakivi T, Ronnemaa T, Raitakari OT: Carotid artery intima-media thickness in children with type 1 diabetes. Diabetes 2002, 51:493-498.
15. Aggoun Y, Tounian P, Dabbas-Tyan M, Massih TA, Girardet JP, Ricour C, Sidi D, Bonnet D: Arterial rigidity and endothelial dysfunction in obese children. Arch Mal Coeur Vaiss 2002, 95:631-635.
16. Matthews DR, Hosker JP, Rudenski AS, Naylor BA, Treacher DF, Turner RC: Homeostasis model assessment: insulin resistance and beta-cell function from fasting plasma glucose and insulin concentrations in man. Diabetologia 1985, 28:412-419.
17. Marshall WA, Tanner JM: Variations in pattern of pubertal changes in girls. Arch Dis Child 1969, 44:291-303.
18. Haller MJ, Stein J, Shuster J, Theriaque D, Silverstein J, Schatz DA, Earing MG, Lerman A, Mahmud FH: Peripheral artery tonometry demonstrates altered endothelial function in children with type 1 diabetes. Pediatr Diabetes 2007, 8:193-198.
19. Selamet Tierney ES, Newburger JW, Gauvreau K, Geva J, Coogan E, Colan SD, de Ferranti SD: Endothelial pulse amplitude testing: feasibility and reproducibility in adolescents. J Pediatr 2009, 154:901-905.
20. Ostberg JE, Donald AE, Halcox JP, Storry C, McCarthy C, Conway GS: Vasculopathy in Turner syndrome: arterial dilatation and intimal thickening without endothelial dysfunction. J Clin Endocrinol Metab 2005, 90:5161-5166.
21. Baguet JP, Douchin S, Pierre H, Rossignol AM, Bost M, Mallion JM: Structural and functional abnormalities of large arteries in the Turner syndrome. Heart 2005, 91:1442-1446.
22. Ross JL, Feuillan P, Long LM, Kowal K, Kushner H, Cutler GB Jr: Lipid abnormalities in Turner syndrome. J Pediatr 1995, 126:242-245.
23. Van PL, Bakalov VK, Bondy CA: Monosomy for the X-chromosome is associated with an atherogenic lipid profile. J Clin Endocrinol Metab 2006, 91:2867-2870.
24. Sas TC, de Muinck Keizer-Schrama SM, Stijnen T, Aanstoot HJ, Drop SL: Carbohydrate metabolism during long-term growth hormone (GH) treatment and after discontinuation of GH treatment in girls with Turner syndrome participating in a randomized dose-response study. Dutch advisory group on growth hormone. J Clin Endocrinol Metab 2000, 85:769-775.
25. Caprio S, Boulware SD, Press M, Sherwin RS, Rubin K, Carpenter TO, Plewe G, Tamborlane WV: Effect of growth hormone treatment on hyperinsulinemia associated with Turner syndrome. J Pediatr 1992, 120:238-243.
26. Radetti G, Pasquino B, Gottardi E, Boscolo Contadin I, Aimaretti G, Rigon F: Insulin sensitivity in Turner's syndrome: influence of GH treatment. Eur J Endocrinol 2004, 151:351-354.
27. Pfeifer M, Verhovec R, Zizek B, Prezelj J, Poredos P, Clayton RN: Growth hormone (GH) treatment reverses early atherosclerotic changes in GH-deficient adults. J Clin Endocrinol Metab 1999, 84:453-457.
28. Lanes R, Soros A, Flores K, Gunczler P, Carrillo E, Bandel J: Endothelial function, carotid artery intima-media thickness, epicardial adipose tissue, and left ventricular mass and function in growth hormone-deficient

adolescents: apparent effects of growth hormone treatment on these parameters. *J Clin Endocrinol Metab* 2005, **90**:3978-3982.

29. Hoffman RP: **Growth hormone (GH) treatment does not restore endothelial function in children with GH deficiency.** *J Pediatr Endocrinol Metab* 2008, **21**:323-328.

30. Capalbo D, Lo Vecchio A, Farina V, Spinelli L, Palladino A, Tiano C, Lettiero T, Lombardi G, Colao A, Salerno M: **Subtle alterations of cardiac performance in children with growth hormone deficiency: results of a two-year prospective, case-control study.** *J Clin Endocrinol Metab* 2009, **94**:3347-3355.

31. Li XP, Zhou Y, Zhao SP, Gao M, Zhou QC, Li YS: **Effect of endogenous estrogen on endothelial function in women with coronary heart disease and its mechanism.** *Clin Chim Acta* 2004, **339**:183-188.

32. Attallah H, Friedlander AL, Hoffman AR: **Visceral obesity, impaired glucose tolerance, metabolic syndrome, and growth hormone therapy.** *Growth Horm IGF Res* 2006, **16 Suppl A**:S62-67.

33. Gravholt CH, Chen JW, Oxvig C, Overgaard MT, Christiansen JS, Frystyk J, Flyvbjerg A: **The GH-IGF-IGFBP axis is changed in Turner syndrome: partial normalization by HRT.** *Growth Horm IGF Res* 2006, **16**:332-339.

34. Ungvari Z, Gautam T, Koncz P, Henthorn JC, Pinto JT, Ballabh P, Yan H, Mitschelen M, Farley J, Sonntag WE, Csiszar A: **Vasoprotective effects of life span-extending peripubertal GH replacement in Lewis dwarf rats.** *J Gerontol A Biol Sci Med Sci* 2010, **65**:1145-1156.

35. Ungvari Z, Sosnowska D, Podlutsky A, Koncz P, Sonntag WE, Csiszar A: **Free radical production, antioxidant capacity, and oxidative stress response signatures in fibroblasts from Lewis dwarf rats: effects of life span-extending peripubertal GH treatment.** *J Gerontol A Biol Sci Med Sci* 2011, **66**:501-510.

36. Gravholt CH, Landin-Wilhelmsen K, Stochholm K, Hjerrild BE, Ledet T, Djurhuus CB, Sylven L, Baandrup U, Kristensen BO, Christiansen JS: **Clinical and epidemiological description of aortic dissection in Turner's syndrome.** *Cardiol Young* 2006, **16**:430-436.

37. Brandenburg H, Steegers EA, Gittenberger-de Groot AC: **Potential involvement of vascular endothelial growth factor in pathophysiology of Turner syndrome.** *Med Hypotheses* 2005, **65**:300-304.

38. Caprio S, Boulware S, Diamond M, Sherwin RS, Carpenter TO, Rubin K, Amiel S, Press M, Tamborlane VV: **Insulin resistance: an early metabolic defect of Turner's syndrome.** *J Clin Endocrinol Metab* 1991, **72**:832-836.

39. Ho VB, Bakalov VK, Cooley M, Van PL, Hood MN, Burklow TR, Bondy CA: **Major vascular anomalies in Turner syndrome: prevalence and magnetic resonance angiographic features.** *Circulation* 2004, **110**:1694-1700.

5

Early diagnosis and treatment referral of children born small for gestational age without catch-up growth are critical for optimal growth outcomes

Christopher P Houk[1] and Peter A Lee[2,3*]

Abstract

Approximately 10% of children born small for their gestational age (SGA) fail to show catch-up growth and may remain short-statured as adults. Despite treatment guidelines for children born SGA that recommend referral for growth hormone (GH) therapy evaluation and initiation by ages 2 to 4 years, the average age of GH treatment initiation is typically much later, at ages 7 to 9 years. Delayed referral for GH treatment is problematic as studies show younger age at GH treatment initiation in children born SGA is an independent predictor for responses such as optimal growth acceleration, normalization of prepubertal height, and most importantly, adult height (AH). This review discusses the importance and associated challenges of early diagnosis of children born SGA who fail to show catch-up growth, contrasts the recommended age of referral for these patients and the average age of GH treatment initiation, and discusses studies showing the significant positive effects of early referral and treatment with GH on AHs in short-statured children born SGA. To optimize the eventual height in short-statured SGA children who fail to manifest catch-up growth, a lowering of the average age of referral for GH therapy evaluation is needed to better align with consensus recommendations for SGA management. The importance of increasing parental and physician awareness that most children born SGA will do well developmentally and will optimally benefit from early initiation of GH treatment when short-statured is addressed, as is the need to shift the age of referral to better align with consensus recommendations.

Keywords: Hormone, GH therapy, Referral age, Short-statured, Optimal height acceleration, Gestational age, Prepubertal height, Adult height

Introduction

Being small for gestational age (SGA) at birth has many causes, including fetal, placental, maternal, and environmental factors [1,2]. SGA is typically diagnosed when birth weight and/or length are at least 2 standard deviations (SDs) below the mean for gestational age, using appropriate reference data [1,3]. Children born SGA comprise a heterogeneous group with a broad spectrum of clinical characteristics [4]. SGA may occur alongside intrauterine growth retardation (IUGR) and/or premature birth, or may be diagnosed at term in the absence of any prenatal complications. The etiology of SGA is frequently unknown, and current estimates suggest that 40% of SGA births will have no identifiable pathology. Of those 60% of SGA infants where an etiology is identified, about 50% involve maternal factors, 5% involve fetal abnormalities, and less than 5% are felt to be due to placental pathology. Maternal factors associated with SGA include inadequate nutrition; hypoxia; diabetes mellitus; drug use and abuse; vascular, hematologic, and renal disorders; infection; and sociodemographic factors. Fetal causes include congenital anomalies; chromosomal abnormalities; infection; and hormone abnormalities involving insulin, leptin, thyroid hormones, and insulin-like growth factors (IGF-1 and IGF-2). Placental factors that may result in SGA include placental insufficiency, infarction, abruption, and vascular abnormalities [1,5-8].

The available SGA incidence and prevalence data are limited due to insufficient or inconsistent records for

* Correspondence: plee@psu.edu

[2]Penn State College of Medicine, Milton S. Hershey Medical Center, PO Box 850, Hershey, PA17033-0850, USA

[3]Indiana University School of Medicine, The Riley Hospital for Children, 702 Barnhill Dr, Indianapolis, IN 46202, USA

Full list of author information is available at the end of the article

birth length and gestational age in national databases [9]. A population-based study including 3650 healthy full-term neonates born in Sweden over a 3-year period found 5.4% (N = 198) were diagnosed SGA, defined as <−2 SDs in birth length and/or weight [10]. Within the group of SGA children, 1.5% were both underweight and short, 2.4% were short only, 1.6% were underweight only. The estimated incidence of SGA births, using the definition of <−2 SDs in length or weight (equivalent to the 2.3 percentile), is 1 in 43, making SGA incidence relatively high compared with other growth disorders [11]. Most children born SGA show catch-up growth, generally defined as growth velocity (cm/year) greater than the median for chronologic age and gender, within the first 2 years of life; however, approximately 10% fail to show catch-up growth and may remain short-statured as adults [1]. Growth hormone (GH) therapy has been approved for long-term therapy of growth failure in short-statured children born SGA who show no evidence of catch-up growth by age 2 to 4 years [1,3,12]. The mechanisms underlying catch-up growth remain unclear [13]. Lack of catch-up growth has not been associated with any specific SGA etiology; however, preterm birth with less than 32 weeks gestation has been associated with a greater risk for no catch-up growth [3,14].

The average age of GH treatment initiation in short-statured children born SGA is typically many years later than the recommended age of 2 to 4 years [3,15-17]. This frequent delay in GH treatment is problematic as older age at GH therapy initiation is associated with significantly reduced growth response [15,18-20]. This review discusses the importance and associated challenges of early diagnosis of SGA with failure of spontaneous catch-up growth. We contrast the recommended age of referral and GH treatment initiation, according to consensus-based guidelines, with the average age(s) reported in treatment studies; we then review the significant positive benefits of early GH treatment on optimal height outcomes in short-statured patients born SGA.

Diagnosis of SGA

Accurate gestational age dating and measurement of birth weight and length are critical for SGA diagnosis [3]. There are several challenges to achieving accurate gestational age dating and accurate birth weight and length measurement. The accuracy of gestational age dating depends on the method used. An estimate based on last menstrual period produces greater error compared with clinical or obstetric estimates using early ultrasound assessment [21-24]. Accurate assessment of growth restriction requires careful and precise neonatal measurements, which are essential to establish size relative to gestational age [25-27]. Additionally, appropriate use of population-relevant reference growth curves is also necessary for accurate diagnosis of SGA [28,29].

Discriminating between pathologic and constitutional SGA is difficult, and guidelines for the selection of appropriate reference comparison data are evolving. The anthropometric definition of SGA does not account for background growth-modifying factors, such as maternal height, weight, ethnicity, and parity [3,30]. These modifying factors can be used to statistically model a corrected birth weight and/or length, and may increase the likelihood of identifying abnormal fetal growth compared with constitutional smallness [30]. This approach to growth assessment adjusts for physiological variation, calculates true growth potential, and creates individually customized fetal, neonatal, and child growth curves and birth weight percentiles [30-33]. Methodology for customized growth assessment is currently being developed and is not yet widely available.

To expedite appropriate early referral to GH treatment, early diagnosis of SGA and recognition of failure of spontaneous catch-up growth are critical [1,3]. Measurements of length, weight, and head circumference should be taken every 3 months in the first year of life and every 6 months thereafter [3]. Diminished head growth, particularly when it occurs both in utero and postnatally, is especially important to follow. Little or no catch-up head growth is a significant risk factor for poor outcome as it has been associated with widespread cognitive impairments [34]. Spontaneous catch-up growth typically occurs by age 2, and is most pronounced in the first 6 to 12 months after birth [1,3]. A child without spontaneous catch-up growth by age 3, or by age 4 in preterm infants, is unlikely to experience it later without therapeutic intervention [1,3]. It has been shown that children born SGA have a 7-fold higher risk of being short at age 18 than do children not born SGA, and children born SGA comprise 22% of adults whose height is below −2 SD scores (SDs) [35].

Indication for GH treatment

GH treatment of short children born SGA has been approved by the US Food and Drug Administration (FDA) since 2001 and the European Medicines Agency (EMA) since 2003 [1,3,11]. Prior to initiating GH treatment, other causes of short stature must be excluded, including growth-inhibiting medication, chronic diseases, endocrine disorders, emotional deprivation, or syndromes associated with short stature. GH stimulation testing or the presence of GH deficiency (GHD) are not required prior to GH treatment of children born SGA as the growth benefit from GH treatment occurs whether GHD is present or not [36-38]. No correlation has been found between spontaneous 24-hour GH profiles or maximal stimulated GH secretion before the start of GH treatment and adult height (AH) SDS or gain in height SDS in children born SGA [37].

Initiation of GH treatment is appropriate when the opportunity for spontaneous catch-up growth has passed [1,3,35,39]. In the US, treatment is indicated in children born SGA who fail to achieve normal growth velocity by age 2. The EMA indication approves GH treatment beginning at age 4 [3]. The International Societies of Pediatric Endocrinology and the Growth Hormone Research Society consensus statement proposes that children born SGA with height below –2.5 SDs at age 2, or with height below –2 SDs at age 4, should be GH treatment eligible [3]. Thus, by age 4, initiation of GH treatment is broadly recommended in SGA children with short stature when the family feels AH is important.

Early referral for GH treatment

The average age of GH treatment initiation in children born SGA is frequently much older than the 2- to 4-year-old age range recommended by consensus guidelines [3,15,40]. Among 360 GH-naïve, born-SGA pediatric patients participating in the American Norditropin Studies: Web-Enabled Research (The ANSWER Program®) registry, the mean age at treatment initiation was 8.4 years [15], and among 1909 children born SGA enrolled in the Pfizer International Growth Database (KIGS; a pharmacoepidemiological survey of children treated with GH) the mean age at start of GH therapy was 9.1 years (range, 3.9-13.3) [17]. Significant variation in age of referral and GH treatment initiation for short-statured SGA patients has been shown among different countries, ranging from a mean age of 6.7 to a mean age of 9.3 [16]. The older-age treatment referral and initiation is problematic as SGA patients beginning GH therapy at ages 9–10 experience lower growth velocity and have shorter AHs compared with those treated earlier [1].

The reasons for the current practice of delayed referral are unclear. One possibility is that parent attitudes and preferences regarding treatment influence physician decision making. For example, physicians were 40% more likely to recommend GH therapy for a child with short stature, not specific to SGA, if the family strongly desired GH treatment compared with a family neutral about treatment [41]. Parental realization of the importance of optimal growth may be delayed due to the presence of other comorbid conditions during the early developmental period of their child born SGA. Parents of children born with extreme SGA, comorbid systemic diseases, and high risk of mortality may feel fortunate for the survival of their child and, comparatively, may not believe short stature is as important an outcome. In particular, among children born SGA with a poor cognitive developmental prognosis, height may be considered unimportant. Parents may simply be pleased to have a reasonably healthy child after a difficult beginning and they may not seek treatment for short stature until the child is older than the optimal referral age. Parents need to be educated that most children born SGA will do well developmentally, that children without spontaneous catch-up growth are highly likely to remain short as adults, and that GH treatment, when initiated at an early age, will improve childhood growth rate and AH.

Alternatively, delayed referral could be due to beliefs of the treating pediatrician or primary care physician. Children born SGA typically leave the care of neonatologists before they are 2 years old and receive care from a pediatrician or primary care physician. Pediatricians and primary care physicians may not consider height to be a concern among patients who are short but healthy until the optimal referral age has passed. It is important to educate families and physicians about the significance of the age of referral because studies show younger age at GH treatment initiation is an important predictor of response to GH therapy [15,18,19].

Younger age and growth response to GH treatment

Effectiveness of GH treatment in short-statured children born SGA has been well demonstrated [12,13,42,43]. A 4-year study of GH treatment in SGA and GHD children enrolled in the NordiNet® international outcome study (IOS) demonstrated similar height improvement in SGA and GHD children, supporting the idea that GH treatment in non-GHD patients is as effective as it is in GHD children [44]. The cumulative mean height standard deviation score (ΔHSDS) was 1.60 in SGA and 1.55 ($P = 0.412$) in GHD children, and height was within the normal range after 4 years of GH treatment in 68% of SGA children and 79% of GHD children.

A 2-year study of GH treatment in children enrolled in the ANSWER Program registry found the largest ΔHSDS at 1 and 2 years occurred in patients with multiple pituitary hormone deficiency (MPHD) (0.85, 1.20; year 1, year 2) and SGA (0.80, 1.18), compared with GHD (0.61, 1.06), idiopathic short stature (ISS) (0.54, 0.90), and Turner Syndrome (TS) (0.50, 0.82) patients [40]. After 2 years of GH treatment among children enrolled in the IOS and ANSWER Program, greater ΔHSDS was found for patients with SGA compared with GHD (1.03 versus 0.97; $P = 0.047$).

However, therapeutic response is variable and age at GH treatment initiation is a critical factor in predicting growth outcome. Mathematical models developed to predict optimal growth following GH therapy in children born SGA show younger age at treatment initiation is a key predictor of growth response [19,45]. The most important determinants of greater first-year growth during GH therapy in short children born SGA were younger age and higher dose of GH [19,45]. The models show growth velocity during the first year of treatment, which is significantly influenced by age at treatment initiation, is the most important predictor of subsequent growth, suggesting AH outcome is indicated by the initial response to GH [19]. Greater long-term growth response observed in AH SDs in children born SGA was shown to depend on the duration of GH treatment, with younger age at treatment initiation and longer phase of treatment producing greater height increases [45].

Younger age at GH treatment initiation is associated with greater short-term height response (see Table 1 [15,16,19,46,47]). A comparison among children born SGA and enrolled in NordiNet IOS from 5 European countries (N = 433) found the greatest changes in height standard deviation score (ΔHSDS) occurring during the first year of GH treatment in countries where children were younger (mean age 6.7) at treatment initiation ($P < 0.0001$) [16]. Among males, the change from baseline ΔHSDS in the first year of GH treatment was significantly greater for patients who started GH treatment at a younger age (ie, younger than age 11 [ΔHSDS = 0.82, N = 101], than it was for patients who were older than age 11 [ΔHSDS = 0.27, N = 30], $P < 0.0001$) [15]. ΔHSDS in years 1–2 of GH treatment was greater in SGA patients enrolled in the NordiNet IOS (N = 423) who were younger at GH treatment initiation [18].

ΔHSDS following 1 year of GH treatment was significantly greater in prepubertal (ΔHSDS = 0.75, N = 24) compared with pubertal (ΔHSDS = 0.40, N = 15, $P = 0.016$) short-statured SGA children [47]. Among very young (ages 2–5) SGA children, the greatest gain in growth velocity during the first 2 years of GH treatment occurred in those younger than age 4 (1.7 SDS, N = 16) compared with children older than 4 (1.2 SDS, N = 23, $P < 0.05$) [46].

Younger age at initiation of GH treatment is also associated with greater long-term height response (see Table 2 [20,36-38,45,48]). In a long-term prediction model of height SDS at the onset of puberty, younger age at GH therapy initiation was associated with greater height outcome at puberty in short-statured SGA children (N = 150) [20]. Younger age at GH treatment initiation was also associated with better AH following long-term GH treatment in short SGA children (N = 38) [49]. Among 77 short-statured, prepubertal children born SGA, better catch-up growth to AH in response to GH treatment was noted in children who were younger at the start of GH treatment (r = –0.56, $P < 0.0001$) [36]. Among children treated for >2 years before puberty, the mean gain in height was 1.7 SDS, compared with 0.9 SDS ($P < 0.001$) when treatment was initiated <2 years before the onset of

Table 1 Age at treatment initiation and short-term GH treatment outcomes in children born SGA

Study	N	Design/Duration	Age[a]/Model	Outcome (ΔHSDS or statistical model)	P Value
Argente 2007 [46]	39[b]	MC, C, R, O/2 years	2 to <4 years	1.7 at 1 year; approximately 2.5 at 2 years	<0.05
			4 to 5 years	1.2 at 1 year; approximately 1.8 at 2 years	
Carvalho-Furtado 2009 [47]	39	Ob/1 year	Prepubertal	0.75	=0.016
			Pubertal	0.40	
Lee 2008 [16]	433	MC, NordiNet IOS/≥1 year	Mean age 6.7 to 9.3	6.7 years = 1.0 and 0.8; 7.6 years = 0.72; 8.3 years = 0.61; 9.3 years = 0.57	<0.0001[c]
Ranke 2003 [19]	613 year 1;	KIGS, clinical trials/2 years	Mean age 6.6/statistical models predicting growth response	Year 1: GH dose (35% of variability), age at treatment start (11% of variability)	<0.0001 <0.0001
	385 year 2			Year 2: HV in year 1 of treatment (29% of variability), age at treatment start (3% of variability), GH dose (2% of variability)	
Ross 2010 [15]	208 year 1;	ANSWER Program registry/2 years	Mean age 8.4/males <11 years vs ≥11 years; females <10 years vs ≥10 years	Year 1 boys: <11 years = 0.82; ≥11 years = 0.27 Year 1 girls: <10 years = 0.58; ≥10 years = 0.41	<0.0001 = 0.093 = 0.0005 = 0.56
	119 year 2			Year 2 boys: <11 years = 1.23; ≥11 years = 0.59 Year 2 girls: <10 years = 1.00; ≥10 years = 0.87	

[a]Age at treatment initiation; [b]Data are reported for study group 1 with 2 years GH treatment; [c]Multivariate analysis showed ΔHSDS was dependent on age at the start of treatment. ANSWER, American Norditropin Studies: Web-enabled Research; C, controlled; GH, growth hormone; ΔHSDS, change in height SDS; HV, height velocity; IOS, international outcome study; KIGS, Pharmacia International Growth Database; MC, multicenter; O, open trial; Ob, observational; R, randomized; SDS, standard deviation score.

Table 2 Age at treatment initiation and long-term GH treatment outcomes in children born SGA

Study	N	Design/Duration	Age[a]/Model	Outcome (ΔHSDS or statistical model)	P Value
Dahlgren 2005 [36]	77	Ob/prepubertal to FH	Prepubertal during >2 years GH therapy vs prepubertal during <2 years GH therapy	Mean gain FH SDS prepubertal for >2 years GH therapy = 1.7; prepubertal for <2 years = 0.9	<0.001
de Ridder 2008 [47]	150	Data from 2 previous GH trials; R, DB/5 years[38]; R, C/3 years[48]	Median age 7.5/Statistical model predicting HSDS at puberty	Age at start (−0.27 estimated coefficient) Other significant predictors: HSDS at start (0.71 estimated coefficient), target height SDS (0.13 estimated coefficient), GH dose X IGF-I SDS at start (−0.29 estimated coefficient), gender (−0.34 estimated coefficient)	<0.0001 = 0.009 to <0.0001
Ranke 2010 [45]	161	KIGS, clinical trials/7.7 years	Median age 7.8 years/ Statistical models predicting AH SDS and ΔHSDS	70% of variability in adult height SDS: HSDS at GH start, ΔHSDS 1st year on GH, years on treatment [younger start, longer phase], maternal HSDS, length SDS at birth, SRS diagnosis	NR
				60% of variability in ΔHSDS: ΔHSDS 1st year GH, H-MPH SDS at GH start, years of GH treatment [younger start, longer phase]	
van Pareren 2003 [37]	54	MC, R, DB/mean 7.8 years	Mean age 8.1/ΔHSDS correlations	ΔHSDS from start of GH treatment to AH negatively correlated with age at treatment start: r = −0.36	<0.01

[a]Age at treatment initiation. AH, adult height; C, controlled; DB, double-blind; FH, final height; GH, growth hormone; HSDS, height SDS; ΔHSDS, change in height SDS; IGF-I, insulin-like growth factor; KIGS, Pharmacia International Growth Database; MC, multicenter; MPH, mid-parental height; NR, not reported; Ob, observational; R, randomized; SDS, standard deviation score; SRS, Silver-Russell syndrome.

puberty [36]. Long-term, continuous GH treatment (mean duration, 7.8 years), in children born SGA (N = 54) resulted in normalization of AH in most, with 98% reaching an AH within their target height range; younger age at the start of GH treatment was significantly associated with greater gain in height SDS from the start of GH treatment until AH (r = −0.36, P <0.01) [37]. Alternatively, GH treatment initiation in short adolescents born SGA (mean age, 12.7 years) has produced a more limited growth response with a mean height gain of 1.1 SDS and 47% of treated patients reaching AH in the normal range for the general population [50].

In addition to better growth outcomes, the greater growth response to GH treatment among younger patients born SGA may result in cost savings. A lower GH dose of approximately 33 mcg/kg/day from treatment initiation to AH is effective in children born SGA not extremely short-statured (eg, height above −3 SD), especially if treatment begins at ages 4–6 [51]. Children beginning GH therapy in late prepuberty or extremely short-statured at treatment initiation often receive a higher dose (≥50 mcg/kg/day) for optimal short-term catch-up growth, and then can be tapered back to 33 mcg/kg/day. Thus, a better cost of GH treatment-to-height benefit outcome ratio may be achieved when GH treatment begins at an early age because a greater growth response occurs at a lower GH dose.

Safety of GH treatment in children born SGA

The long-term safety of GH treatment in childhood has been under intense recent discussion due to the Safety and Appropriateness of Growth hormone treatments in Europe (SAGhE) mortality data from France suggesting increased all-cause, bone tumor-related, and circulatory system disease-related mortality over the mean 17.3-year follow-up period among adults who had received GH treatment as children (N = 6928) for the diagnoses of idiopathic isolated GHD, neurosecretory dysfunction, idiopathic short stature or born SGA [52]. However, the preliminary data from Belgium, The Netherlands, and Sweden (N = 2543) contrasted with the report from France in that the majority of the 21 deaths that occurred over the follow-up period were due to accidents or suicide and not a single case of death was related to cancer or cardiovascular disease [53]. Questions have been raised about the SAGhE data from France due to methodological limitations of the study, including the lack of an ideal control group of untreated patients, and in August 2011, the FDA stated the evidence of increased risk of death is inconclusive [54,55].

Additionally, multiple reports have demonstrated GH is safe for use at currently recommended doses in short-statured children born SGA [17,37]. GH treatment has been shown safe across heterogeneous groups of children born SGA, including very young (ages 2–5) children born SGA, preterm (gestation ≤36 weeks) children born SGA, and in children born SGA who were both preterm and very young [46,56,57]. Continuous GH treatment over 6 years was well tolerated in 54 children with short stature born SGA [37]. Relative insulin resistance occurred but there was no adverse effect on glucose levels or development of diabetes and no GH related adverse events were detected [37]. Similarly, among 84 SGA children participating in the US SGA trial from the KIGS Database, a reduction in insulin sensitivity occurred during GH treatment, but no patients developed impaired glucose tolerance or overt diabetes mellitus [17].

The International SGA Advisory Board states that because insulin resistance may increase during GH therapy, reviewing for a family history of type 2 diabetes mellitus (T2DM) is important [1]. Annual screening of carbohydrate status, such as hemoglobin A1c, a fasting or postprandial glucose, and insulin levels, is suitable in lean children without a family history of diabetes. If pubertal children are obese, have a family history of T2DM, or have acanthosis nigricans, glucose homeostasis should be monitored more frequently and intensely (using A1c in addition to oral glucose tolerance test with insulin measurements when indicated). Additionally, fasting serum lipids and blood pressure should be periodically monitored during long-term GH therapy.

Conclusions

SGA diagnosis is challenging, and guidelines for the selection of appropriate reference comparison data continue to evolve. Early diagnosis of SGA with failure to show catch-up growth and early referral to GH therapy are needed. In short-statured children born SGA without catch-up growth, early referral for GH evaluation and therapy is critical for optimal growth acceleration, normalization of prepubertal height, and improvements in AH. The average age of treatment referral varies, and often exceeds the International Societies of Pediatric Endocrinology and Growth Hormone Research Society consensus guidelines (that recommend referral at ages 2–4) by many years. The reasons for this referral delay are not known but likely involve parental and physician attitudes about the importance of early growth in children born SGA. Most children born SGA will do well developmentally, and it is essential that parents understand the benefits of GH treatment for short stature that accrue at a younger age of treatment initiation. Optimizing eventual height in short-statured patients born SGA without catch-up growth is most efficiently done by lowering the age of referral for GH evaluation and treatment to a time in childhood where initiation of treatment provides optimal benefit and aligns with consensus recommendations for SGA management.

Abbreviations

AH: adult height; ANSWER: American Norditropin Studies: Web-Enabled Research; EMA: European Medicines Agency; GH: growth hormone; GHD: GH deficiency; HSDS: height standard deviation score; ΔHSDS: change in height standard deviation score; IGF-1, IGF-2: insulin-like growth factors; IOS: international outcome study; ISS: idiopathic short stature; IUGR: intrauterine growth retardation; KIGS: Pfizer International Growth Database; MPHD: multiple pituitary hormone deficiency; SD: standard

deviation; SDS: SD score; SGA: small for gestational age; TS: Turner Syndrome; T2DM: type 2 diabetes mellitus.

Competing interests

Dr. Houk has no competing interests to declare. Dr. Lee has served as an advisory board member for Novo Nordisk Inc., and his institution has received grant funding from Novo Nordisk Inc. as part of the American Norditropin® Studies Web-Enabled Research (ANSWER) Program. Dr. Lee is also a member of the Editorial Board for the *International Journal of Pediatric Endocrinology*.

Authors' contributions

CH & PL were the primary investigators, interpreted the data, critically reviewed and provided final approval of this manuscript.

Acknowledgement

Funding to support the preparation of this manuscript was provided by Novo Nordisk Inc. We wish to thank Lynanne McGuire, PhD, of MedVal Scientific Information Services, LLC for providing medical writing and editorial assistance, including composing the first draft of the manuscript. MedVal received payment for these services. This manuscript was prepared according to the International Society for Medical Publication Professionals' "Good Publication Practice for Communicating Company-Sponsored Medical Research: the GPP2 Guidelines."

Author details

¹Medical College of Georgia, 1120 15th Street, Room BG1007, Augusta, GA 30912, USA. ²Penn State College of Medicine, Milton S. Hershey Medical Center, PO Box 850, Hershey, PA 17033-0850, USA. ³Indiana University School of Medicine, The Riley Hospital for Children, 702 Barnhill Dr, Indianapolis, IN 46202, USA.

References

1. Lee PA, Chernausek SD, Hokken-Koelega AC, Czernichow P: **International Small for Gestational Age Advisory Board consensus development conference statement: management of short children born small for gestational age, April 24-October 1, 2001.** *Pediatrics* 2003, 111(6 Pt 1): 1253–1261.
2. McCowan L, Horgan RP: **Risk factors for small for gestational age infants.** *Best Pract Res Clin Obstet Gynaecol* 2009, 23(6):779–793.
3. Clayton PE, Cianfarani S, Czernichow P, Johannsson G, Rapaport R, Rogol A: **Management of the child born small for gestational age through to adulthood: a consensus statement of the International Societies of Pediatric Endocrinology and the Growth Hormone Research Society.** *J Clin Endocrinol Metab* 2007, 92(3):804–810.
4. Ester W, Bannink E, van Dijk M, Willemsen R, van der Kaay D, de Ridder M, Hokken-Koelega A: **Subclassification of small for gestational age children with persistent short stature: growth patterns and response to GH treatment.** *Horm Res* 2008, 69(2):89–98.
5. Neerhof MG: **Causes of intrauterine growth restriction.** *Clin Perinatol* 1995, 22(2):375–385.
6. Wollmann HA: **Intrauterine growth restriction: definition and etiology.** *Horm Res* 1998, 49(Suppl 2):1–6.
7. Heinrich UE: **Intrauterine growth retardation and familial short stature.** *Baillieres Clin Endocrinol Metab* 1992, 6(3):589–601.
8. Pollack RN, Divon MY: **Intrauterine growth retardation: definition, classification, and etiology.** *Clin Obstet Gynecol* 1992, 35(1):99–107.
9. Loftus J, Heatley R, Walsh C, Dimitri P: **Systematic review of the clinical effectiveness of Genotropin (somatropin) in children with short stature.** *J Pediatr Endocrinol Metab* 2010, 23(6):535–551.
10. Albertsson-Wikland K, Karlberg J: **Natural growth in children born small for gestational age with and without catch-up growth.** *Acta Paediatr Suppl* 1994, 399:64–70.
11. Saenger P, Czernichow P, Hughes I, Reiter EO: **Small for gestational age: short stature and beyond.** *Endocr Rev* 2007, 28(2):219–251.
12. Chatelain P, Carrascosa A, Bona G, Ferrandez-Longas A, Sippell W: **Growth hormone therapy for short children born small for gestational age.** *Horm Res* 2007, 68(6):300–309.

13. Jung H, Rosilio M, Blum WF, Drop SL: Growth hormone treatment for short stature in children born small for gestational age. *Adv Ther* 2008, 25 (10):951–978.

14. Itabashi K, Mishina J, Tada H, Sakurai M, Nanri Y, Hirohata Y: Longitudinal follow-up of height up to five years of age in infants born preterm small for gestational age; comparison to full-term small for gestational age infants. *Early Hum Dev* 2007, 83(5):327–333.

15. Ross J, Lee PA, Gut R, Germak J: Factors influencing the one- and two-year growth response in children treated with growth hormone: analysis from an observational study. *Int J Pediatr Endocrinol* 2010, 2010:494656.

16. Lee PA, Gruters A, Tauber M, Pienkowski C, Pedersen BT, Rakov V: One year growth hormone (GH) treatment response in short children born small for gestational age (SGA) dependent on baseline characteristics: data from the NordiNet international outcome study (IOS). Poster presented at the 90th Annual Meeting of the Endocrine Society, San Francisco, CA. 2008.

17. Cutfield WS, Lindberg A, Rapaport R, Wajnrajch MP, Saenger P: Safety of growth hormone treatment in children born small for gestational age: the US trial and KIGS analysis. *Horm Res* 2006, 65(Suppl 3):153–159.

18. Lee PA, Gruters A, Tauber M, Oliver I, Pienkowski C, Snajderova M, Tonnes Peterson B, Rakov R: Similar change in height standard deviation scores during the first 2 years of growth hormone therapy for children with growth hormone deficiency, multiple pituitary hormone deficiencies and short children born small for gestational age: data from the NordiNet® international outcome study (IOS) [abstract]. *Horm Res* 2009, 72(Suppl 3):443.

19. Ranke MB, Lindberg A, Cowell CT, Wikland KA, Reiter EO, Wilton P, Price DA: Prediction of response to growth hormone treatment in short children born small for gestational age: analysis of data from KIGS (Pharmacia International Growth Database). *J Clin Endocrinol Metab* 2003, 88(1):125–131.

20. de Ridder MA, Stijnen T, Hokken-Koelega AC: Prediction model for adult height of small for gestational age children at the start of growth hormone treatment. *J Clin Endocrinol Metab* 2008, 93(2):477–483.

21. Ananth CV: Menstrual versus clinical estimate of gestational age dating in the United States: temporal trends and variability in indices of perinatal outcomes. *Paediatr Perinat Epidemiol* 2007, 21(Suppl 2):22–30.

22. Dietz PM, England LJ, Callaghan WM, Pearl M, Wier ML, Kharrazi M: A comparison of LMP-based and ultrasound-based estimates of gestational age using linked California livebirth and prenatal screening records. *Paediatr Perinat Epidemiol* 2007, 21(Suppl 2):62–71.

23. Lynch CD, Zhang J: The research implications of the selection of a gestational age estimation method. *Paediatr Perinat Epidemiol* 2007, 21(Suppl 2):86–96.

24. Callaghan WM, Dietz PM: Differences in birth weight for gestational age distributions according to the measures used to assign gestational age. *Am J Epidemiol* 2010, 171(7):826–836.

25. Lawrence EJ: Part 1: a matter of size: evaluating the growth-restricted neonate. *Adv Neonatal Care* 2006, 6(6):313–322.

26. Sifianou P: Small and growth-restricted babies: drawing the distinction. *Acta Paediatr* 2006, 95(12):1620–1624.

27. Zhang J, Merialdi M, Platt LD, Kramer MS: Defining normal and abnormal fetal growth: promises and challenges. *Am J Obstet Gynecol* 2010, 202(6): 522–528.

28. Olsen IE, Groveman SA, Lawson ML, Clark RH, Zemel BS: New intrauterine growth curves based on United States data. *Pediatrics* 2010, 125(2): e214–e224.

29. Marconi AM, Ronzoni S, Bozzetti P, Vailati S, Morabito A, Battaglia FC: Comparison of fetal and neonatal growth curves in detecting growth restriction. *Obstet Gynecol* 2008, 112(6):1227–1234.

30. Gardosi J: New definition of small for gestational age based on fetal growth potential. *Horm Res* 2006, 65(Suppl 3):15–18.

31. Figueras F, Gardosi J: Should we customize fetal growth standards? *Fetal Diagn Ther* 2009, 25(3):297–303.

32. Mamelle N, Boniol M, Riviere O, Joly MO, Mellier G, Maria B, Rousset B, Claris O: Identification of newborns with Fetal Growth Restriction (FGR) in weight and/or length based on constitutional growth potential. *Eur J Pediatr* 2006, 165(10):717–725.

33. Narchi H, Skinner A: Infants of diabetic mothers with abnormal fetal growth missed by standard growth charts. *J Obstet Gynaecol* 2009, 29(7):609–613.

34. Frisk V, Amsel R, Whyte HE: The importance of head growth patterns in predicting the cognitive abilities and literacy skills of small-for-gestational-age children. *Dev Neuropsychol* 2002, 22(3):565–593.

35. Karlberg J, Albertsson-Wikland K: Growth in full-term small-for-gestational-age infants: from birth to final height. *Pediatr Res* 1995, 38(5):733–739.

36. Dahlgren J, Wikland KA: Final height in short children born small for gestational age treated with growth hormone. *Pediatr Res* 2005, 57(2): 216–222.

37. Van Pareren Y, Mulder P, Houdijk M, Jansen M, Reeser M, Hokken-Koelega A: Adult height after long-term, continuous growth hormone (GH) treatment in short children born small for gestational age: results of a randomized, double-blind, dose-response GH trial. *J Clin Endocrinol Metab* 2003, 88(8):3584–3590.

38. Sas T, de Waal W, Mulder P, Houdijk M, Jansen M, Reeser M, Hokken-Koelega A: Growth hormone treatment in children with short stature born small for gestational age: 5-year results of a randomized, double-blind, dose-response trial. *J Clin Endocrinol Metab* 1999, 84(9):3064–3070.

39. Hokken-Koelega AC, De Ridder MA, Lemmen RJ, Den Hartog H, De Muinck Keizer-Schrama SM, Drop SL: Children born small for gestational age: do they catch up? *Pediatr Res* 1995, 38(2):267–271.

40. Lee PA, Germak J, Gut R, Khutoryansky N, Ross J: Identification of factors associated with good response to growth hormone therapy in children with short stature: results from the ANSWER Program®. *Int J Pediatr Endocrinol* 2011, 2011:6.

41. Finkelstein BS, Singh J, Silvers JB, Marrero U, Neuhauser D, Cuttler L: Patient attitudes and preferences regarding treatment: GH therapy for childhood short stature. *Horm Res* 1999, 51(Suppl 1):67–72.

42. Maiorana A, Cianfarani S: Impact of growth hormone therapy on adult height of children born small for gestational age. *Pediatrics* 2009, 124(3): e519–e531.

43. Labarta JI, Ruiz JA, Molina I, De Arriba A, Mayayo E, Longas AF: Growth and growth hormone treatment in short stature children born small for gestational age. *Pediatr Endocrinol Rev* 2009, 6(Suppl 3):350–357.

44. Blankenstein O, Oliver I, Snajderova M, Christesen HT, Lee PA, Rakov V, Pederson BT, Saevendahl L: Long-term GH treatment response in short children born SGA in GHD children: data from the NordiNet® IOS. *Endocr Rev* 2011, 32(Suppl 3):P1–P750.

45. Ranke MB, Lindberg A: Height at start, first-year growth response and cause of shortness at birth are major determinants of adult height outcomes of short children born small for gestational age and Silver-Russell syndrome treated with growth hormone: analysis of data from KIGS. *Horm Res Paediatr* 2010, 74(4):259–266.

46. Argente J, Gracia R, Ibanez L, Oliver A, Borrajo E, Vela A, Lopez-Siguero JP, Moreno ML, Rodriguez-Hierro F: Improvement in growth after two years of growth hormone therapy in very young children born small for gestational age and without spontaneous catch-up growth: results of a multicenter, controlled, randomized, open clinical trial. *J Clin Endocrinol Metab* 2007, 92(8):3095–3101.

47. Carvalho-Furtado AC, Naves LA: Clinical predictors of response in the first year of recombinant growth hormone treatment in short children born small for gestational age [abstract]. *Horm Res* 2009, 72(Suppl 3):341.

48. Arends NJ, Boonstra VH, Mulder PG, Odink RJ, Stokvis-Brantsma WH, Rongen-Westerlaken C, Mulder JC, Delemarre-Van de Waal H, Reeser HM, Jansen M, Waelkens JJ, Hokken-Koelega AC: GH treatment and its effect on bone mineral density, bone maturation and growth in short children born small for gestational age: 3-year results of a randomized, controlled GH trial. *Clin Endocrinol (Oxf)* 2003, 59(6):779–787.

49. Xatzipsalti M, Maggina P, Panagiotou E, Polychroni I, Delis D, Stamogiannou LN: Final height and body composition in growth hormone-treated short Greek children born small for gestational age [abstract]. *Horm Res* 2009, 72(Suppl 3):378.

50. Carel JC, Chatelain P, Rochiccioli P, Chaussain JL: Improvement in adult height after growth hormone treatment in adolescents with short stature born small for gestational age: results of a randomized controlled study. *J Clin Endocrinol Metab* 2003, 88(4):1587–1593.

51. de Zegher F, Hokken-Koelega A: Growth hormone therapy for children born small for gestational age: height gain is less dose dependent over the long term than over the short term. *Pediatrics* 2005, 115(4):e458–e462.

52. Carel JC, Ecosse E, Landier F, Meguellati-Hakkas D, Kaguelidou F, Rey G, Coste J: Long-term mortality after recombinant growth hormone treatment for isolated growth hormone deficiency or childhood short stature: preliminary report of the French SAGhE Study. *J Clin Endocrinol Metab* 2012, 97(2):416–425.

53. Savendahl L, Maes M, Albertsson-Wikland K, Borgstrom B, Carel JC, Henrard S, Speybroeck N, Thomas M, Zandwijken G, Hokken-Koelega A: **Long-term mortality and causes of death in isolated GHD, ISS, and SGA patients treated with recombinant growth hormone during childhood in Belgium, the Netherlands, and Sweden: preliminary report of 3 countries participating in the EU SAGhE Study.** *J Clin Endocrinol Metab* 2012, **97**(2): E213–E217.
54. Rosenfeld RG, Cohen P, Robison LL, Bercu BB, Clayton P, Hoffman AR, Radovick S, Saenger P, Savage MO, Wit JM: **Long-term surveillance of growth hormone therapy.** *J Clin Endocrinol Metab* 2012, **97**(1):68–72.
55. Malozowski S: **Reports of increased mortality and GH: will this affect current clinical practice?** *J Clin Endocrinol Metab* 2012, **97**(2):380–383.
56. de Kort SW, Willemsen RH, van der Kaay DC, Duivenvoorden HJ, Hokken-Koelega AC: **Does preterm birth influence the response to growth hormone treatment in short, small for gestational age children?** *Clin Endocrinol (Oxf)* 2009, **70**(4):582–587.
57. Garcia RA, Longui CA, Kochi C, Arruda M, Faria CD, Calliari LE, Monte O, Pachi PR, Saenger P: **First two years' response to growth hormone treatment in very young preterm small for gestational age children.** *Horm Res* 2009, **72**(5):275–280.

6

State of the Art Review: *Emerging Therapies: The Use of Insulin Sensitizers in the Treatment of Adolescents with Polycystic Ovary Syndrome (PCOS)*

David H Geller[1*], Danièle Pacaud[2], Catherine M Gordon[3] and Madhusmita Misra[4], for
of the Drug and Therapeutics Committee of the Pediatric Endocrine Society

Abstract

PCOS, a heterogeneous disorder characterized by cystic ovarian morphology, androgen excess, and/or irregular periods, emerges during or shortly after puberty. Peri- and post-pubertal obesity, insulin resistance and consequent hyperinsulinemia are highly prevalent co-morbidities of PCOS and promote an ongoing state of excess androgen. Given the relationship of insulin to androgen excess, reduction of insulin secretion and/or improvement of its action at target tissues offer the possibility of improving the physical stigmata of androgen excess by correction of the reproductive dysfunction and preventing metabolic derangements from becoming entrenched. While lifestyle changes that concentrate on behavioral, dietary and exercise regimens should be considered as first line therapy for weight reduction and normalization of insulin levels in adolescents with PCOS, several therapeutic options are available and in wide use, including oral contraceptives, metformin, thiazolidenediones and spironolactone. Overwhelmingly, the data on the safety and efficacy of these medications derive from the adult PCOS literature. Despite the paucity of randomized control trials to adequately evaluate these modalities in adolescents, their use, particularly that of metformin, has gained popularity in the pediatric endocrine community. In this article, we present an overview of the use of insulin sensitizing medications in PCOS and review both the adult and (where available) adolescent literature, focusing specifically on the use of metformin in both mono- and combination therapy.

Background

Recognition of the highly prevalent association between PCOS and insulin resistance (IR) has stimulated research into the mechanism(s) behind this relationship, defining the metabolic, cardiovascular, and reproductive consequences of the IR, and evaluating therapies that target IR. Much of the current therapeutic paradigm incorporating insulin sensitization is derived from studies in adult women; application to the adolescent requires critical evaluation of the data supporting insulin sensitizer use in this age group. Although not intended as a comprehensive review of PCOS therapy, this report will discuss the options available for the treatment of adolescents with PCOS, with focus on the possible efficacy and costs of insulin sensitizing agents in comparison to more traditional therapies for PCOS.

PCOS is a heterogeneous condition affecting 7-10% of women worldwide [1,2], irrespective of ethnic background [3], making it the most common endocrine disorder among reproductive-aged women. The 2003 Androgen Excess Society (AES) consensus required two of the following three criteria as necessary for the diagnosis: hyperandrogenism, ovarian dysfunction (oligo- or anovulation), and/or a polycystic ovary [4]. Summarizing the report of the recent 4th annual meeting of the Androgen Excess and PCOS Society [5], Yildiz and Azziz noted the difficulty in defining certain sub-phenotypes of PCOS, such as women with irregular menstrual cycling and polycystic ovarian morphology without evidence of hyperandrogenism (previously considered essential for the diagnosis).

While hyperandrogenism is central to classically defined PCOS pathophysiology [6-8], and testosterone

* Correspondence: david.geller@cshs.org
[1]Division of Pediatric Endocrinology, Cedars-Sinai Medical Center, David Geffen-UCLA School of Medicine 8700 Beverly Blvd., Rm 4220, Los Angeles, CA 90048, USA
Full list of author information is available at the end of the article

and DHEA-S are increased in up to 75% of PCOS patients, obesity and IR are frequently associated [9-11]. As many as 60% of women with PCOS have BMI values in the overweight or obese range [2] and 70% demonstrate IR and diabetes beyond that predicted by weight alone [12-14]. Hyperinsulinemia consequent to obesity and IR places women with PCOS at far greater risk to develop type 2 diabetes (T2DM) than healthy controls [15]: 15-36% of all T2DM reported in women, irrespective of age, is found in association with PCOS [14,16-19]. While most PCOS women demonstrate preserved or even exaggerated insulin secretory responsiveness, many PCOS women, particularly those with a family history of T2DM, manifest secretory impairment and glucose intolerance. In addition, the typically gradual transition from impaired glucose tolerance (IGT) to overt T2DM may be accelerated 5 to 10-fold in women with PCOS [20,21]. Legro demonstrated that 40% of women with PCOS had glucose intolerance, and 7.5% of these women manifested frank T2DM, prevalence rates 5-7 fold higher than those reported in population-based studies of women aged 20-44 [22]. 1/3 of women with PCOS fulfill criteria for the diagnosis of the metabolic syndrome (MBS) [11]. These associated metabolic derangements greatly increase a woman's lifetime risk to develop T2DM and cardiovascular co-morbidities [23,24]. Underscoring concerns about the strong association between IR and PCOS, the AES recently recommended that all patients with PCOS be tested for IGT with a 2-h oral glucose tolerance test every 2 years, and annually if evidence of IGT or additional risk factors for emergence of T2DM is identified. Moreover, the AES position statement proposed that PCOS patients with IGT be treated with intensive lifestyle modification and weight loss, and considered for treatment with insulin-sensitizing agents, even before the onset of overt T2DM [25].

The association between insulin and androgen excesses: history and cellular mechanisms

The association between disordered carbohydrate metabolism and excessive androgen action in women was first reported in 1921 [26] as "the diabetes of bearded women (*diabète des femmes à barbe*)", preceding Stein and Leventhal's formal description of PCOS [27]. A half-century later, researchers described a group of adolescent girls with the constellation of hyperandrogenism, severe IR, and *acanthosis nigricans*, a dermatologic manifestation of hyperinsulinemia (HAIR-AN, or "type A" IR) [28]. A subset of these patients was shown to have mutations of the insulin receptor [29-31]. A second, distinct form of insulin insensitivity associated with androgen excess in post-menopausal women, designated "type B" IR, results from anti-insulin receptor antibodies [32]. Nevertheless,

population analyses of PCOS women consistently fails to demonstrate either of these forms of IR as common to the disorder [33].

Burghen and colleagues observed a positive correlation between basal and glucose-stimulated insulin and androgen levels in PCOS, independent of weight, suggesting a causal relationship between hyperinsulinism and hyperandrogenism [34]. An abundant literature corroborates strong associations between insulin and various circulating androgens in PCOS [35-37], particularly free testosterone levels [38-40]. Emphasizing the apparently singular nature of the abnormalities of insulin action in PCOS, a significant inverse relationship exists between insulin sensitivity and testosterone levels for women with PCOS-associated metabolic derangements a relationship independent of BMI [41-43] whose underlying mechanism remains poorly defined.

More recent reports [37,44] confirm a degree of IR in non-obese women with PCOS not found in lean controls. Ehrmann demonstrated that the striking relationship between PCOS androgen excess and MBS can be linked causally to hyperinsulinemia and thus underlying IR [11]; oscillatory glucose infusions verified concurrent defects in β-cell entrainment in women with PCOS [45]. Insulin secretory defects are more pronounced in PCOS women having first-degree relatives with T2DM [21,45], and appear to develop earlier in the evolution of glucose intolerance in women with PCOS than in the general population. Despite these quantitative defects in β-cell function, women with PCOS generally maintain normal glucose tolerance, in contrast to that observed in classical T2DM [46]. That weight reduction alone often fails to resolve the insulin secretory defects in PCOS further emphasizes the uniqueness of the metabolic derangements in this syndrome [36]. The impairment of insulin dynamics found in PCOS thus appears to differ from that observed in T2DM, both with respect to peripheral insulin sensitivity and β-cell secretory capability.

The hyperinsulinemic response to peripheral IR observed in women with PCOS is frequently modest [47,48]. Corroborating data involving more exacting measures of insulin sensitivity are less consistent, with some studies reporting decreased insulin sensitivity in obese, but not lean PCOS, despite comparably elevated insulin levels [47,49]. These discrepancies may reflect differences in methodology used to quantify insulin sensitivity (*e.g.,* fasting measures of glucose and insulin [HOMA, QUICKI]), insulin sensitivity index [ISI], minimal modeling of frequently-sampled IV glucose tolerance testing [FSIGT], insulin clamps). Surrogate measures based on fasting insulin and glucose correlate poorly with gold standard techniques such as the euglycemic clamp in the assessment of insulin dynamics in adult PCOS [50], 2-hr glucose levels in adolescents with PCOS [51], and FSIGT in healthy children [52]. Moreover, the excess abdominal fat mass observed in both obese and lean PCOS likely contributes to attenuated insulin sensitivity [53-57].

In response to whole body insulin insensitivity, a more permissive transduction of the insulin signal at the ovarian thecal level may contribute to the pathogenesis of the androgen excess [reviewed in [16]], amplified even in the absence of markedly elevated circulating levels of insulin. Human theca cells possess the full complement of insulin signaling elements and insulin increases thecal testosterone biosynthesis in dose-dependent fashion [58,59]; thus, insulin exerts a direct effect on androgen synthesis. In both obese and lean PCOS, insulin augments *CYP17* activity, increasing androgen production [60,61]. Serine phosphorylation of both the insulin receptor and regulatory steroidogenic enzymes by as-yet unidentified serine kinase has been proposed to underlie both cellular IR and increased ovarian androgenesis in women with PCOS [62]. Insulin also suppresses hepatic sex hormone binding globulin (SHBG) production [63,64], with a consequent increase in free androgen levels. Centrally, androgen excess may reduce hypothalamic feedback inhibition, resulting in increased GnRH pulsatility, particularly during puberty [65-67]. Increased insulin does not appear to govern gonadotropin secretion directly: PCOS women treated with pioglitazone demonstrate improved insulin sensitivity without alterations in LH pulse frequency or amplitude, or gonadotropin responses to GnRH [68]. Conversely, some data support a blunting of baseline LH and LH pulse amplitude in obese PCOS women, suggesting perhaps that the effect of IR (and consequent insulin excess) is to inhibit LH secretion [69-72].

The Heritability of PCOS and IR
A genetic etiology for PCOS has been established on the basis of familial clustering [6,21,43-45], with heritability estimates as high as 0.79 [73]. Genetic studies of PCOS typically extend preliminary genome-wide association studies (GWAS), seeking correlations between specific allelic variants of GWAS-nominated genes and PCOS and/or its co-morbidities (*e.g.*, IR) [74]. An exhaustive discussion of the candidate genes identified is beyond the scope of this review and few genes have been broadly accepted as causative, due to lack of replication in larger studies [75-80]. The success of these studies has been limited by the lack of consensus in diagnostic criteria resulting in broad phenotypic heterogeneity (described above), the limited sample sizes of many studies, and the difficulty in identifying among kindreds a PCOS phenotype in males and late adolescent women. Concurrent variation at multiple genetic loci (characteristic of the inheritance patterns of many common complex disorders) and lifestyle/environmental factors exerting

epigenetic influences on emerging disease further confound efforts to define PCOS heritability.

Family studies of adult female first-degree relatives of PCOS probands demonstrate that the prevalence of PCOS and associated abnormalities of insulin dynamics are increased, consistent with a dominant mode of transmission [81-83]. Kahsar-Miller [84] determined the prevalence of PCOS in first-degree relatives of women with PCOS to be as high as 35% (mothers) and 40% (sisters), 5 times that observed in the general population. Both IR and T2DM are increased in the parents of women with PCOS compared to the parents of women in the general population [85]. Mothers [86] and sisters [87] of PCOS probands exhibit menstrual irregularities, androgen excess, aberrant lipoprotein profiles, and MBS, with profound defects in insulin secretory function and sensitivity [88]. First-degree male relatives of PCOS women also demonstrate increased adrenal androgens (DHEA-S), IR, endothelial dysfunction and MBS [89-91]. Recent cross-sectional studies by Sir-Peterman demonstrated that daughters of women with PCOS manifest increased 2-hr insulin concentrations (despite preserved glucose tolerance) vs. controls across the entirety of pubertal maturation [92,93]. Conversely, Kent observed only late pubertal hyperinsulinemia in girls predisposed to PCOS [94]. Neither of these studies tracked subjects longitudinally into young adulthood; thus, the causal relationship between disordered insulin action and a permanent, post-pubertal state of androgen excess remains unproven.

Adolescent IR and post-pubertal androgen excess
Although biochemical evidence of ovarian hyperandrogenism in PCOS is detectable shortly after pubertal onset [95], consequent menstrual irregularity is often underappreciated, masked by the frequent acyclicity of postmenarchal adolescence. Thus, oligomenorrhea may escape recognition as pathologic until young adulthood. The physiological IR that typifies mid-pubertal maturation delays timely recognition of metabolic derangements that precede and promote hyperandrogenism [38]. Peripubertal metabolic dysfunction is one of the first phenotypic traits observed in adolescent girls who develop PCOS [96,97]. Lewy demonstrated ~ 50% reduction in insulin sensitivity in adolescents with PCOS and concluded that profound metabolic derangements must already exist early in puberty [98]. Apter reported that adolescents with functional ovarian hyperandrogenism (FOH) exhibit disproportionate, early pubertal increases in mean serum insulin levels [99]. Abnormal insulin dynamics are frequently established by the time phenotypic features of PCOS (hirsutism, cystic acne) emerge in late adolescence, irrespective of subject BMI [100]. Studying a cohort of girls with premature adrenarche, whose androgen profiles are reminiscent of PCOS, Ibanez

[101-105] observed increased insulin levels and glucose intolerance throughout maturation. Ovarian hyperandrogenism consistently follows menarche, subsequent to the emergence of IR, supporting the premise that IR promotes dysregulated ovarian androgen production [106,107]. In girls predisposed to PCOS hyperinsulinemia precedes androgen excess [92], suggesting the primacy of metabolic dysregulation in the ontogeny of hyperandrogenism. Overweight and obese adolescent girls, possessing higher circulating insulin levels than lean counterparts [54,66,108], also exhibit elevated androgens, further predisposing them to PCOS [109,110].

Earlier recognition of permanent states of hyperandrogenism necessitates consideration of treatment algorithms proposing earlier intervention to prevent establishment of metabolic, cardiovascular, and reproductive *sequelae* that manifest in young adulthood. However, long-term outcomes data to support the most cost-effective management, especially in the adolescent population, are lacking. A variety of therapeutic modalities are currently employed in the treatment of PCOS: oral contraceptives (OCPs), insulin sensitizing medications (metformin, thiazolidenediones), and agents that exert anti-androgen effects (both androgen receptor blockade and 5α-reductase inhibition), alone or in combination (Table 1). Therapy aimed at reducing androgen over-production in PCOS fails to ameliorate co-morbid IR: no significant improvement in insulin dynamics is observed following long-term treatment of adolescents with PCOS with GnRH analogues [111-114]. Similarly, treatment with anti-androgens fails to rectify metabolic derangements in PCOS patients treated [115-117]. Reduction of hyperandrogenemia thus has little effect on IR. Conversely, as will be discussed below, insulin sensitization decreases both androgen and insulin excess,

suggesting that, in selected patients with PCOS, insulin excess may be fundamental to the development of hyperandrogenemia.

Adolescents with emerging PCOS face considerable life-long morbidity: i) 2/3 of late adolescents with menstrual irregularity due to FOH remain oligomenorrheic into adulthood [118]; (ii) adolescents with PCOS are 4-5 fold more likely to develop MBS than age- and BMI-matched control girls [96]; and (iii) potentially life-threatening cardiovascular dysfunction has its origins during pubertal maturation, and demonstrable by young adulthood [119-121]. The abundant evidence suggesting that IR and resultant hyperinsulinemia facilitate ovarian hyperandrogenism is central to the argument for the use of insulin sensitizers to treat adolescents with PCOS [122], when treatment might preclude adverse metabolic, reproductive and cardiovascular outcomes.

The remainder of this document will: 1) discuss the primary modalities available for the treatment of PCOS; 2) review the literature that compares and contrasts their efficacy, alone or in combination; 3) where available, evaluate the data concerning treatment of a late adolescent PCOS population; and 4) consider whether insulin sensitization, given the role insulin may play in promoting androgen production, should be considered as first-line therapy for the treatment of adolescents with PCOS.

Modalities for Treatment of PCOS
Therapy for PCOS becomes necessary in adults in order to induce ovulatory cycles and fertility, and to improve cosmetic appearance (*i.e.,* reduction of hirsutism and acne). At the same time, it is important to address obesity and associated metabolic complications, which include: 1) endothelial dysfunction and inflammation, 2) an

Table 1 Treatment modalities for Polycystic Ovary Syndrome: mechanism of action and desired clinical impact

Therapy	Mechanism of Action	Regular menses	↓ Androgen levels or effects	Improves insulin sensitivity	Contraception	Metabolic Effects
Combination E+P pills	Endometrial changes ↓ GnRH frequency, ↓ LH and FSH ↑ SHBG ↓ androgens (↓ free (active) androgen)	√√	√		√	May be associated with worsened lipid profile, hypertension, decreased glucose tolerance, and prothrombotic effects
Androgen blockers	↓ androgen action		√			May be associated with improved lipid profile and blood pressure control
Weight loss ± insulin sensitizers	↑ insulin sensitivity ↑ SHBG ↓ androgens (↓ free (active) androgen)	√	√	√		Associated with improved glucose tolerance, lipid profile, and blood pressure control

(Adapted from personal communication from Paul Boepple, M.D.)

atherogenic serum lipoprotein profile, 3) increased coronary artery calcification, 4) nonalcoholic fatty liver disease and nonalcoholic steatohepatitis, and 5) obstructive sleep apnea. Therapeutic options include lifestyle modification, combine oral contraceptive pills, androgen receptor antagonists, insulin-lowering medications (e.g., metformin and thiazolidinediones) (Table 1). In adolescents with PCOS, induction of ovulatory cycles and fertility is of lesser importance, although it is important to induce some element of menstrual cyclicity in order to optimize endometrial health. Improving cosmetic appearance and reduction of weight and obesity- associated metabolic complications are important therapeutic targets.

Lifestyle modification and weight loss

The first line of therapy in obese adolescents with PCOS is lifestyle modification and weight loss. In addition to an improvement in metabolic co-morbidities of obesity, this would be expected to reduce insulin levels and increase insulin sensitivity, resulting in a decrease in LH and androgen levels. Behavioral, exercise and dietary modifications should therefore be encouraged from the initial encounter, particularly in adolescents, to optimize healthy habits before adulthood, and while these changes are still possible and preventive.

Adult women with PCOS

Salmi reported improvement in almost every clinical variable associated with PCOS after weight loss [123], and studies have demonstrated that even modest reductions in weight in the range of 2-7% are successful in improving ovulatory function in at least some adult women with this condition [124-126]. Modest weight reductions with improved fitness are as effective as more drastic reductions in weight to reverse metabolic dysfunction associated with PCOS and ovulatory function in adult women [127]. Recently, Palomba reported a decrease in IR with associated improvement in menstrual cyclicity, fertility, SHBG, and androgen levels in adults with PCOS randomized to either a structured training program or a hypocaloric hyperproteinemic diet [128]. The authors posited that improved insulin sensitivity was integral to these changes albeit brought about by different mechanisms and interventions. In contrast, Hoeger reported increases in ovulation rates only after weight loss [124]. Kiddy similarly reported that weight loss of at least 5% (with a 1000 calorie, low fat diet for 6-7 months) was necessary to increase SHBG, decrease insulin levels and improve reproductive function in adults with PCOS [126]. Whereas the degree of IR in PCOS is greater than that predicted by BMI alone, nearly half of PCOS women are not obese [129] and the degree of visceral adiposity alone is inadequate to explain differences in insulin sensitivity between PCOS and normal women, suggesting that weight loss by itself may be insufficient to improve ovarian function in the sub-population of lean women with PCOS[130].

Adolescents with PCOS

Consistent with studies in adults, pediatric studies have demonstrated decreases in adrenal and ovarian androgens with weight loss in both obese pre-pubertal and pubertal girls [131,132], and a 59% reduction in free androgen index with a 122% increase in SHBG levels in obese adolescent girls with PCOS [133]. In the last study, changes were observed despite only modest weight reductions. Importantly, increases in SHBG were much greater in girls who lost weight compared to those who did not.

However, lifestyle modifications are difficult to sustain and are associated with high degrees of recidivism. One study reported a drop out rate of almost 40% in adult subjects enrolled in a study that included intensive lifestyle modification [124]. In a study of adolescents with PCOS, 30% of subjects enrolled into an intensive lifestyle modification program dropped out; 40% attended less than 50% of the sessions and demonstrated no weight change [133]. Therefore, in most instances, pharmacological therapy for PCOS becomes necessary. Available data indicate that in adult women with PCOS, the addition of metformin therapy to lifestyle modification appears more effective than lifestyle changes alone in maintaining weight loss and in ameliorating metabolic complications of obesity [134,135]. In addition, marked improvements in androgen profiles on the basis of a regimented diet and exercise program would be less anticipated in those adolescents with PCOS and normal body composition.

A potential alternative to pharmacological therapy, which we discuss subsequently, particularly in extremely overweight adolescents, is weight reduction surgery. Surgical weight loss procedures have the advantage of more extensive and persistent weight loss than dietary or exercise programs. With the emerging popularity of bariatric surgery to reduce weight in very obese adults, studies have examined the effectiveness of the surgical approach in reducing the severity of clinical features associated with PCOS in these patients. Two studies reported that all adult women with PCOS undergoing gastric bypass surgery resumed menses in the subsequent months, with a significant improvement in hirsutism scores [136,137] and reductions in androgen levels [137]. In one study, about 77% of women reported moderate to complete resolution of hirsutism [136] and in another study, a 48% reduction in hirsutism scores and a 62.5% reduction in free testosterone levels was reported [138]. Bariatric surgery has been successfully implemented in a few hundred adolescents [139]; as more adolescents undergo these procedures, the necessary data regarding their effectiveness in treating associated PCOS will become available. At this time, the possible morbidity associated with this type of surgery limits weight loss surgery to select adolescents with extremely high BMI and associated complications, and centers with an appropriate team-centered approach.

Use of Oral Contraceptive Pills (OCPs) in PCOS

OCPs are considered to be among the primary treatment options for both adult and adolescent women with PCOS, particularly for those who did not wish to become pregnant [140]. These agents produce regular menstrual cyclicity, lower the risk of endometrial hyperplasia, and dramatically improve acne and hirsutism. Most commonly used OCPs contain both an estrogenic component (typically ethinyl estradiol, in doses ranging from 15 to 50 μg) and a progestin with variable potency and androgenicity [141]. Oral contraceptives improve symptoms through a variety of mechanisms. Estrogens increase the production of SHBG, resulting in a decrease of circulating free androgens, as well as their bioavailability [142]. Progestins protect the endometrium against hyperplasia induced by unopposed estrogen stimulation. The androgenicity of the progestins, mediated through differential androgen receptor binding and blockade [143] or inhibition of 5α-reductase activity [144,145], varies depending on the dosage used and on androgen measurement indices. Some progestins, such as drospirenone and cyproterone acetate, have proven anti-androgenic effects and therefore may yield added benefit in PCOS [146]. Finally combined OCPs suppress luteinizing and follicular stimulating hormones, resulting in reduced ovarian stimulation and androgen production. However, none of these mechanisms directly affect IR [147].

Despite the popularity of OCP use and the number of available combinations, studies contrasting the different agents in head to head comparison are few, their results often equivocal (and contradictory), and few have included an adolescent population. The outcome measures assessed among different studies vary considerably, making the comparison of results difficult. Van der Vange [148] randomized 70 healthy adult women to 7 different OCPs preparations for 6 months; and because the absolute free testosterone levels were similar in all 7 groups, they concluded that these preparations would be of equal benefit in the treatment of hyperandrogenic symptoms. A more recent study compared the effect of 4 OCPs with different progestins on hormonal parameters in 40 women with PCOS over 3 months [149]. They found that all 4 progestins combined with the same dose of ethinylestradiol resulted in significant decrease in testosterone (total and free), androsteredione, dehydroepiandrosterone sulfate; but drospirenone and chlormadinone had more pronounced effects than desogestrel and gestodene. However, clinical effect was not assessed. In a 12-month randomized control trial of adolescents with PCOS testing the efficacy

of combined pills with desogestrol or cyproterone acetate as the progestin, the preparations were found to have similar effects on hirsutism and androgen levels [150]. Finally, the benefit of combining GnRH analog with OCPs to suppress LH pulsatility and androgen production has been investigated, particularly with respect to moderate-severe hirsutism (see below); little added benefit was observed despite the marked increase in cost over OCPs alone [39,151].

Independent of their effect in improving the signs and symptoms of PCOS, OCPs possess additional benefits that may support a decision for their use in this age group. The contraceptive potential of birth control pills is a paramount consideration: 1/3 of teenage girls with PCOS reported being sexually active in one recent study [152]. Women with PCOS may be at increased risk of developing gynecologic cancers [153-155], and the use of OCPs reduces the risk of both ovarian [156] and uterine cancer [157] in the general population of women. Conversely, a recent Cochrane review on the treatment options for women with PCOS found insufficient data for the efficacy of OCP in preventing endometrial cancers in this adult population [158].

Regardless of their potential benefits, use of OCPs fails to diminish IR in PCOS and may actually be associated with long-term metabolic derangements, such as glucose intolerance, abnormal lipid profiles and cardiovascular disease. Recent work by Mastorakos showed that a 12-month use of newer OCPs containing either desogestrel or cyproterone as progestin was associated with decreased insulin sensitivity and increase total, LDL and HDL cholesterol and variable changes in triglycerides in adolescents with PCOS [150,159]. Two recent meta-analyses have linked current use of low dose OCPs in women without PCOS to more than a doubling of the risk of myocardial infarction (risk estimates 2.12 (95% confidence interval (CI) = 1.56, 2.86) [160] and 2.48 (95% CI: 1.91-3.22) [161]. Although the use of OCPs is associated with an overall increased risk of adverse cardiovascular events (e.g., venous thrombosis and myocardial infarction) among all users, the absolute risk remains minimal in adolescents, even in the subpopulation using tobacco [162,163]. While newer OCPs containing less androgenic progestin agents have the potential for less deleterious impact on IR and lipid profile, an insufficient number of adolescent subjects receiving OCPs (and anti-androgen) monotherapy have been studied to draw definitive conclusions about their long-term safety. Moreover, longitudinal studies have not yet been conducted among the population of women with PCOS receiving OCPs, adult or adolescent; thus, the potential exists for the excessive use of OCPs to exacerbate the underlying metabolic derangements prevalent in PCOS, thereby augmenting the subsequent risk for adverse cardiovascular outcomes. Finally, there may be social, ethnic and/or religious stigmata associated with the use of OCPs in some adolescent populations. These concerns have led to a consideration of other approaches for adolescents with PCOS, and specifically, treatment that concurrently targets IR.

Studies of Insulin Sensitizers and Insulin Lowering Drugs in Adolescents with PCOS

These medications act to reduce insulin levels (metformin) and increase insulin sensitivity (metformin and thiazolidenediones), thus treating the metabolic co-morbidities associated with PCOS and obesity. Reductions in insulin levels effect a concurrent reduction in androgen levels (discussed subsequently) and induce menstrual cyclicity and ovulatory cycles in a majority of those treated. However, recent guidelines recommend that (i) clomiphene (rather than metformin) should be used to induce ovulatory cycles in adult women with PCOS desiring fertility, and (ii) hyperandrogenism causing hirsutism should be treated with estrogen-progestin combination pills, with addition of an androgen receptor blocker after six months if the former are not effective in reducing hirsutism (reviewed in [164]). The role of insulin-lowering agents and sensitizers such as metformin in PCOS may be limited to optimizing weight loss when used with lifestyle modification, and in treatment or amelioration of metabolic complications including hyperlipidemia and reduction of levels of pro-inflammatory cytokines, Additional reasons to consider the use of metformin or thiazolidenediones rather than combined oral contraceptive pills may include the presence of Factor V Leiden mutations, which increase the risk of thromboembolic episodes with estrogen use, or an intolerance, non-adherence, or refusal to use estradiol-progesterone (E_2-P) combination pills. The paucity of randomized controlled studies of the various therapeutic options in adolescents with PCOS makes it difficult to develop therapeutic guidelines in this younger population. In subsequent sections, we review available data in adolescents, and some data from adults with PCOS, that compare the efficacy of metformin and thiazolidinediones versus combined OCPs in inducing menstrual cyclicity, reducing hyperandrogenism and hirsutism, and effects of these medications on lipid levels and levels of cardiovascular risk markers.

1. Metformin

Metformin increases insulin sensitivity in the liver by: 1) reducing gluconeogenic enzyme activities (PEPCK, FBPase, glucose-6-phosphatase), 2) inhibiting hepatic uptake of lactate and alanine, 3) increasing the conversion of pyruvate to alanine, and 4) inhibiting glucose output. The cellular consequence of these AMP-activated protein kinase (AMPK)-mediated effects is alterations in the AMP/ATP ratio. In addition, metformin increases peripheral glucose

uptake, decreases fatty acid oxidation and decreases glucose absorption from the gut. Molecularly, metformin-induced phosphorylation modulates the activities of both α1 and α2 catalytic subunits of AMPK, resulting in improved muscle glucose uptake in the presence of insulin. Metformin-induced activation of AMPK may also augment hepatic fatty acid oxidation and improve hepatic insulin sensitivity. In human muscle biopsies, metformin's effect is transduced by phsophorylation of the α2 subunit threonine residue 172, an effect maintained after discontinuation of the medication. However, in mouse skeletal muscle cell lines, metformin-induced phosphorylation of (primarily) α1 Thr172 had no effect on AMP/ATP ratios. Thus, the actual mechanism by which metformin activates AMPK to sensitize target tissues to insulin, or even whether the metformin effect requires AMPK in humans, remains unproven [165].

Knowledge of the effects of insulin on free androgen levels has prompted multiple trials of the efficacy of drugs that increase insulin sensitivity or reduce insulin levels, including metformin, in the treatment of PCOS [166-171]. Most of these studies targeted adult women with this disorder, often yielding promising results with respect to resumption of menstrual cyclicity (in 50-60%), improved percentage of ovulatory cycles, and fertility [reviewed in [170]]. However, a recent large randomized study of more than 600 women reported no improvement in fertility (as assessed by live birth rates) with use of extended release metformin in women with PCOS compared with clomiphene [172,173]. In adults with PCOS, increased abdominal fat, decreased insulin sensitivity, and endothelial dysfunction also contribute to increased cardiovascular risk, and are associated with alterations in circulating levels of adipocytokines; cardiovascular risk markers such as endothelin-1, plasminogen activator-1 (PAI-1), and lipoprotein (a); pro-inflammatory markers such as IL-1, TNF-α, and CRP; and higher neutrophil counts [174-186]. The contribution of decreased insulin sensitivity to increased cardiovascular risk makes a strong case for the use of insulin sensitizers in PCOS in adults for benefits beyond those associated with reproductive integrity. Metformin has been used successfully in adult obese and non-obese women to decrease levels of markers of cardiovascular risk in studies lasting an average of six months [174,176,181,185-188].

Studies in adolescents with PCOS have been limited, and data on the benefits of therapeutic intervention on restoration of menstrual cyclicity less convincing than in adults [174,189-191]. Longitudinal data are sparse regarding the effects of decreased insulin sensitivity and increased abdominal fat on long-term cardiovascular outcomes in teenagers with PCOS, and few studies have examined the relationship between cardiovascular risk factors and the use of metformin in this younger population.

Recent work by Ibanez indicates that relatively lean girls with hyperinsulinemic hyperandrogenism have a dyslipidemic profile, with high levels of triglycerides and other atherogenic lipids [192]. Similarly, an increased prevalence of the metabolic syndrome in adolescent girls with PCOS compared with weight matched controls reported by Coviello included evidence of abnormal lipid profiles [96].

A recent survey indicated that 30% of pediatric endocrinologists consider metformin appropriate treatment for adolescents with PCOS, and 68% for obese adolescents with PCOS [193]. The following sections briefly review some adult and available adolescent data regarding efficacy of insulin sensitizers in treating those with PCOS. The bulk of available data in adolescents derives from studies by Ibanez in relatively lean girls with a history of precocious pubarche, hyperinsulinemic hyperandrogenism, and post-pubertal features consistent with PCOS, studies which remain to be replicated [55,189,192,194-197].

Androgen-lowering effects of metformin

In both lean and obese women with PCOS, metformin (i) decreases insulin levels in association with decreases in clinical indices of ovarian cytochrome P450c17 activity, and (ii) increases SHBG levels, resulting in decreases in free testosterone [60,61,63,64]. Long-term metformin therapy may also decrease the activity of several other adrenal steroidogenic pathway elements [198,199]. In addition, metformin use is associated with increases levels of IGFBP-1 (which may be a consequence of a reduction in insulin levels), with the resultant decrease in IGF-1 bioavailability possibly decreasing the stimulatory effects of IGF-1 on ovarian steroidogenesis. However, Munir demonstrated that modulation of human theca P450c17 *in vitro* is transduced exclusively through insulin receptors, rather than IGF-1 receptors [59], making less clear the role of IGF-1 in governing thecal androgen production at the whole body level.

Studies indicate that the degree to which metformin therapy is effective in improving the androgenic and metabolic profile in adolescents with PCOS may be related to (i) dose used, particularly when metformin is used as monotherapy, necessitating higher doses [191,200-202]; (ii) the agent with which metformin is combined, estrogen-progestin combination pills or anti-androgenic agents such as flutamide, spironolactone, and cyproterone acetate [115,116,203-210]; and (iii) the characteristics of the PCOS patient being treated, whether obese or lean, hyperinsulinemic, or normoinsulinemic [191,194,200,202,211,212]. We will consider each of these aspects individually:

Metformin monotherapy

A dose of 1.5-2 g per day appears necessary for clinical effectiveness when metformin is used alone [201], the efficacy dependent on the outcome measure chosen. Arslanian reported decreased insulin sensitivity in fifteen obese adolescents with PCOS in whom metformin therapy (850 mg, twice daily) was associated with an improvement in glucose tolerance and a decrease in testosterone levels [191]. Six of the study subjects had simultaneous improvements in menstrual cyclicity. Of note, these girls also had significant decreases in BMI (mean decrease of 1.4 kg/m^2) over the three-month study period. In another study of eleven obese girls with PCOS, metformin use was associated with a downward trend in circulating testosterone concentrations and a decrease in total cholesterol levels, even after adjusting for weight loss [213]. Although a daily metformin dose of 1.5 g (500 mg three times daily) was effective in two of the eleven girls, nine required an increase to 2.55 g (850 mg three times a day) after 8-10 weeks on the lower dose. Ninety percent of those treated resumed regular menses, and in 39% of the follow up visits in girls with regular menses, the cycles were ovulatory, based on luteal phase (day 21) progesterone levels. The proportion of girls resuming menses in this study was higher than that observed in other studies of women with PCOS receiving metformin, in which menstrual cyclicity was restored in fewer than 50% overall [202,204,214,215]. A third uncontrolled study in 18 adolescent girls 15-18 years old similarly reported a reduction in levels of androgens and resumption of menstrual cyclicity and ovulatory cycles in all 16 girls who tolerated 1700 mg of metformin daily. Girls in this study also had a reduction in BMI that was maintained (along with regular and ovulatory menstrual cycles) six months after the end of metformin treatment [216]. The absence of a control group and significant weight loss in subjects in these studies make these data difficult to interpret in terms of metformin's efficacy independent of weight loss.

Similar results from a placebo-controlled study by Bridger appear to confirm beneficial effects of metformin monotherapy, at least in the short term [200]. In this study, 22 obese adolescents with hyperinsulinemia and PCOS were randomized to receive metformin (1.5 g per day) or placebo for a twelve-week period. The group receiving metformin had significant decreases in levels of testosterone and increases in HDL-cholesterol, in the absence of changes in insulin sensitivity or BMI. Because insulin sensitivity did not significantly change with metformin, a direct effect of metformin on androgen secretion could not be ruled out. However, in an uncontrolled study, Glueck reported that metformin therapy associated with caloric restriction for 12 months in 35 adolescents with PCOS was associated with a 4.4% decrease in weight, as well as decreases in insulin, HOMA-IR (an index of insulin sensitivity derived from fasting glucose and insulin values), cholesterol and TG, and improved menstrual function, with regular monthly cycles increasing from 22% to 74% [217].

Lower doses of metformin have proven effective in non-obese adolescents with PCOS. Ibanez and colleagues reported decreased ovarian hyperandrogenism, hyperinsulinemia, and hirsutism, as well as improved menstrual cyclicity and lipid profiles in ten non-obese girls with hyperinsulinemic hyperandrogenism treated with as little as 1.25 g of metformin daily [197]. Leukocytosis, another pro-inflammatory surrogate marker observed in adolescents with hyperinsulinemic hyperandrogenism, also normalizes with metformin monotherapy (vs. no medication) in a randomized study design [174].

Metformin use is associated with gastrointestinal side effects, which can be minimized by slow titration of the medication to the desired dose over a one-month period. In none of the studies presented above were severe adverse effects with metformin observed; specifically, lactic acidosis has not been reported in this population. Compliance with the higher doses required in some teenagers may be an obstacle to efficacy of metformin therapy, given the potential for initial gastrointestinal side effects [200]. Extended-release metformin may be useful in such instances.

Metformin (with or without anti-androgens) versus estrogen-progestin combination pills)

E_2-P combination pills are the treatment of first choice in adolescents with PCOS (see above), particularly when efforts at weight loss, including reduction in caloric intake and increased physical activity, fail. Although exogenous estrogen decreases free androgen levels by increasing levels of SHBG and suppressing ovarian secretion of gonadal steroids (both estrogen and androgen), it neither increases insulin sensitivity nor decreases inflammatory mediators, adipose tissue or adipose-derived adipocytokines, based on studies in adults [55,150,189,210,218,219], and may cause an increase in lipids. In adolescent girls with PCOS, Mastorakos demonstrated an increase in levels of total, LDL- and HDL-associated cholesterol with combined E_2-P containing pills, and a tendency towards increasing triglyceride levels with use of cyproterone acetate-containing combination pills [150]. The same group later reported increased IR after 12 months of both E_2-P- and cyproterone acetate-containing combination pills. The later formulation also resulted in hyperinsulinemia [159].

An important question is whether metformin can improve menstrual cyclicity and hirsutism scores in PCOS without predisposing to the deleterious metabolic effects attributed to use of combined oral contraceptive agents. To answer this question, Hoeger randomized 43 adolescent girls with PCOS to either lifestyle intervention, estrogen-progestin (ethinyl estradiol + desogestrel) combination pills, metformin (1700 mg daily), or placebo for a six-month period, and demonstrated that groups randomized to lifestyle intervention and the combination pills (but not metformin) had increases in SHBG levels and reductions in free androgen index and in PAI-1 [133] despite only non-significant changes in weight in

all groups. Hirsutism scores did not change in any group. Among girls not receiving OCPs, the frequency of menses did not differ between groups; observed menses were ovulatory 75% of the time in the metformin group, as opposed to 60% of the time in the group receiving combined pills and 50% of the time in the group randomized to placebo. However, use of OCPs was associated with a 14% increase in total cholesterol and 40% increase in high-sensitivity CRP, whereas, these adverse metabolic effects were not observed in the other groups, with the metformin group demonstrating a 25% decrease in triglyceride levels. Unlike the previous study, use of combined pills did not result in hyperinsulinemia. Metformin use was associated with a significant decrease in glucose levels, but insulin levels did not change. These data suggest that in obese adolescents with PCOS, OCPs and lifestyle intervention have beneficial effects on androgen levels. However, combination pills affect cardiovascular risk markers adversely, while metformin has beneficial effects on both lipids and glucose levels.

In contrast to these data, Allen found concurrent decreases in both IR (measured by fasted baseline glucose/insulin ratios and QUICKI derivation) and testosterone levels in 35 obese PCOS girls randomized to either metformin or an OCP for six months [220]. Significantly, both cohorts lost weight (mean BMI decrease of 1.5 kg/m^2 in the estrogen/progestin group and 1 kg/m^2 in the metformin group). The authors concluded that the two drugs produced similar benefits for the cardinal features of PCOS in adolescents.

Other data comparing combine OCPs and metformin derive from Ibanez' studies of non-obese hyperinsulinemic, hyperandrogenic adolescents. In 32 such adolescents with a mean age of 15 years and a BMI of 22 kg/m^2, Ibanez and de Zegher [189] found low baseline adiponectin levels and increased abdominal fat. Over 3-9 months in a randomized study design, E_2-P (ethinyl estradiol + drospirenone) combination pills further decreased adiponectin levels while increasing both triglyceride levels and central adiposity. Conversely, metformin (850 mg/day) in combination with low-dose flutamide (62.5 mg/day) reversed these values towards normal, with a 4-kg mean decrease in fat mass and a commensurate increase in lean mass. These authors also observed that metformin attenuated the pro-inflammatory state in young women with hyperinsulinemic hyperandrogenism, resulting in reductions in IL-6 and CRP levels and neutrophil counts, whereas use of E_2-P combination pills aggravated the pro-inflammatory state [174,189,221,222]. Whereas metformin alone did not significantly reduce the free androgen index in obese adolescents, the combination of metformin and flutamide was as effective as E_2-P combination pills in reducing the hyperandrogenism associated with PCOS [133]. In addition, metformin was superior to E_2-P in increasing insulin sensitivity, while decreasing dyslipidemia, anovulation, body adiposity, and the pro-inflammatory state associated with PCOS. It should be noted that the population of girls studied by Ibanez and colleagues all had histories of precocious adrenarche, perhaps suggestive of a unique sub-class of PCOS patients.

Further studies are necessary to determine whether or not metformin exerts beneficial effects beyond those of combined OCPs alone, in the population of adolescent girls with PCOS. Although definitive data from well-controlled trials are lacking, reports suggest the cosmetic result achieved with OCPs may be superior to that of metformin in the treatment of hirsutism in adolescents with PCOS, at least over a prolonged period. It remains to be definitively determined whether the superior metabolic effects achieved with metformin (in contrast with combination pills) in adolescents with PCOS can be sustained and over what duration these effects persist. The re-emergence of phenotypic and metabolic abnormalities following discontinuation of medication is an important consideration, as recent data suggest a loss of the benefits of metformin almost immediately after cessation of therapy [195,197,223]. This may be of particular importance in adolescents in whom compliance with medical therapy is often problematic.

Metformin in combination with estrogen-progestin combination pills or anti-androgens

In adult women with PCOS, adding metformin to a combination OCP decreases IR, as well as androgen levels. However, the anticipated correction of deranged lipid profiles and abdominal obesity through metformin use appears to be blunted [209,224,225]. In 36 adolescent obese girls with PCOS randomized for six months to a combined pill (ethinyl estradiol + drosperinone) with lifestyle intervention and metformin (2000 mg daily) or to an OCP with lifestyle intervention and placebo, weight reductions, increases in SHBG, and decreases in free androgen index, and decreases in hirsutism scores occurred in both groups, but did not differ between groups [133]. Total cholesterol increased in both groups, but the metformin group had greater increases in HDL. No changes in insulin or glucose occurred in either group. Data from this study suggest only modest metabolic benefits of adding metformin to a regime of a combined pill with lifestyle intervention in obese adolescents with PCOS.

In contrast, in 31 non-obese girls with hyperinsulinemic hyperandrogenism (average age, 16 years), random assignment to metformin-treated or not to a protocol consisting of flutamide and ethinyl estradiol + drosperinone over a 3-month period resulted in a decrease in IL-6 and an increase in adiponectin levels in the group receiving metformin [222]. The authors examined the effects of randomly withdrawing metformin use or not in 42 lean young women (average age, 19 years), and again observed beneficial effects of metformin. Similarly, addition of metformin-flutamide led to normalization of leukocyte and neutrophil counts in 41 young women (average age, 18 years), in whom prior use of ethinyl estradiol-drospirenone had effected an increase in these inflammatory markers [174]. These women had improvements in insulin sensitivity, dyslipidemia, ovulatory patterns, and adiposity indices as a consequence of the addition of metformin-flutamide to a regimen of OCP monotherapy. These data suggest greater benefit when metformin is added to a regime that includes combination pills in non-obese adolescents and young women with PCOS.

The type of progesterone in the E_2-P combination pill used in conjunction with insulin sensitizers may also exert variable effects on body composition. Ibanez and de Zegher reported on 29 non-obese young women with PCOS (~ 20 years of age) receiving metformin+flutamide combination therapy. When switched from a combination pill with gestodene to one containing drospirenone, these patients exhibited decreased abdominal fat mass and increased lean mass without changes in overall body weight [221]. Of note, both gestodene and drospirenone are newer synthetic progestins. As a class, progestins bind weakly to the androgen receptor, resulting in variable androgenic effects. Whereas gestodene has minimal androgenic properties, drospirenone exerts no androgenic effects, and in fact antagonizes the androgen receptor after binding (although in doses higher than those used in combination pills). Drospirenone also has anti-mineralocorticoid effects and is therefore thought to minimize the water retention and breast tenderness associated with combination pills.

Anti-androgens such as spironolactone, cyproterone acetate, and flutamide are commonly administered to address the androgen excess features of PCOS. The anti-androgenic effects of flutamide, a non-steroidal androgen receptor antagonist, appear superior to those of spironolactone or cyproterone acetate (the latter not available in the U.S. at present) [203,226]. The combination of metformin with anti-androgens appears promising based on a handful of recent studies in lean [206] and obese [205] young adult women with PCOS, as well as in lean adolescent girls with hyperinsulinemic hyperandrogenism [174,189,190]. This combination effectively decreases abdominal obesity and levels of inflammatory markers in these limited studies. When used alone and in high doses, flutamide can be hepatotoxic; however, flutamide has a good safety profile when used in polytherapy and in lower dosages [116,227]. A combination of low-dose flutamide (62.5 mg) and metformin (850 mg) appears both safe and effective in adolescents and young women, in durations ranging from 3-54 months (mean, 19 months), with preservation of normal liver function [228]. Thus, data from the Ibanez group suggest that low-dose polytherapy provides both an enhanced safety profile and an expanded spectrum of clinical benefit, when contrasted with high-dose monotherapy, owing to the metabolic corrections exerted by the metformin [190]. Lastly, some have endorsed the use of finasteride, a 5-α reductase inhibitor that blocks conversion of testosterone to its dihydrotestosterone metabolite in skin target tissue, to ameliorate the dermatologic effects of androgen excess in adults. This medication remains off-label for adolescents, alone or in combination with metformin or other insulin sensitizers. It is mandatory to exclude pregnancy in those adolescents whose treatment regimen includes the use of anti-androgens, due to their potential for precluding proper virilization of male fetuses. Even more important is the need to emphasize ongoing use of contraception, given the increase in ovulatory rates as a result of metformin use.

Metformin use in obese versus lean, and hyperinsulinemic versus normoinsulinemic PCOS

Silfen [100] observed that lean adolescents with PCOS had lower insulin levels, increased insulin sensitivity, and a more favorable lipid profile than did obese adolescents with PCOS. Conversely, levels of adrenal androgens were higher in the lean PCOS subjects. Given these differences, one might anticipate differences in individual responses to metformin as a function of body composition. However, all studies to date report beneficial effects of metformin in lean as well as obese adolescents with PCOS [55,191,195,213].

Regrettably, there is a paucity of data regarding the use of metformin in hyperinsulinemic versus normoinsulinemic adolescents with PCOS, and it remains unclear whether metformin use should be restricted to adolescents with PCOS (both obese and lean) with biochemical or phenotypic (i.e., acanthosis nigricans) evidence of hyperinsulinemia. Ibanez and colleagues define hyperinsulinemia as a peak insulin of > 150 μU/mL during a 2-hr oral glucose tolerance test and/or mean serum insulin levels of > 84 μIU/mL during standard oral glucose tolerance testing [54,55,104,189,190,192,195,206,221-223,229-232]. Vuguin [233] and Silfen [234] demonstrated good correlation between fasting glucose:insulin ratios of < 7 mg/10^{-4} IU and IVGTT measures of IR in adolescents with premature adrenarche, substantially greater than the figure determined for IR associated with adult PCOS (approximately, 4.5 mg/10^{-4} IU) [235].

Significant effects of metformin on hirsutism scores and ovulation were found in lean, hyperinsulinemic women with PCOS, and a decrease in DHEA-S levels in lean PCOS, regardless of insulin levels [211]. In overweight and obese women with PCOS, significant effects were observed on waist-hip ratio in the normoinsulinemic overweight women, and on menstrual cyclicity in normoinsulinemic obese women. Although these data suggest beneficial effects of metformin on body composition and menstrual function in normoinsulinemic

overweight and obese adults, it is not known whether these data can be extrapolated to adolescents, and in particular to lean normoinsulinemic adolescents. Further studies will be necessary to address these specific questions in adolescents with PCOS. In conclusion, use of low-dose polytherapy may be superior to high-dose monotherapy with respect to efficacy and safety profile; however, further studies in adolescents with PCOS are necessary before definitive recommendations can be developed.

Prevention of PCOS with metformin (earlier intervention)

Girls at higher risk to develop PCOS, such as those with low birth weight and precocious pubarche [196,236], have a slowing of progression of endocrine-metabolic perturbations associated with PCOS when metformin is started during either the pre-pubertal or early postmenarchal period [223,237]. This observation has been exploited to propose a benefit to early intervention in high-risk groups predisposed to PCOS. Of greater concern are data suggesting that these benefits are lost almost immediately following discontinuation of metformin [195,197,223].

2. Thiazolidenediones

Thiazolidenediones act as insulin sensitizers through their activation of the nuclear receptor PPAR-γ, leading to increased production of insulin-sensitive adipocytes and increased glucose uptake in these cells, increased secretion of adiponectin, and decreased secretion of pro-inflammatory cytokines. Recent data in adult women with PCOS suggest that thiazolidinediones exert additional benefit with respect to hyperandrogenism, IR, anovulation, and inflammatory mediator levels, in both lean and obese women with PCOS [212,238-242]. These benefits are observed despite increases in weight, BMI, and waist to hip ratio in those treated [239]. Seto-Young and colleagues have proposed that the effects of thiazolideindiones may be independent of the effects on insulin secretion [243]. These authors reported that PPARγ-agonists stimulate IGFBP-1 and progesterone production, directly decrease estrogen and testosterone secretion, and concurrently antagonize the insulin-induced enhancement of estrogen and testosterone secretion in cultured human ovarian cells. The thiazolidenedione, pioglitazone, has been shown to ameliorate the signs and symptoms of PCOS in a cohort of women who failed a previous trial of metformin [244]. These medications have not been rigorously studied in adolescents, in either traditional states of IR or in late adolescent girls with unambiguous PCOS; thus, they remain "off label" for use in this age group. Despite proven efficacy in mitigating both IR and androgen excess while restoring menstrual cyclicity in adult women with PCOS [245,246], FDA concerns led to the removal of the vanguard thiazolidenedione, troglitazone, from the market.

Concerns regarding potential adverse cardiovascular events in T2DM patients taking thaizolidenediones (*e.g.*, Avandia, [rosiglitazone]) resulted in the recent addition of a black box warning to the package inserts for that agent, thus reinforcing the need for caution when considering use of this class of medication, in both adolescents and women with PCOS. Concerns about hepatotoxicity and peripheral lipogenetic effects must be addressed before the use of these medications in adolescent girls can be endorsed without reservation [241,243]. Of note, one case report has indicated efficacy of pioglitazone, but not metformin, in ameliorating insulin resistance, hyperinsulinemia, and hyperandrogenism, and in resumption of menses in two sisters with Dunnigan-type familial partial lipodystrophy [247].

Conclusion

PCOS is a multi-phenotypic disorder characterized by androgen excess and menstrual acyclicity, with demonstrable biochemical aberrations during pubertal maturation, and clinical manifestations shortly after pubertal completion. A variety of therapies may rectify both the biochemical derangements and clinical features (Table 1) of PCOS, and many patients are treated with polytherapy to address the multiple facets of the syndrome. Women with PCOS have abnormalities of insulin secretion and action, and underlying IR has been proposed to be fundamental to the development of ovarian hyperandrogenism. Application of therapies to diminish IR and consequent hyperinsulinemia has gained increasing support as first-line therapy. As listed in Table 2, arguments can be made in support of and against the use of insulin sensitizers in the treatment of adolescent PCOS. Studies demonstrating long-term efficacy and safety of metformin and the thiazolidenediones in the adolescent age group are lacking, having been chiefly limited to adult women with PCOS, particularly those with impaired glucose tolerance and overt T2DM [248]: these are clearly essential in order to promote their use as therapeutic options for adolescents with PCOS. The paucity of data on the effects of these modalities in the treatment of adolescent PCOS highlights the need for well-designed, controlled studies to optimize treatment algorithms for this disorder in the late teen and young adult. The variability of phenotypic expression within the syndrome further confounds advocacy of a single treatment regimen, the determination of which requires individualization to address the specific presenting complaint(s) of the adolescent patient. Additionally, future individualization of treatment options will rely increasingly on pharmacogenomic models that evaluate putative genetic determinants of metformin response (as described in adult type 2 DM patients) [249-252], to improve prediction of therapeutic efficacy. To date, large-scale studies targeting the prevalence of specific metformin response elements have not been undertaken in either adolescent or adult PCOS populations. Finally, when treating teenagers, a comprehensive approach is imperative, one that considers important ancillary issues such as prevention of pregnancy in those who are sexually active, as well as the need to stress lifestyle counseling for those with significant obesity and/or IR. Although beyond the scope of this review, the use of cosmetic measures to combat hirsutism and dermatological approaches to address acne are common practice and serve as useful adjuncts to the specific medical therapies for PCOS. Other cosmetic concerns, particularly regarding the increased BMI, are of paramount importance in this adolescent patient cohort, with serious negative effect on an affected teenager's quality of life [253,254]. The insufficiency of validated data concerning the use of the insulin sensitizers in adolescent PCOS justifies the continued designation of these medications as "off label" in this age group, which thus cannot be recommended as first-line therapy at the present time.

Summary

Background

1. PCOS, a heterogeneous disorder characterized by cystic ovarian morphology, androgen excess, and/or irregular periods, emerges during or shortly after puberty.

2. Insulin resistance and consequent hyperinsulinemia are highly prevalent and facilitate the formation of excess androgen.

Lifestyle Changes

1. Lifestyle changes involving behavioral, dietary, and exercise regimens should be considered as first line therapy for weight reduction and improvement of insulin levels in obese adolescents with PCOS.

OCPs

1. OCPs, the traditional treatment option for both adult and adolescent women with PCOS not wishing to become pregnant, restore menstrual cyclicity and reduce signs of androgen excess without improving IR.

2. Studies on the risk-benefit profiles for different OCPs provide equivocal results with regard to hirsutism, acne, and menstrual dysfunction, and lack sufficient data on their efficacy and safety in the adolescent population.

3. Cardiovascular risk markers, often high in the PCOS population, may be increased by OCPs.

Metformin

1. Several, although not all, studies of adult women with PCOS treated with metformin demonstrate promising results for resumption of menstrual cyclicity and ovulation, restoration of fertility, improved insulin dynamics,

Table 2 Pros and cons of insulin sensitizer therapy in PCOS

PROS	CONS
Reduces insulin resistance and addresses an important component of the pathophysiology of PCOS Useful for treating hyperglycemia in patients with PCOS-associated type 2 DM	Insulin-sensitizing effect may not persist after discontinuing medication
Metformin may cause weight reduction and is associated with improvement in lipid profile	Weight reduction is minor with metformin; TZDs may cause weight gain and peripheral lipogenesis
	Cosmetic improvements with insulin sensitizers may be less marked than with E_2-P combination pills
	Insulin sensitizers may induce ovulation with risk of unwanted pregnancy unless used with contraception
An option in patients with Factor V Leiden mutations and other risk factors for coagulopathy in whom E_2-P combination pills may be contraindicated	
Potential for use in adolescents with lean PCOS in whom lifestyle modification is likely to be ineffective	Lean PCOS responds well to conventional E_2-P combination pills in conjunction with anti-androgen medications
Excellent safety profile for metformin, with few side effects reported	Insulin sensitizers are potential teratogens Select patients may require frequent monitoring of liver and renal function TZDs have been associated with adverse cardiovascular events in adult patients
	Insufficient studies of efficacy and long term safety of insulin sensitizers in adolescents

adipocytokine and inflammatory mediator profiles, and cardiovascular indices.

2. The benefits to adults with PCOS in improving hirsutism scores, menstrual cyclicity, and metabolic status depends on whether metformin is used as monotherapy or in combination with anti-androgen and/or OCP, as well as the insulin sensitivity status of the patient.

3. In adolescents with PCOS, little is known about the safety and efficacy of metformin, either in mono- or combination therapy.

Other

1. Thiazolidinediones may provide reproductive, metabolic, and cardiovascular function benefits to adult women with PCOS in whom previous metformin therapy failed.

2. Thiazolidinediones remain off-label in adolescents, due to lack of evidence on efficacy and safety.

Acknowledgements
The authors would like to thank the Pediatric Endocrine Society (PES) Drug and Therapeutics Committee for its careful review of the manuscript and constructive comments. We would also like to acknowledge the Board of Directors of the PES for their review and endorsement of this manuscript.

Author details
[1]Division of Pediatric Endocrinology, Cedars-Sinai Medical Center, David Geffen-UCLA School of Medicine 8700 Beverly Blvd., Rm 4220, Los Angeles, CA 90048, USA. [2]Division of Pediatric Endocrinology, Alberta Children's Hospital, University of Calgary, 2888 Hospital Drive NW, Calgary, Alberta T2N 4Z6, Canada. [3]Divisions of Adolescent Medicine and Endocrinology, Children's Hospital and Harvard Medical School, 300 Longwood Avenue, 333 Longwood-6, Boston, MA 02115, USA. [4]Pediatric Endocrine Unit, Mass General Hospital for Children and Harvard Medical School, 55 Fruit Street, Boston, MA 02114, USA.

Authors' contributions
DHG participated in the planning, implementation, writing, review and editing of the manuscript. DP participated in the planning, implementation, writing, review and editing of the manuscript. CMG participated in the review and editing of the manuscript. MM participated in the conception, planning, implementation, writing, review and editing of the manuscript. All authors have read and approved the final manuscript.

Competing interests
The authors have no competing financial or other interests to declare in relation to this manuscript.

References
1. Asuncion M, Calvo RM, San Millan JL, et al: A prospective study of the prevalence of the polycystic ovary syndrome in unselected Caucasian women from Spain. J Clin Endocrinol Metab 2000, 85(7):2434-8.
2. Azziz R, Woods KS, Reyna R, et al: The prevalence and features of the polycystic ovary syndrome in an unselected population. J Clin Endocrinol Metab 2004, 89(6):2745-9.
3. Goodarzi MO, Quinones MJ, Azziz R, et al: Polycystic ovary syndrome in Mexican-Americans: prevalence and association with the severity of insulin resistance. Fertil Steril 2005, 84(3):766-9.
4. Rotterdam E: Revised 2003 consensus on diagnostic criteria and long-term health risks related to polycystic ovary syndrome. Fertility and Sterility 2004, 81(1):19-25.
5. Yildiz BO, Azziz R: Ovarian and adipose tissue dysfunction in polycystic ovary syndrome: report of the 4th special scientific meeting of the Androgen Excess and PCOS Society. Fertil Steril 2010, 94(2):690-3.
6. Gilling-Smith C, Story H, Rogers V, et al: Evidence for a primary abnormality of thecal cell steroidogenesis in the polycystic ovary syndrome. Clin Endocrinol (Oxf) 1997, 47(1):93-9.
7. Nelson VL, Legro RS, Strauss JF, et al: Augmented androgen production is a stable steroidogenic phenotype of propagated theca cells from polycystic ovaries. Mol Endocrinol 1999, 13(6):946-57.
8. Franks S, Stark J, Hardy K: Follicle dynamics and anovulation in polycystic ovary syndrome. Hum Reprod Update 2008, 14(4):367-78.
9. Huang A, Brennan K, Azziz R: Prevalence of hyperandrogenemia in the polycystic ovary syndrome diagnosed by the National Institutes of Health 1990 criteria. Fertil Steril 2010, 93(6):1938-41.

10. Kiddy DS, Sharp PS, White DM, et al: Differences in clinical and endocrine features between obese and non-obese subjects with polycystic ovary syndrome: an analysis of 263 consecutive cases. Clin Endocrinol (Oxf) 1990, 32(2):213-20.

11. Ehrmann DA, Liljenquist DR, Kasza K, et al: Prevalence and predictors of the metabolic syndrome in women with polycystic ovary syndrome. J Clin Endocrinol Metab 2006, 91(1):48-53.

12. Carmina E, Lobo RA: Use of fasting blood to assess the prevalence of insulin resistance in women with polycystic ovary syndrome. Fertil Steril 2004, 82(3):661-5.

13. DeUgarte CM, Bartolucci AA, Azziz R: Prevalence of insulin resistance in the polycystic ovary syndrome using the homeostasis model assessment. Fertil Steril 2005, 83(5):1454-60.

14. Yildiz BO, Knochenhauer ES, Azziz R: Impact of obesity on the risk for polycystic ovary syndrome. J Clin Endocrinol Metab 2008, 93(1):162-8.

15. Azziz R: Controversy in clinical endocrinology: diagnosis of polycystic ovarian syndrome: the Rotterdam criteria are premature. J Clin Endocrinol Metab 2006, 91(3):781-5.

16. Dunaif A: Insulin resistance and the polycystic ovary syndrome: mechanism and implications for pathogenesis. Endocr Rev 1997, 18(6):774-800.

17. Azziz R, Marin C, Hoq L, et al: Health care-related economic burden of the polycystic ovary syndrome during the reproductive life span. J Clin Endocrinol Metab 2005, 90:4650-4658.

18. Talbott EO, Zborowski JV, Rager JR, et al: Polycystic ovarian syndrome (PCOS): a significant contributor to the overall burden of type 2 diabetes in women. J Womens Health (Larchmt) 2007, 16(2):191-7.

19. Alvarez-Blasco F, Botella-Carretero JI, San Millan JL, et al: Prevalence and characteristics of the polycystic ovary syndrome in overweight and obese women. Arch Intern Med 2006, 166(19):2081-6.

20. Ehrmann DA, Barnes RB, Rosenfield RL, et al: Prevalence of impaired glucose tolerance and diabetes in women with polycystic ovary syndrome. Diabetes Care 1999, 22(1):141-6.

21. Ehrmann DA, Kasza K, Azziz R, et al: Effects of race and family history of type 2 diabetes on metabolic status of women with polycystic ovary syndrome. J Clin Endocrinol Metab 2005, 90(1):66-71.

22. Legro RS, Kunselman AR, Dodson WC, et al: Prevalence and predictors of risk for type 2 diabetes mellitus and impaired glucose tolerance in polycystic ovary syndrome: a prospective, controlled study in 254 affected women. J Clin Endocrinol Metab 1999, 84(1):165-9.

23. Moran LJ, Misso ML, Wild RA, et al: Impaired glucose tolerance, type 2 diabetes and metabolic syndrome in polycystic ovary syndrome: a systematic review and meta-analysis. Hum Reprod Update 2010, 16(4):347-63.

24. Wild RA, Carmina E, Diamanti-Kandarakis E, et al: Assessment of cardiovascular risk and prevention of cardiovascular disease in women with the polycystic ovary syndrome: a consensus statement by the Androgen Excess and Polycystic Ovary Syndrome (AE-PCOS) Society. J Clin Endocrinol Metab 2010, 95(5):2038-49.

25. Salley KE, Wickham EP, Cheang KI, et al: Glucose intolerance in polycystic ovary syndrome–a position statement of the Androgen Excess Society. J Clin Endocrinol Metab 2007, 92(12):4546-56.

26. Achard EC, Thiers J: Le virilisme pilaire et son association a l'insuffisance glycolitique (diabète des femmes à barbe). Bulletin Acad Nat Med, Paris 1921, 86:51-85.

27. Stein I, Leventhal M: Amenorrhea associated with bilateral polycystic ovaries. Am J Obstet Gynecol 1935, 29:181-91.

28. Barbieri RL, Ryan KJ: Hyperandrogenism, insulin resistance, and acanthosis nigricans syndrome: a common endocrinopathy with distinct pathophysiologic features. Am J Obstet Gynecol 1983, 147(1):90-101.

29. Kahn CR, Flier JS, Bar RS, et al: The syndromes of insulin resistance and acanthosis nigricans. Insulin-receptor disorders in man. N Engl J Med 1976, 294(14):739-45.

30. O'Rahilly S, Choi WH, Patel P, et al: Detection of mutations in insulin-receptor gene in NIDDM patients by analysis of single-stranded conformation polymorphisms. Diabetes 1991, 40(6):777-82.

31. Taylor SI, Cama A, Accili D, et al: Mutations in the insulin receptor gene. Endocr Rev 1992, 13(3):566-95.

32. Flier JS, Kahn CR, Roth J, et al: Antibodies that impair insulin receptor binding in an unusual diabetic syndrome with severe insulin resistance. Science 1975, 190(4209):63-5.

33. Flier JS, Eastman RC, Minaker KL, et al: Acanthosis nigricans in obese women with hyperandrogenism. Characterization of an insulin-resistant state distinct from the type A and B syndromes. Diabetes 1985, 34(2):101-7.

34. Burghen GA, Givens JR, Kitabchi AE: Correlation of hyperandrogenism with hyperinsulinism in polycystic ovarian disease. J Clin Endocrinol Metab 1980, 50(1):113-6.

35. Franks S: Polycystic ovary syndrome. N Engl J Med 1995, 333(13):853-61.

36. Holte J: Disturbances in insulin secretion and sensitivity in women with the polycystic ovary syndrome. Baillieres Clin Endocrinol Metab 1996, 10(2):221-47.

37. Toprak S, Yonem A, Cakir B, et al: Insulin resistance in nonobese patients with polycystic ovary syndrome. Horm Res 2001, 55(2):65-70.

38. Homburg R, Lambalk CB: Polycystic ovary syndrome in adolescence–a therapeutic conundrum. Hum Reprod 2004, 19(5):1039-42.

39. Acien P, Quereda F, Matallin P, et al: Insulin, androgens, and obesity in women with and without polycystic ovary syndrome: a heterogeneous group of disorders. Fertil Steril 1999, 72(1):32-40.

40. Ciampelli M, Fulghesu AM, Cucinelli F, et al: Impact of insulin and body mass index on metabolic and endocrine variables in polycystic ovary syndrome. Metabolism 1999, 48(2):167-72.

41. Dunaif A, Segal KR, Futterweit W, et al: Profound peripheral insulin resistance, independent of obesity, in polycystic ovary syndrome. Diabetes 1989, 38(9):1165-74.

42. Chang RJ, Nakamura RM, Judd HL, et al: Insulin resistance in nonobese patients with polycystic ovarian disease. J Clin Endocrinol Metab 1983, 57(2):356-9.

43. Dunaif A, Hoffman AR, Scully RE, et al: Clinical, biochemical, and ovarian morphologic features in women with acanthosis nigricans and masculinization. Obstet Gynecol 1985, 66(4):545-52.

44. Mather KJ, Kwan F, Corenblum B: Hyperinsulinemia in polycystic ovary syndrome correlates with increased cardiovascular risk independent of obesity. Fertil Steril 2000, 73(1):150-6.

45. Ehrmann DA, Sturis J, Byrne MM, et al: Insulin secretory defects in polycystic ovary syndrome. Relationship to insulin sensitivity and family history of non-insulin-dependent diabetes mellitus. J Clin Invest 1995, 96(1):520-7.

46. Dunaif A, Finegood DT: Beta-cell dysfunction independent of obesity and glucose intolerance in the polycystic ovary syndrome. J Clin Endocrinol Metab 1996, 81(3):942-7.

47. Vrbikova J, Cibula D, Dvorakova K, et al: Insulin sensitivity in women with polycystic ovary syndrome. J Clin Endocrinol Metab 2004, 89(6):2942-2945.

48. Morales AJ, Laughlin GA, Butzow T, et al: Insulin, somatotropic, and luteinizing hormone axes in lean and obese women with polycystic ovary syndrome: common and distinct features. J Clin Endocrinol Metab 1996, 81(8):2854-64.

49. Ovesen P, Moller J, Ingerslev HJ, et al: Normal basal and insulin-stimulated fuel metabolism in lean women with the polycystic ovary syndrome. J Clin Endocrinol Metab 1993, 77(6):1636-40.

50. Diamanti-Kandarakis E, Kouli C, Alexandraki K, et al: Failure of mathematical indices to accurately assess insulin resistance in lean, overweight, or obese women with polycystic ovary syndrome. J Clin Endocrinol Metab 2004, 89(3):1273-6.

51. Palmert MR, Gordon CM, Kartashov AI, et al: Screening for abnormal glucose tolerance in adolescents with polycystic ovary syndrome. J Clin Endocrinol Metab 2002, 87(3):1017-23.

52. Cutfield WS, Jefferies CA, Jackson WE, et al: Evaluation of HOMA and QUICKI as measures of insulin sensitivity in prepubertal children. Pediatr Diabetes 2003, 4(3):119-25.

53. Kirchengast S, Huber J: Body composition characteristics and body fat distribution in lean women with polycystic ovary syndrome. Hum Reprod 2001, 16(6):1255-60.

54. Ibanez L, Ong K, de Zegher F, et al: Fat distribution in non-obese girls with and without precocious pubarche: central adiposity related to insulinaemia and androgenaemia from prepuberty to postmenarche. Clin Endocrinol (Oxf) 2003, 58(3):372-9.

55. Ibanez L, De Zegher F: Flutamide-metformin therapy to reduce fat mass in hyperinsulinemic ovarian hyperandrogenism: effects in adolescents and in women on third-generation oral contraception. J Clin Endocrinol Metab 2003, 88(10):4720-4.

56. Puder JJ, Varga S, Kraenzlin M, et al: Central fat excess in polycystic ovary syndrome: relation to low-grade inflammation and insulin resistance. J Clin Endocrinol Metab 2005, 90(11):6014-21.

57. Morin-Papunen LC, Vauhkonen I, Koivunen RM, et al: Insulin sensitivity, insulin secretion, and metabolic and hormonal parameters in healthy women and women with polycystic ovarian syndrome. Hum Reprod 2000, 15(6):1266-74.

58. Nestler JE, Jakubowicz DJ, Falcon de Vargas A, et al: Insulin stimulates testosterone biosynthesis by human thecal cells from women with polycystic ovary syndrome by activating its own receptor and using inositolglycan mediators as the signal transduction system. J Clin Endocrinol Metab 1998, 83(6):2001-2005.

59. Munir I, Yen HW, Geller DH, et al: Insulin augmentation of 17alpha-hydroxylase activity is mediated by phosphatidyl inositol 3-kinase but not extracellular signal-regulated kinase-1/2 in human ovarian theca cells. Endocrinology 2004, 145(1):175-83.

60. Nestler JE, Jakubowicz DJ: Decreases in ovarian cytochrome P450c17 alpha activity and serum free testosterone after reduction of insulin secretion in polycystic ovary syndrome. N Engl J Med 1996, 335(9):617-23.

61. Nestler JE, Jakubowicz DJ: Lean women with polycystic ovary syndrome respond to insulin reduction with decreases in ovarian P450c17 alpha activity and serum androgens. J Clin Endocrinol Metab 1997, 82(12):4075-9.

62. Zhang LH, Rodriguez H, Ohno S, et al: Serine phosphorylation of human P450c17 increases 17,20-lyase activity: implications for adrenarche and the polycystic ovary syndrome. Proc Natl Acad Sci U S A 1995, 92(23):10619-23.

63. Plymate SR, Matej LA, Jones RE, et al: Inhibition of sex hormone-binding globulin production in the human hepatoma (Hep G2) cell line by insulin and prolactin. J Clin Endocrinol Metab 1988, 67(3):460-4.

64. Nestler JE, Powers LP, Matt DW, et al: A direct effect of hyperinsulinemia on serum sex hormone-binding globulin levels in obese women with polycystic ovary syndrome. J Clin Endocrinol Metab 1991, 72(1):83-9.

65. Blank SK, McCartney CR, Marshall JC: The origins and sequelae of abnormal neuroendocrine function in polycystic ovary syndrome. Hum Reprod Update 2006, 12(4):351-61.

66. Chhabra S, McCartney CR, Yoo RY, et al: Progesterone inhibition of the hypothalamic gonadotropin-releasing hormone pulse generator: evidence for varied effects in hyperandrogenemic adolescent girls. J Clin Endocrinol Metab 2005, 90(5):2810-5.

67. Marshall JC, Eagleson CA: Neuroendocrine aspects of polycystic ovary syndrome. Endocrinol Metab Clin North Am 1999, 28(2):295-324.

68. Mehta RV, Patel KS, Coffler MS, et al: Luteinizing hormone secretion is not influenced by insulin infusion in women with polycystic ovary syndrome despite improved insulin sensitivity during pioglitazone treatment. J Clin Endocrinol Metab 2005, 90(4):2136-41.

69. Pagan YLea: Inverse relationship between luteinizing hormone and body mass index in polycystic ovarian syndrome: investigation of hypothalamic and pituitary contributions. J Clin Endocrinol Metab 2006, 91:1309-16.

70. Srouji SSea: Pharmacokinetic factors contribute to the inverse relationship between luteinizing hormone and body mass index in polycystic ovarian syndrome. J Clin Endocrinol Metab 2007, 92:1347-52.

71. Hall JE, Taylor AE, Hayes RJ, et al: Insights into hypothalamic-pituitary dysfunction in polycystic ovary syndrome. J Endocrinol Invest 1998, 21:602-11.

72. Taylor AEea: Determinants of abnormal gonadotropin secretion in clinically defined women with polycystic ovary syndrome. J Clin Endocrinol Metab 1997, 82:2248-56.

73. Vink JM, Sadrzadeh S, Lambalk CB, et al: Heritability of polycystic ovary syndrome in a Dutch twin-family study. J Clin Endocrinol Metab 2006, 91(6):2100-4.

74. Goodarzi MO: Looking for polycystic ovary syndrome genes: rational and best strategy. Semin Reprod Med 2008, 26(1):5-13.

75. Gaasenbeek M, Powell BL, Sovio U, et al: Large-scale analysis of the relationship between CYP11A promoter variation, polycystic ovarian syndrome, and serum testosterone. J Clin Endocrinol Metab 2004, 89(5):2408-13.

76. Goodarzi MO, Jones MR, Antoine HJ, et al: Nonreplication of the type 5 17beta-hydroxysteroid dehydrogenase gene association with polycystic ovary syndrome. J Clin Endocrinol Metab 2008, 93(1):300-3.

77. Powell BL, Haddad L, Bennett A, et al: Analysis of multiple data sets reveals no association between the insulin gene variable number tandem repeat element and polycystic ovary syndrome or related traits. J Clin Endocrinol Metab 2005, 90(5):2988-93.

78. Urbanek M, Woodroffe A, Ewens KG, et al: Candidate gene region for polycystic ovary syndrome on chromosome 19p13.2. J Clin Endocrinol Metab 2005, 90(12):6623-9.

79. Jones MR, Mathur R, Cui J, et al: Independent confirmation of association between metabolic phenotypes of polycystic ovary syndrome and variation in the type 6 17beta-hydroxysteroid dehydrogenase gene. J Clin Endocrinol Metab 2009, 94(12):5034-8.

80. Ewens KGea: Family-based analysis of candidate genes for polycystic ovary syndrome. J Clin Endocrinol Metab 2010, 95:2306-15.

81. Govind A, Obhrai MS, Clayton RN: Polycystic ovaries are inherited as an autosomal dominant trait: analysis of 29 polycystic ovary syndrome and 10 control families. J Clin Endocrinol Metab 1999, 84(1):38-43.

82. Legro RS, Driscoll D, Strauss JF, et al: Evidence for a genetic basis for hyperandrogenemia in polycystic ovary syndrome. Proc Natl Acad Sci U S A 1998, 95(25):14956-60.

83. Lunde O, Magnus P, Sandvik L, et al: Familial clustering in the polycystic ovarian syndrome. Gynecol Obstet Invest 1989, 28(1):23-30.

84. Kahsar-Miller MD, Nixon C, Boots LR, et al: Prevalence of polycystic ovary syndrome (PCOS) in first-degree relatives of patients with PCOS. Fertil Steril 2001, 75(1):53-8.

85. Sir-Petermann T, Angel B, Maliqueo M, et al: Prevalence of Type II diabetes mellitus and insulin resistance in parents of women with polycystic ovary syndrome. Diabetologia 2002, 45(7):959-64.

86. Sam S, Legro RS, Essah PA, et al: Evidence for metabolic and reproductive phenotypes in mothers of women with polycystic ovary syndrome. Proc Natl Acad Sci U S A 2006, 103(18):7030-5.

87. Sam S, Legro RS, Bentley-Lewis R, et al: Dyslipidemia and metabolic syndrome in the sisters of women with polycystic ovary syndrome. J Clin Endocrinol Metab 2005, 90(8):4797-802.

88. Colilla S, Cox NJ, Ehrmann DA: Heritability of insulin secretion and insulin action in women with polycystic ovary syndrome and their first degree relatives. J Clin Endocrinol Metab 2001, 86(5):2027-31.

89. Legro RS, Kunselman AR, Demers L, et al: Elevated dehydroepiandrosterone sulfate levels as the reproductive phenotype in the brothers of women with polycystic ovary syndrome. J Clin Endocrinol Metab 2002, 87(5):2134-8.

90. Kaushal R, Parchure N, Bano G, et al: Insulin resistance and endothelial dysfunction in the brothers of Indian subcontinent Asian women with polycystic ovaries. Clin Endocrinol (Oxf) 2004, 60(3):322-8.

91. Coviello AD, Sam S, Legro RS, et al: High prevalence of metabolic syndrome in first-degree male relatives of women with polycystic ovary syndrome is related to high rates of obesity. J Clin Endocrinol Metab 2009, 94(11):4361-6.

92. Sir-Petermann T, Codner E, Perez V, et al: Metabolic and reproductive features before and during puberty in daughters of women with polycystic ovary syndrome. J Clin Endocrinol Metab 2009, 94(6):1923-30.

93. Sir-Petermann T, Maliqueo M, Codner E, et al: Early metabolic derangements in daughters of women with polycystic ovary syndrome. J Clin Endocrinol Metab 2007, 92(12):4637-42.

94. Kent SC, Gnatuk CL, Kunselman AR, et al: Hyperandrogenism and hyperinsulinism in children of women with polycystic ovary syndrome: a controlled study. J Clin Endocrinol Metab 2008, 93(5):1662-9.

95. Francis GL, Getts A, McPherson JC: Preliminary results suggesting exaggerated ovarian androgen production early in the course of polycystic ovary syndrome. J Adolesc Health Care 1990, 11(6):480-4.

96. Coviello AD, Legro RS, Dunaif A: Adolescent girls with polycystic ovary syndrome have an increased risk of the metabolic syndrome associated with increasing androgen levels independent of obesity and insulin resistance. J Clin Endocrinol Metab 2006, 91(2):492-7.

97. Marshall JC: Obesity in adolescent girls: is excess androgen the real bad actor? J Clin Endocrinol Metab 2006, 91(2):393-5.

98. Lewy VD, Danadian K, Witchel SF, et al: Early metabolic abnormalities in adolescent girls with polycystic ovarian syndrome. J Pediatr 2001, 138(1):38-44.

99. Apter D, Butzow T, Laughlin GA, et al: Metabolic features of polycystic ovary syndrome are found in adolescent girls with hyperandrogenism. J Clin Endocrinol Metab 1995, 80(10):2966-73.

100. Silfen ME, Denburg MR, Manibo AM, et al: Early endocrine, metabolic, and sonographic characteristics of polycystic ovary syndrome (PCOS): comparison between nonobese and obese adolescents. J Clin Endocrinol Metab 2003, 88(10):4682-8.

101. Ibanez L, Potau N, Zampolli M, et al: Hyperinsulinemia in postpubertal girls with a history of premature pubarche and functional ovarian hyperandrogenism. J Clin Endocrinol Metab 1996, 81(3):1237-43.

102. Ibanez L, Potau N, Zampolli M, et al: Hyperinsulinemia and decreased insulin-like growth factor-binding protein-1 are common features in prepubertal and pubertal girls with a history of premature pubarche. J Clin Endocrinol Metab 1997, 82(7):2283-8.

103. Ibanez L, Castell C, Tresserras R, et al: Increased prevalence of type 2 diabetes mellitus and impaired glucose tolerance in first-degree relatives of girls with a history of precocious pubarche. Clin Endocrinol (Oxf) 1999, 51(4):395-401.

104. Ibanez L, de Zegher F, Potau N: Anovulation after precocious pubarche: early markers and time course in adolescence. J Clin Endocrinol Metab 1999, 84(8):2691-5.

105. Ibanez L, Potau N, De Zegher F: Endocrinology and metabolism after premature pubarche in girls. Acta Paediatr Suppl 1999, 88(433):73-7.

106. Oppenheimer E, Linder B, DiMartino-Nardi J: Decreased insulin sensitivity in prepubertal girls with premature adrenarche and acanthosis nigricans. J Clin Endocrinol Metab 1995, 80(2):614-8.

107. Richards GE, Cavallo A, Meyer WJ, et al: Obesity, acanthosis nigricans, insulin resistance, and hyperandrogenemia: pediatric perspective and natural history. J Pediatr 1985, 107(6):893-7.

108. McCartney CR, Prendergast KA, Chhabra S, et al: The association of obesity and hyperandrogenemia during the pubertal transition in girls: obesity as a potential factor in the genesis of postpubertal hyperandrogenism. J Clin Endocrinol Metab 2006, 91(5):1714-22.

109. Rosenfield RL: Clinical review: Identifying children at risk for polycystic ovary syndrome. J Clin Endocrinol Metab 2007, 92(3):787-96.

110. Zumoff B, Freeman R, Coupey S, et al: A chronobiologic abnormality in luteinizing hormone secretion in teenage girls with the polycystic-ovary syndrome. N Engl J Med 1983, 309(20):1206-9.

111. Dale PO, Tanbo T, Djoseland O, et al: Persistence of hyperinsulinemia in polycystic ovary syndrome after ovarian suppression by gonadotropin-releasing hormone agonist. Acta Endocrinol (Copenh) 1992, 126(2):132-6.

112. Dunaif A, Green G, Futterweit W, et al: Suppression of hyperandrogenism does not improve peripheral or hepatic insulin resistance in the polycystic ovary syndrome. J Clin Endocrinol Metab 1990, 70(3):699-704.

113. Geffner ME, Kaplan SA, Bersch N, et al: Persistence of insulin resistance in polycystic ovarian disease after inhibition of ovarian steroid secretion. Fertil Steril 1986, 45(3):327-33.

114. Lasco A, Cucinotta D, Gigante A, et al: No changes of peripheral insulin resistance in polycystic ovary syndrome after long-term reduction of endogenous androgens with leuprolide. Eur J Endocrinol 1995, 133(6):718-22.

115. Diamanti-Kandarakis E, Mitrakou A, Hennes MM, et al: Insulin sensitivity and antiandrogenic therapy in women with polycystic ovary syndrome. Metabolism 1995, 44(4):525-31.

116. Diamanti-Kandarakis E, Mitrakou A, Raptis S, et al: The effect of a pure antiandrogen receptor blocker, flutamide, on the lipid profile in the polycystic ovary syndrome. J Clin Endocrinol Metab 1998, 83(8):2699-705.

117. Sahin I, Serter R, Karakurt F, et al: Metformin versus flutamide in the treatment of metabolic consequences of non-obese young women with polycystic ovary syndrome: a randomized prospective study. Gynecol Endocrinol 2004, 19(3):115-24.

118. Apter D: How possible is the prevention of polycystic ovary syndrome development in adolescent patients with early onset of hyperandrogenism. J Endocrinol Invest 1998, 21(9):613-7.

119. Carmina E, Orio F, Palomba S, et al: Endothelial dysfunction in PCOS: role of obesity and adipose hormones. Am J Med 2006, 119(4):356 e1-6.

120. Lakhani K, Hardiman P, Seifalian AM: Intima-media thickness of elastic and muscular arteries of young women with polycystic ovaries. Atherosclerosis 2004, 175(2):353-9.

121. Vryonidou A, Papatheodorou A, Tavridou A, et al: Association of hyperandrogenemic and metabolic phenotype with carotid intima-media thickness in young women with polycystic ovary syndrome. J Clin Endocrinol Metab 2005, 90(5):2740-6.

122. Goodarzi MO, Korenman SG: The importance of insulin resistance in polycystic ovary syndrome. Fertil Steril 2003, 80(2):255-8.

123. Salmi DJ, Zisser HC, Jovanovic L: Screening for and treatment of polycystic ovary syndrome in teenagers. Exp Biol Med (Maywood) 2004, 229(5):369-77.

124. Hoeger KM, Kochman L, Wixom N, et al: A randomized, 48-week, placebo-controlled trial of intensive lifestyle modification and/or metformin therapy in overweight women with polycystic ovary syndrome: a pilot study. Fertil Steril 2004, 82(2):421-9.

125. Huber-Buchholz MM, Carey DG, Norman RJ: Restoration of reproductive potential by lifestyle modification in obese polycystic ovary syndrome: role of insulin sensitivity and luteinizing hormone. J Clin Endocrinol Metab 1999, 84(4):1470-4.

126. Kiddy DS, Hamilton-Fairley D, Bush A, et al: Improvement in endocrine and ovarian function during dietary treatment of obese women with polycystic ovary syndrome. Clin Endocrinol (Oxf) 1992, 36(1):105-11.

127. Hoeger KM: Obesity and lifestyle management in polycystic ovary syndrome. Clin Obstet Gynecol 2007, 50(1):277-94.

128. Palomba S, Giallauria F, Falbo A, et al: Structured exercise training programme versus hypocaloric hyperproteic diet in obese polycystic ovary syndrome patients with anovulatory infertility: a 24-week pilot study. Hum Reprod 2008, 23(3):642-50.

129. Azziz R, Carmina E, Dewailly D, et al: The Androgen Excess and PCOS Society criteria for the polycystic ovary syndrome: the complete task force report. Fertil Steril 2009, 91(2):456-88.

130. Carmina E, Bucchieri S, Esposito A, et al: Abdominal fat quantity and distribution in women with polycystic ovary syndrome and extent of its relation to insulin resistance. J Clin Endocrinol Metab 2007, 92(7):2500-5.

131. Wabitsch M, Hauner H, Heinze E, et al: Body fat distribution and steroid hormone concentrations in obese adolescent girls before and after weight reduction. J Clin Endocrinol Metab 1995, 80(12):3469-75.

132. Reinehr T, de Sousa G, Roth CL, et al: Androgens before and after weight loss in obese children. J Clin Endocrinol Metab 2005, 90(10):5588-95.

133. Hoeger K, Davidson K, Kochman L, et al: The impact of metformin, oral contraceptives, and lifestyle modification on polycystic ovary syndrome in obese adolescent women in two randomized, placebo-controlled clinical trials. J Clin Endocrinol Metab 2008, 93(11):4299-306.

134. Otta CF, Wior M, Iraci GS, et al: Clinical, metabolic, and endocrine parameters in response to metformin and lifestyle intervention in women with polycystic ovary syndrome: a randomized, double-blind, and placebo control trial. Gynecol Endocrinol 2010, 26(3):173-8.

135. Pasquali R, Gambineri A, Biscotti D, et al: Effect of long-term treatment with metformin added to hypocaloric diet on body composition, fat distribution, and androgen and insulin levels in abdominally obese women with and without the polycystic ovary syndrome. J Clin Endocrinol Metab 2000, 85(8):2767-74.

136. Eid GM, Cottam DR, Velcu LM, et al: Effective treatment of polycystic ovarian syndrome with Roux-en-Y gastric bypass. Surg Obes Relat Dis 2005, 1(2):77-80.

137. Escobar-Morreale HF, Botella-Carretero JI, Alvarez-Blasco F, et al: The polycystic ovary syndrome associated with morbid obesity may resolve after weight loss induced by bariatric surgery. J Clin Endocrinol Metab 2005, 90(12):6364-9.

138. Escobar-Morreale HF: Polycystic ovary syndrome: treatment strategies and management. Expert Opin Pharmacother 2008, 9(17):2995-3008.

139. Schilling PL, Davis MM, Albanese CT, et al: National trends in adolescent bariatric surgical procedures and implications for surgical centers of excellence. J Am Coll Surg 2008, 206(1):1-12.

140. Martin KA, Chang RJ, Ehrmann DA, et al: Evaluation and treatment of hirsutism in premenopausal women: an endocrine society clinical practice guideline. J Clin Endocrinol Metab 2008, 93(4):1105-20.

141. Nader S, Diamanti-Kandarakis E: Polycystic ovary syndrome, oral contraceptives and metabolic issues: new perspectives and a unifying hypothesis. Hum Reprod 2007, 22(2):317-22.

142. Ehrmann DA: Polycystic ovary syndrome. N Engl J Med 2005, 352(12):1223-36.

143. Schindler AE: Differential effects of progestins on hemostasis. Maturitas 2003, 46(Suppl 1):S31-7.

144. Cassidenti DL, Paulson RJ, Serafini P, et al: Effects of sex steroids on skin 5 alpha-reductase activity in vitro. Obstet Gynecol 1991, 78(1):103-7.

145. Hammond GL, Rabe T, Wagner JD: Preclinical profiles of progestins used in formulations of oral contraceptives and hormone replacement therapy. *Am J Obstet Gynecol* 2001, **185**(2 Suppl):S24-31.

146. Franks S, Layton A, Glasier A: Cyproterone acetate/ethinyl estradiol for acne and hirsutism: time to revise prescribing policy. *Hum Reprod* 2008, **23**(2):231-2.

147. Givens JR, Andersen RN, Wiser WL, et al: Dynamics of suppression and recovery of plasma FSH, LH, androstenedione and testosterone in polycystic ovarian disease using an oral contraceptive. *J Clin Endocrinol Metab* 1974, **38**(5):727-35.

148. van der Vange N, Blankenstein MA, Kloosterboer HJ, et al: Effects of seven low-dose combined oral contraceptives on sex hormone binding globulin, corticosteroid binding globulin, total and free testosterone. *Contraception* 1990, **41**(4):345-52.

149. De Leo V, Di Sabatino A, Musacchio MC, et al: Effect of oral contraceptives on markers of hyperandrogenism and SHBG in women with polycystic ovary syndrome. *Contraception* 2010, **82**(3):276-80.

150. Mastorakos G, Koliopoulos C, Creatsas G: Androgen and lipid profiles in adolescents with polycystic ovary syndrome who were treated with two forms of combined oral contraceptives. *Fertil Steril* 2002, **77**(5):919-27.

151. Heiner JS, Greendale GA, Kawakami AK, et al: Comparison of a gonadotropin-releasing hormone agonist and a low dose oral contraceptive given alone or together in the treatment of hirsutism. *J Clin Endocrinol Metab* 1995, **80**(12):3412-8.

152. Trent ME, Rich M, Austin SB, et al: Fertility concerns and sexual behavior in adolescent girls with polycystic ovary syndrome: implications for quality of life. *J Pediatr Adolesc Gynecol* 2003, **16**(1):33-7.

153. Dahlgren E, Friberg LG, Johansson S, et al: Endometrial carcinoma; ovarian dysfunction–a risk factor in young women. *Eur J Obstet Gynecol Reprod Biol* 1991, **41**(2):143-50.

154. Iatrakis G, Tsionis C, Adonakis G, et al: Polycystic ovarian syndrome, insulin resistance and thickness of the endometrium. *Eur J Obstet Gynecol Reprod Biol* 2006, **127**(2):218-21.

155. Pillay OC, Te Fong LF, Crow JC, et al: The association between polycystic ovaries and endometrial cancer. *Hum Reprod* 2006, **21**(4):924-9.

156. Lurie G, Thompson P, McDuffie KE, et al: Association of estrogen and progestin potency of oral contraceptives with ovarian carcinoma risk. *Obstet Gynecol* 2007, **109**(3):597-607.

157. Grimes DA, Economy KE: Primary prevention of gynecologic cancers. *Am J Obstet Gynecol* 1995, **172**(1 Pt 1):227-35.

158. Costello M, Shrestha B, Eden J, et al: Insulin-sensitising drugs versus the combined oral contraceptive pill for hirsutism, acne and risk of diabetes, cardiovascular disease, and endometrial cancer in polycystic ovary syndrome. *Cochrane Database Syst Rev* 2007, , 1: CD005552.

159. Mastorakos G, Koliopoulos C, Deligeoroglou E, et al: Effects of two forms of combined oral contraceptives on carbohydrate metabolism in adolescents with polycystic ovary syndrome. *Fertil Steril* 2006, **85**(2):420-7.

160. Baillargeon JP, McClish DK, Essah PA, et al: Association between the current use of low-dose oral contraceptives and cardiovascular arterial disease: a meta-analysis. *J Clin Endocrinol Metab* 2005, **90**(7):3863-70.

161. Khader YS, Rice J, John L, et al: Oral contraceptives use and the risk of myocardial infarction: a meta-analysis. *Contraception* 2003, **68**(1):11-7.

162. Burkman RT: Hormone replacement therapy. Current controversies. *Minerva Ginecol* 2003, **55**(2):107-16.

163. Keeling D: Combined oral contraceptives and the risk of myocardial infarction. *Ann Med* 2003, **35**(6):413-8.

164. Barbieri RL: Update in female reproduction: a life-cycle approach. *J Clin Endocrinol Metab* 2008, **93**(7):2439-46.

165. Fryer LG, Parbu-Patel A, Carling D: The Anti-diabetic drugs rosiglitazone and metformin stimulate AMP-activated protein kinase through distinct signaling pathways. *J Biol Chem* 2002, **277**(28):25226-32.

166. Checa MA, Requena A, Salvador C, et al: Insulin-sensitizing agents: use in pregnancy and as therapy in polycystic ovary syndrome. *Hum Reprod Update* 2005, **11**(4):375-90.

167. Kashyap S, Wells GA, Rosenwaks Z: Insulin-sensitizing agents as primary therapy for patients with polycystic ovarian syndrome. *Hum Reprod* 2004, **19**(11):2474-83.

168. la Marca A, Egbe TO, Morgante G, et al: Metformin treatment reduces ovarian cytochrome P-450c17alpha response to human chorionic gonadotrophin in women with insulin resistance-related polycystic ovary syndrome. *Hum Reprod* 2000, **15**(1):21-3.

169. La Marca A, Artensio AC, Stabile G, et al: Metformin treatment of PCOS during adolescence and the reproductive period. *Eur J Obstet Gynecol Reprod Biol* 2005, **121**(1):3-7.

170. Lord JM, Flight IH, Norman RJ: Metformin in polycystic ovary syndrome: systematic review and meta-analysis. *BMJ* 2003, **327**(7421):951-3.

171. Velazquez EM, Mendoza S, Hamer T, et al: Metformin therapy in polycystic ovary syndrome reduces hyperinsulinemia, insulin resistance, hyperandrogenemia, and systolic blood pressure, while facilitating normal menses and pregnancy. *Metabolism* 1994, **43**(5):647-54.

172. Legro RS, Barnhart HX, Schlaff WD, et al: Clomiphene, metformin, or both for infertility in the polycystic ovary syndrome. *N Engl J Med* 2007, **356**(6):551-66.

173. Vanky E, Stridsklev S, Heimstad R, et al: Metformin versus placebo from first trimester to delivery in polycystic ovary syndrome: a randomized, controlled multicenter study. *J Clin Endocrinol Metab* 2010, **95**(12):E448-55.

174. Ibanez L, Jaramillo AM, Ferrer A, et al: High neutrophil count in girls and women with hyperinsulinaemic hyperandrogenism: normalization with metformin and flutamide overcomes the aggravation by oral contraception. *Hum Reprod* 2005, **20**(9):2457-62.

175. Kelly CC, Lyall H, Petrie JR, et al: Low grade chronic inflammation in women with polycystic ovarian syndrome. *J Clin Endocrinol Metab* 2001, **86**(6):2453-5.

176. Morin-Papunen L, Rautio K, Ruokonen A, et al: Metformin reduces serum C-reactive protein levels in women with polycystic ovary syndrome. *J Clin Endocrinol Metab* 2003, **88**(10):4649-54.

177. Rexrode KM, Pradhan A, Manson JE, et al: Relationship of total and abdominal adiposity with CRP and IL-6 in women. *Ann Epidemiol* 2003, **13**(10):674-82.

178. Boulman N, Levy Y, Leiba R, et al: Increased C-reactive protein levels in the polycystic ovary syndrome: a marker of cardiovascular disease. *J Clin Endocrinol Metab* 2004, **89**(5):2160-5.

179. Goldstein BJ, Scalia R: Adiponectin: A novel adipokine linking adipocytes and vascular function. *J Clin Endocrinol Metab* 2004, **89**(6):2563-8.

180. Orio F Jr, Palomba S, Cascella T, et al: Early impairment of endothelial structure and function in young normal-weight women with polycystic ovary syndrome. *J Clin Endocrinol Metab* 2004, **89**(9):4588-93.

181. Orio F Jr, Palomba S, Cascella T, et al: Improvement in endothelial structure and function after metformin treatment in young normal-weight women with polycystic ovary syndrome: results of a 6-month study. *J Clin Endocrinol Metab* 2005, **90**(11):6072-6.

182. Orio F Jr, Palomba S, Cascella T, et al: The increase of leukocytes as a new putative marker of low-grade chronic inflammation and early cardiovascular risk in polycystic ovary syndrome. *J Clin Endocrinol Metab* 2005, **90**(1):2-5.

183. Tarkun I, Arslan BC, Canturk Z, et al: Endothelial dysfunction in young women with polycystic ovary syndrome: relationship with insulin resistance and low-grade chronic inflammation. *J Clin Endocrinol Metab* 2004, **89**(11):5592-6.

184. Vural B, Caliskan E, Turkoz E, et al: Evaluation of metabolic syndrome frequency and premature carotid atherosclerosis in young women with polycystic ovary syndrome. *Hum Reprod* 2005, **20**(9):2409-13.

185. Diamanti-Kandarakis E, Spina G, Kouli C, et al: Increased endothelin-1 levels in women with polycystic ovary syndrome and the beneficial effect of metformin therapy. *J Clin Endocrinol Metab* 2001, **86**(10):4666-73.

186. Velazquez EM, Mendoza SG, Wang P, et al: Metformin therapy is associated with a decrease in plasma plasminogen activator inhibitor-1, lipoprotein(a), and immunoreactive insulin levels in patients with the polycystic ovary syndrome. *Metabolism* 1997, **46**(4):454-7.

187. Diamanti-Kandarakis E, Paterakis T, Alexandraki K, et al: Indices of low-grade chronic inflammation in polycystic ovary syndrome and the beneficial effect of metformin. *Hum Reprod* 2006, **21**(6):1426-31.

188. Diamanti-Kandarakis E, Alexandraki K, Protogerou A, et al: Metformin administration improves endothelial function in women with polycystic ovary syndrome. *Eur J Endocrinol* 2005, **152**(5):749-56.

189. Ibanez L, de Zegher F: Ethinylestradiol-drospirenone, flutamide-metformin, or both for adolescents and women with hyperinsulinemic hyperandrogenism: opposite effects on adipocytokines and body adiposity. *J Clin Endocrinol Metab* 2004, **89**(4):1592-7.

190. Ibanez L, de Zegher F: Low-dose flutamide-metformin therapy for hyperinsulinemic hyperandrogenism in non-obese adolescents and women. *Hum Reprod Update* 2006, **12**(3):243-52.

191. Arslanian SA, Lewy V, Danadian K, et al: Metformin therapy in obese adolescents with polycystic ovary syndrome and impaired glucose tolerance: amelioration of exaggerated adrenal response to adrenocorticotropin with reduction of insulinemia/insulin resistance. J Clin Endocrinol Metab 2002, 87(4):1555-9.

192. Ibanez L, Potau N, Chacon P, et al: Hyperinsulinaemia, dyslipaemia and cardiovascular risk in girls with a history of premature pubarche. Diabetologia 1998, 41(9):1057-63.

193. Guttmann-Bauman I: Approach to adolescent polycystic ovary syndrome (PCOS) in the pediatric endocrine community in the U.S.A. J Pediatr Endocrinol Metab 2005, 18(5):499-506.

194. Ibanez L, Valls C, Ferrer A, et al: Sensitization to insulin induces ovulation in nonobese adolescents with anovulatory hyperandrogenism. J Clin Endocrinol Metab 2001, 86(8):3595-8.

195. Ibanez L, Ong K, Ferrer A, et al: Low-dose flutamide-metformin therapy reverses insulin resistance and reduces fat mass in nonobese adolescents with ovarian hyperandrogenism. J Clin Endocrinol Metab 2003, 88(6):2600-6.

196. Ibanez L, Potau N, Francois I, et al: Precocious pubarche, hyperinsulinism, and ovarian hyperandrogenism in girls: relation to reduced fetal growth. J Clin Endocrinol Metab 1998, 83(10):3558-62.

197. Ibanez L, Valls C, Potau N, et al: Sensitization to insulin in adolescent girls to normalize hirsutism, hyperandrogenism, oligomenorrhea, dyslipidemia, and hyperinsulinism after precocious pubarche. J Clin Endocrinol Metab 2000, 85(10):3526-30.

198. Vrbikova J, Hill M, Starka L, et al: The effects of long-term metformin treatment on adrenal and ovarian steroidogenesis in women with polycystic ovary syndrome. Eur J Endocrinol 2001, 144(6):619-28.

199. la Marca A, Morgante G, Paglia T, et al: Effects of metformin on adrenal steroidogenesis in women with polycystic ovary syndrome. Fertil Steril 1999, 72(6):985-9.

200. Bridger T, MacDonald S, Baltzer F, et al: Randomized placebo-controlled trial of metformin for adolescents with polycystic ovary syndrome. Arch Pediatr Adolesc Med 2006, 160(3):241-6.

201. Nestler JE: Metformin and the polycystic ovary syndrome. J Clin Endocrinol Metab 2001, 86(3):1430.

202. Glueck CJ, Wang P, Fontaine R, et al: Metformin-induced resumption of normal menses in 39 of 43 (91%) previously amenorrheic women with the polycystic ovary syndrome. Metabolism 1999, 48(4):511-9.

203. Cusan L, Dupont A, Gomez JL, et al: Comparison of flutamide and spironolactone in the treatment of hirsutism: a randomized controlled trial. Fertil Steril 1994, 61(2):281-7.

204. Diamanti-Kandarakis E, Kouli C, Tsianateli T, et al: Therapeutic effects of metformin on insulin resistance and hyperandrogenism in polycystic ovary syndrome. Eur J Endocrinol 1998, 138(3):269-74.

205. Gambineri A, Pelusi C, Genghini S, et al: Effect of flutamide and metformin administered alone or in combination in dieting obese women with polycystic ovary syndrome. Clin Endocrinol (Oxf) 2004, 60(2):241-9.

206. Ibanez L, Valls C, Ferrer A, et al: Additive effects of insulin-sensitizing and anti-androgen treatment in young, nonobese women with hyperinsulinism, hyperandrogenism, dyslipidemia, and anovulation. J Clin Endocrinol Metab 2002, 87(6):2870-4.

207. Ganie MA, Khurana ML, Eunice M, et al: Comparison of efficacy of spironolactone with metformin in the management of polycystic ovary syndrome: an open-labeled study. J Clin Endocrinol Metab 2004, 89(6):2756-62.

208. Rautio K, Tapanainen JS, Ruokonen A, et al: Effects of metformin and ethinyl estradiol-cyproterone acetate on lipid levels in obese and non-obese women with polycystic ovary syndrome. Eur J Endocrinol 2005, 152(2):269-75.

209. Mitkov M, Pehlivanov B, Terzieva D: Combined use of metformin and ethinyl estradiol-cyproterone acetate in polycystic ovary syndrome. Eur J Obstet Gynecol Reprod Biol 2005, 118(2):209-13.

210. Morin-Papunen L, Vauhkonen I, Koivunen R, et al: Metformin versus ethinyl estradiol-cyproterone acetate in the treatment of nonobese women with polycystic ovary syndrome: a randomized study. J Clin Endocrinol Metab 2003, 88(1):148-56.

211. Onalan G, Goktolga U, Ceyhan T, et al: Predictive value of glucose-insulin ratio in PCOS and profile of women who will benefit from metformin therapy: obese, lean, hyper or normoinsulinemic? Eur J Obstet Gynecol Reprod Biol 2005, 123(2):204-11.

212. Yilmaz M, Biri A, Karakoc A, et al: The effects of rosiglitazone and metformin on insulin resistance and serum androgen levels in obese and lean patients with polycystic ovary syndrome. J Endocrinol Invest 2005, 28(11):1003-8.

213. Glueck CJ, Wang P, Fontaine R, et al: Metformin to restore normal menses in oligo-amenorrheic teenage girls with polycystic ovary syndrome (PCOS). J Adolesc Health 2001, 29(3):160-9.

214. Velazquez E, Acosta A, Mendoza SG: Menstrual cyclicity after metformin therapy in polycystic ovary syndrome. Obstet Gynecol 1997, 90(3):392-5.

215. Morin-Papunen LC, Koivunen RM, Ruokonen A, et al: Metformin therapy improves the menstrual pattern with minimal endocrine and metabolic effects in women with polycystic ovary syndrome. Fertil Steril 1998, 69(4):691-6.

216. De Leo V, Musacchio MC, Morgante G, et al: Metformin treatment is effective in obese teenage girls with PCOS. Hum Reprod 2006, 21(9):2252-6.

217. Glueck CJ, Aregawi D, Winiarska M, et al: Metformin-diet ameliorates coronary heart disease risk factors and facilitates resumption of regular menses in adolescents with polycystic ovary syndrome. J Pediatr Endocrinol Metab 2006, 19(6):831-42.

218. Diamanti-Kandarakis E, Baillargeon JP, Iuorno MJ, et al: A modern medical quandary: polycystic ovary syndrome, insulin resistance, and oral contraceptive pills. J Clin Endocrinol Metab 2003, 88(5):1927-32.

219. Vrbikova J, Cibula D: Combined oral contraceptives in the treatment of polycystic ovary syndrome. Hum Reprod Update 2005, 11(3):277-91.

220. Allen HF, Mazzoni C, Heptulla RA, et al: Randomized controlled trial evaluating response to metformin versus standard therapy in the treatment of adolescents with polycystic ovary syndrome. J Pediatr Endocrinol Metab 2005, 18(8):761-8.

221. Ibanez L, De Zegher F: Flutamide-metformin plus an oral contraceptive (OC) for young women with polycystic ovary syndrome: switch from third- to fourth-generation OC reduces body adiposity. Hum Reprod 2004, 19(8):1725-7.

222. Ibanez L, de Zegher F: Flutamide-metformin plus ethinylestradiol-drospirenone for lipolysis and antiatherogenesis in young women with ovarian hyperandrogenism: the key role of metformin at the start and after more than one year of therapy. J Clin Endocrinol Metab 2005, 90(1):39-43.

223. Ibanez L, Valls C, Marcos MV, et al: Insulin sensitization for girls with precocious pubarche and with risk for polycystic ovary syndrome: effects of prepubertal initiation and postpubertal discontinuation of metformin treatment. J Clin Endocrinol Metab 2004, 89(9):4331-7.

224. Elter K, Imir G, Durmusoglu F: Clinical, endocrine and metabolic effects of metformin added to ethinyl estradiol-cyproterone acetate in non-obese women with polycystic ovarian syndrome: a randomized controlled study. Hum Reprod 2002, 17(7):1729-37.

225. Cibula D, Fanta M, Vrbikova J, et al: The effect of combination therapy with metformin and combined oral contraceptives (COC) versus COC alone on insulin sensitivity, hyperandrogenaemia, SHBG and lipids in PCOS patients. Hum Reprod 2005, 20(1):180-4.

226. Poyet P, Labrie F: Comparison of the antiandrogenic/androgenic activities of flutamide, cyproterone acetate and megestrol acetate. Mol Cell Endocrinol 1985, 42(3):283-8.

227. Muderris II, Bayram F, Guven M: Treatment of hirsutism with lowest-dose flutamide (62.5 mg/day). Gynecol Endocrinol 2000, 14(1):38-41.

228. Ibanez L, Jaramillo A, Ferrer A, et al: Absence of hepatotoxicity after long-term, low-dose flutamide in hyperandrogenic girls and young women. Hum Reprod 2005, 20(7):1833-6.

229. Ibanez L, Potau N, Marcos MV, et al: Treatment of hirsutism, hyperandrogenism, oligomenorrhea, dyslipidemia, and hyperinsulinism in nonobese, adolescent girls: effect of flutamide. J Clin Endocrinol Metab 2000, 85(9):3251-5.

230. Ibanez L, Potau N, Ferrer A, et al: Anovulation in eumenorrheic, nonobese adolescent girls born small for gestational age: insulin sensitization induces ovulation, increases lean body mass, and reduces abdominal fat excess, dyslipidemia, and subclinical hyperandrogenism. J Clin Endocrinol Metab 2002, 87(12):5702-5.

231. Ibanez L, de Zegher F: Low-dose combination of flutamide, metformin and an oral contraceptive for non-obese, young women with polycystic ovary syndrome. Hum Reprod 2003, 18(1):57-60.

232. Ibanez L, Valls C, Cabre S, et al: Flutamide-metformin plus ethinylestradiol-drospirenone for lipolysis and antiatherogenesis in young women with ovarian hyperandrogenism: the key role of early, low-dose flutamide. *J Clin Endocrinol Metab* 2004, **89**(9):4716-20.

233. Vuguin P, Saenger P, DiMartino-Nardi J: Fasting glucose insulin ratio: a useful measure of insulin resistance in girls with premature adrenarche. *J Clin Endocrinol Metab* 2001, **86**(10):4618-21.

234. Silfen ME, Manibo AM, McMahon DJ, et al: Comparison of simple measures of insulin sensitivity in young girls with premature adrenarche: the fasting glucose to insulin ratio may be a simple and useful measure. *J Clin Endocrinol Metab* 2001, **86**(6):2863-8.

235. Legro RS, Finegood DT, Dunaif A: A fasting glucose to insulin ratio is a useful measure of insulin sensitivity in women with polycystic ovary syndrome. *J Clin Endocrinol Metab* 1998, **83**(8):2694-8.

236. Ibanez L, Valls C, Potau N, et al: Polycystic ovary syndrome after precocious pubarche: ontogeny of the low-birthweight effect. *Clin Endocrinol (Oxf)* 2001, **55**(5):667-72.

237. Ibanez L, Ferrer A, Ong K, et al: Insulin sensitization early after menarche prevents progression from precocious pubarche to polycystic ovary syndrome. *J Pediatr* 2004, **144**(1):23-9.

238. Baillargeon J, Jakubowicz DJ, Iuorno MJ, et al: Effects of metformin and rosiglitazone, along and in combination, in nonobese women with polycystic ovary syndrome and normal indices of insulin sensitivity. *Fertil Steril* 2004, **82**(4):893-902.

239. Ortega-Gonzalez C, Luna S, Hernandez L, et al: Responses of serum androgen and insulin resistance to metformin and pioglitazone in obese, insulin-resistant women with polycystic ovary syndrome. *J Clin Endocrinol Metab* 2005, **90**(3):1360-5.

240. Ehrmann DA, Schneider DJ, Sobel BE, et al: Troglitazone improves defects in insulin action, insulin secretion, ovarian steroidogenesis, and fibrinolysis in women with polycystic ovary syndrome. *J Clin Endocrinol Metab* 1997, **82**(7):2108-16.

241. Tarkun I, Cetinarslan B, Turemen E, et al: Effect of rosiglitazone on insulin resistance, C-reactive protein and endothelial function in non-obese young women with polycystic ovary syndrome. *Eur J Endocrinol* 2005, **153**(1):115-21.

242. Dereli D, Dereli T, Bayraktar F, et al: Endocrine and metabolic effects of rosiglitazone in non-obese women with polycystic ovary disease. *Endocr J* 2005, **52**(3):299-308.

243. Seto-Young D, Paliou M, Schlosser J, et al: Direct thiazolidinedione action in the human ovary: insulin-independent and insulin-sensitizing effects on steroidogenesis and insulin-like growth factor binding protein-1 production. *J Clin Endocrinol Metab* 2005, **90**(11):6099-105.

244. Glueck CJ, Moreira A, Goldenberg N, et al: Pioglitazone and metformin in obese women with polycystic ovary syndrome not optimally responsive to metformin. *Hum Reprod* 2003, **18**(8):1618-25.

245. Dunaif A, Scott D, Finegood D, et al: The insulin-sensitizing agent troglitazone improves metabolic and reproductive abnormalities in the polycystic ovary syndrome. *J Clin Endocrinol Metab* 1996, **81**(9):3299-306.

246. Hasegawa I, Murakawa H, Suzuki M, et al: Effect of troglitazone on endocrine and ovulatory performance in women with insulin resistance-related polycystic ovary syndrome. *Fertil Steril* 1999, **71**(2):323-7.

247. Gambineri A, Semple RK, Forlani G, et al: Monogenic polycystic ovary syndrome due to a mutation in the lamin A/C gene is sensitive to thiazolidinediones but not to metformin. *Eur J Endocrinol* 2008, **159**(3):347-53.

248. Franks S: When should an insulin sensitizing agent be used in the treatment of polycystic ovary syndrome? *Clin Endocrinol (Oxf)* 2011, **74**(2):148-51.

249. Shu Y, Sheardown SA, Brown C, et al: Effect of genetic variation in the organic cation transporter 1 (OCT1) on metformin action. *J Clin Invest* 2007, **117**(5):1422-31.

250. Ahlin G, Chen L, Lazorova L, et al: Genotype-dependent effects of inhibitors of the organic cation transporter, OCT1: predictions of metformin interactions. *Pharmacogenomics J* 2010.

251. Becker ML, Visser LE, van Schaik RH, et al: Genetic variation in the organic cation transporter 1 is associated with metformin response in patients with diabetes mellitus. *Pharmacogenomics J* 2009, **9**(4):242-7.

252. Kajiwara M, Terada T, Ogasawara K, et al: Identification of multidrug and toxin extrusion (MATE1 and MATE2-K) variants with complete loss of transport activity. *J Hum Genet* 2009, **54**(1):40-6.

253. Trent M, Austin SB, Rich M, et al: Overweight status of adolescent girls with polycystic ovary syndrome: body mass index as mediator of quality of life. *Ambul Pediatr* 2005, **5**(2):107-11.

254. Trent ME, Rich M, Austin SB, et al: Quality of life in adolescent girls with polycystic ovary syndrome. *Arch Pediatr Adolesc Med* 2002, **156**(6):556-60.

7

Growth hormone significantly increases the adult height of children with idiopathic short stature: comparison of subgroups and benefit

Juan F Sotos[1*] and Naomi J Tokar[2]

Abstract

Background: Children with Idiopathic Short Stature do not attain a normal adult height. The improvement of adult height with treatment with recombinant human growth hormone (rhGH), at doses of 0.16 to 0.28 mg/kg/week is modest, usually less that 4 cm, and they remain short as adults. The benefit obtained seems dose dependent and benefits of 7.0 to 8.0 cm have been reported with higher doses of 0.32 to 0.4 mg/kg/week, but the number of studies is limited. The topic has remained controversial.

Objective: The objective was to conduct a retrospective analysis of our experience with 123 children with ISS treated with 0.32 ± 0.03 mg/kg/week of rhGH, with the aim of comparing the different subgroups of non-familial short stature, familial short stature, normal puberty, and delayed puberty and to assess the benefit by comparison with 305 untreated historical controls, from nine different randomized and nonrandomized controlled studies.

Results: Eighty eight of our children (68 males and 20 females) attained an adult height or near adult height of −0.71 SDS (0.74 SD) (95% CI, −0.87 to −0.55) with a benefit over untreated controls of 9.5 cm (7.4 to 11.6 cm) for males and 8.6 cm (6.7 to 10.5 cm) for females.

In the analysis of the subgroups, the adult height and adult height gain of children with non-familial short stature were significantly higher than of familial short stature. No difference was found in the cohorts with normal or delayed puberty in any of the subgroups, except between the non-familial short stature and familial short stature puberty cohorts. This has implications for the interpretation of the benefit of treatment in studies where the number of children with familial short stature in the controls or treated subjects is not known.

The treatment was safe. There were no significant adverse events. The IGF-1 values were essentially within the levels expected for the stages of puberty.

Conclusion: Our experience was quite positive with normalization of the heights and growth of the children during childhood and the attainment of normal adult heights, the main two aims of treatment.

Keywords: Idiopathic short stature, Growth hormone, Short children, Short stature

Introduction

Children with idiopathic short stature (ISS) do not attain a normal adult height. In the three randomized controlled studies (Cochran Central Register Control Trials), the adult height of the controls was −2.4 SDS (0.56 SD) [1], −2.37 SDS (0.46 SD) [2] and −2.2 SDS (0.75 SD) [3]. In an additional 6 non-randomized controlled studies

the adult height of the controls ranged between −2.4 SDS (0.8 SD) and −1.88 SDS (0.57 SD) [4-9].

Growth hormone treatment significantly improves the growth velocity and the adult height of children with ISS [10-13] and is considered safe [14-16]. The United States (US) Food and Drug Administration (FDA) approved growth hormone treatment for children with ISS in 2003.

Nevertheless, the use of growth hormone has remained controversial [17-19], mainly because of the modest benefit [20,21] and high cost [22,23]. As Wit JM and Dunkel L stated [24], few topics in pediatric endocrinology provoked

* Correspondence: Juan.Sotos@NationwideChildrens.org
[1]Nationwide Children's Hospital, The Ohio State University – College of Medicine, 700 Children's Drive, Columbus, OH 43205, USA
Full list of author information is available at the end of the article

more discussion and dissent than ISS. The impression is that despite the significant gain in height, growth hormone treated children remain short as adults, in the lower level of the normal range; an improvement in adult height after years of treatment in the order of 4 cm and a benefit that is less than in other conditions for which GH has been licensed [20,21]. Many of the studies, however, used GH doses of 0.16 to 0.26 mg/kg/week, which may not have been adequate. Furthermore, some of the studies included children with intrauterine growth retardation or with familial short stature, which may have affected the results.

The benefit obtained seems dose dependent and mean benefits of 7.0 to 8.0 cm have been reported with higher doses of 0.32 to 0.4 mg/kg/week [2,3,9].

There have been also ethical issues raised [25] and considerations expressed as to whether ISS should be considered a disease, whether the degree of psychosocial morbidity warrants treatment [26-28], whether it is enhancement or endo-cosmetology rather than treatment [29], and whether treatment has any effect in health related quality of life [30-32].

As the name idiopathic indicates, the cause is unknown. A variety of genes affecting growth, of genes along the growth hormone IGF-I axis [33-38], polygenic traits determined by polymorphisms [39], heterozygous GHR mutations, a dominant negative mutation of the GHR causing familial short stature [40] and mutations in other genes have now been demonstrated in children previously classified as ISS [41-43]. So the label of normal short children may not be appropriate.

All these concerns have been extensively discussed in a number of publications [44] and taken in consideration in the Consensus of the International Pediatric Endocrine Societies [45]. The interest of the child is the primary concern. The main goal of the treatment is the normalization of the height during childhood and improvement of the adult height. Children with a height of less than –2 SDS [45] or a height of more than 2 SDS below their midparental target height, warrant consideration for treatment.

Idiopathic short stature describes a heterogeneous group of children of unknown etiology with variable response to growth hormone [46]. It is defined as short children with a height below –2 SD (2.3 percentile) (and by some authors below the 5th percentile (–1.65 SD)) for age, sex and population group, normal stimulated growth hormone levels and absence of comorbid conditions (systemic disease, bone dysplasias, hormonal deficiencies, dysmorphic syndromes, chromosomal disorders, malnutrition), intrauterine growth retardation or treatment with medications that affect growth (i.e. Ritalin) [45,47].

Specifically, the children with ISS have normal birth weight, and no growth hormone deficiency [45].

The criteria do not include midparental height (MPH). Thus, studies of idiopathic short stature have included two groups of children: those affected with nonfamilial short stature (NFSS) and those with familial short stature (FSS), who may be different in their response to treatment, adult heights, and attainment of MPH. Children with FSS, without treatment, may attain an adult height near or equal to midparental height, but shorter than the normal population [48,49]. It is possible, also, that the modest or small benefit obtained by growth hormone treatment in a number of studies was because many of the children were affected with familial short stature.

After the Consensus on the definition of idiopathic short stature in 1996 [50], ISS also includes what previously was known as constitutional delay of growth and puberty (CDGP). A number of studies have indicated that the adult height attained in children with CDGP, with heights below –2 SDS, is less than the MPH and that they remain somewhat shorter than normal [51,52], some with average heights in the 10th percentile [53] or 5th percentile [54,55].

As the result of the aforementioned, there is consideration of the need to subcategorize the children into different groups: NFSS and FSS and in both, normal puberty and delayed puberty [45,56].

We conducted a retrospective analysis of our experience with 123 children with ISS treated with rhGH, with the aim of comparing the different subgroups and assessing the benefit by comparison with historical controls. As far as we are aware, there are only 2 studies comparing NFSS and FSS [3,9] and no studies of treated children identifying the different subgroups of NFSS, FSS, normal and delayed puberty. The study was approved by the Institutional Review Board of the Hospital and consent and assent approvals were obtained.

Subjects
Of the 123 children with idiopathic short stature treated with rhGH (0.32 ± 0.03 mg/kg/week – 6 days per week), from the late 80's to 2012, 88 attained adult or near adult height, 68 males and 20 females. Twenty-seven of the children were lost to follow-up (22 males out of 98, 22%, and 5 females out of 25, 20%). Eight males with NFSS and delayed puberty, who were treated with depotestosterone with 50 mg a month for 6 months or 100 mg for 3 months to induce pubertal changes, were not included in the results reported, to avoid questions in the interpretation of results, even though it is known that testosterone increases the growth velocity but does not improve adult height [57,58], if any it may decrease the adult height if treatment is prolonged or with higher doses, by advancing bone age (123 children –27-8 = 88).

Of the 68 males, forty-seven were classified as NFSS and 21 (30%) as FSS; 16 females were classified as NFSS and 4 as FSS. The groups were further divided into those with normal puberty and delayed puberty. The duration of treatment was 5.2 ± 2.7 years for the 68 males and 3.5 ± 0.9 for the 20 females, with a range of 2 to 8 years.

All the children met the criteria for ISS with the height below −2.0 SD (except for 1 female who was −1.81), normal stimulated growth hormone levels, normal birth weight and length, and absence of comorbid conditions.

The age at start of treatment ranged between 4.7 years and 16 years, 11.9 ± 3.3 years for the 68 males and 12 ± 1.9 years for the 20 females. The children were seen every 3 months and the rhGH dose was adjusted at each visit. The beginning dose of GH in the late 80's was 0.22 mg/kg/week 3 times a week, but the dose was increased to 0.3 mg/kg/week or more, because the response was not as good as expected. With the normal weight gain the dose would decrease to 0.28 mg/kg/week and adjustments were made. The dose ranged from 0.28 to 0.4 mg/kg/week with adjustments, for a calculated average dose, throughout the years, of 0.32 ± 0.03 mg/kg/week. The dose was not increased for puberty.

A number of determinations were obtained before the onset of treatment; bone age, CBC, sedimentation rate, chemistry panel, anti-endomysial antibodies, tissue trans-glutaminase antibodies, glucose, hemoglobin A_{1C}, TSH, free T_4, IGF-I, IGFBP-3 and cortisol; and most of them annually. An MRI of the brain was obtained at the time of the growth hormone stimulation testing on many of them in the past. This is no longer felt needed. Karyotypes were obtained in many. Bone age was determined by Greulich and Pyle standards and adult height predicted by Bayley-Pinneau tables.

Heights were measured by a wall-mounted stadiometer. The heights at the onset of treatment were expressed as SDS for chronologic age. The height SDS was calculated in the usual manner: height of the subject in cm minus the mean height for age or adults divided by the SD in cm from the mean. Adult heights were obtained at 19 ± 2.45 years, range 15.7 to 27.53, for males and at 18.3 ± 2.34 years, range 15 to 24 years, for females. Sixty-seven of the adult heights were obtained by us (76%) and 9 in a doctor's office (10%). Twelve (14%) were obtained at home, following detailed instructions and were consistent with predicted heights. The last bone age available in our records was 16.0 ± 1.0 years for males and 14.1 ± 0.46 for females, but some adult heights were obtained later. To obtain final adult heights, the potential remaining growth of some children whose heights were obtained before closure of the epiphyses (near adult height) was calculated. These numbers for calculated final adult heights were not included in the numbers reported and it will be addressed later (Additional file 1: Table S1).

Pubertal development was assessed by the method of Tanner. Males with testicular volume of less than 4.0 ml

by the age of 14.0 years and females with no breast development by the age of 13 years were classified as delayed onset of puberty. Children whose heights were below the midparental height SDS target range of −1.6 SD were classified as NFSS and those within the target range as FSS. Children whose fathers or mothers were below −2.0 SDS were also classified as FSS. Of the 25 subjects (males and females) with FSS, 9 (36%) had a father or a mother with a height below −2 SD (−2.25 to −2.87 SD). The classification of delayed onset of puberty includes the previously used definition of constitutional delay of growth and puberty (CDGP) in accordance with the international consensus [45].

Target height (MPH) was calculated from the self-reported parental heights by the method of Tanner: (height of the father + height of the mother + 13)/2 for the males and (height of the father + height of the mother − 13)/2 for females and expressed in cm [47]. No addition for secular trend was needed, since there was no or minimal increase in secular trend in the United States National Health Statistics between 1977 and 2000. Midparental height SDS was calculated by the following equation: (father's height SDS + mother's height SDS)/√2(1 + r (M,F); r is the correlation between the parent's height which is 0.3 [50]. The SDS was based on the US National Center Health Statistics of 1977. The values for MPHs SDSs were not different than those calculated by target height, by the method of Tanner, when corrected for assortative mating (correlation between the parent's heights). The characteristics of NFSS and FSS children treated to adult height are illustrated in Table 1.

Lost to follow-up
Twenty-two males (22% of the total of 98) were lost to follow-up: 6 were treated for less than 6 months and 16 were lost at 10 to 14.4 years of age. Five females (20% of the total of 25) were lost to follow-up: 2 were treated for less than 6 months and 3 were lost at 9.4 to 12.5 years of age. All had a good response to rhGH treatment. An analysis of intent to treat to adult height was conducted.

Methods
Growth hormone from stimulations tests was assayed by monoclonal antibody (Hybritech IRMA or Immulite chemiluminescent) methods that measure selectively the 22 kDa GH and yields values of 64 to 68% of those obtained with polyclonal antibody RIA methods (Additional file 2: Figure S1). All children had values of serum growth hormone of more than 7 ng/ml in one or both stimulation tests or more than 10 ng/ml when a polyclonal antibody RIA method was used (a few were measured by the Kallestad RIA method at the beginning of the study).

Table 1 Idiopathic short stature treated with GH, non-familial short stature (NFSS) & familial short stature (FSS)

Characteristic	NFSS Mean (SD)		FSS Mean (SD)		Reference mean (SD)
	Males (#47)	Females (#16)	Males (#21)	Females (#4)	Normal
Age start – yr	11.96 (3.50)	12.08 (1.39)	11.96 (2.81)	12.07 (0.88)	
BA start – yr	9.00 (3.20)	9.39 (1.51)	9.10 (2.91)	10.30 (1.38)	
GH stim peak mean	12.4	10.8	13.1	14.8	>7 ng/ml
range – ng/ml	7.04 to 28.0	7.0 to 19.8	7.1 to 38.5	8.8 to 20.9	>7 ng/ml
GH Freq Samp 12	2.53 (1.08) (#31)		2.49 (1.46) (#11)		M = 2.54 (0.84)
hr mean ng/ml		1.78 (0.64) (#8)		3.02 (#1)	F = 1.96 (0.85)
SMC – U/ml	0.79 (0.43) (#27)	0.87 (0.22) (#6)	1.09 (0.60) (#11)	1.55 (0.04) (#2)	T-I = 1.04 (0.66)
IGF-1 – ng/ml	144 (101) (#19)	166 (63) (#10)	158 (69) (#11)	205 (9) (#2)	T-I = 109–485
					T-II = 174-512
Duration Rx – yr	5.21 (2.69)	3.59 (0.94)	5.30 (2.30)	3.17 (0.88)	

Abbreviations: *GH* serum growth hormone, *BA* bone age, *(#)* number, *M* males, *F* females, *T* Tanner stage.

Growth hormone secretion was evaluated by 12-hours overnight frequent sampling on a number of the children in the 1990s; we no longer do that.

Plasma levels of IGF-I were obtained by RIA after acid alcohol extraction (Nichol's Institute Diagnostic, San Juan Capistrano, CA). This method was not available early in the study and a number of the determinations were made as Somadomedin C. Laboratory determinations for CBC, sedimentation rate, glucose, hemoglobin A$_{1C}$, TSH, free T$_4$, cortisol and others were performed by standard laboratory procedures.

Statistics

Paired and unpaired, two-tailed Student *T* test was used to compare the means of the different groups. A p value of 0.05 or less was considered significant. The 95% confidence intervals (CI) of the different results and groups were calculated. Correlations to assess the factors influencing AHs (young age, delayed bone age, distance to MPH, etc.) have been reported by others and were beyond the scope of this presentation.

Results

A few growth charts in Figure 1 illustrate what we observed in many children: a catch up growth for the first 3 or more years of treatment to a level expected for the midparental height, a subsequent normal growth, the growth spurt with puberty and the attainment of a normal adult height.

Figure 2 provides information on the means ± standard deviations and range of the height at the beginning of

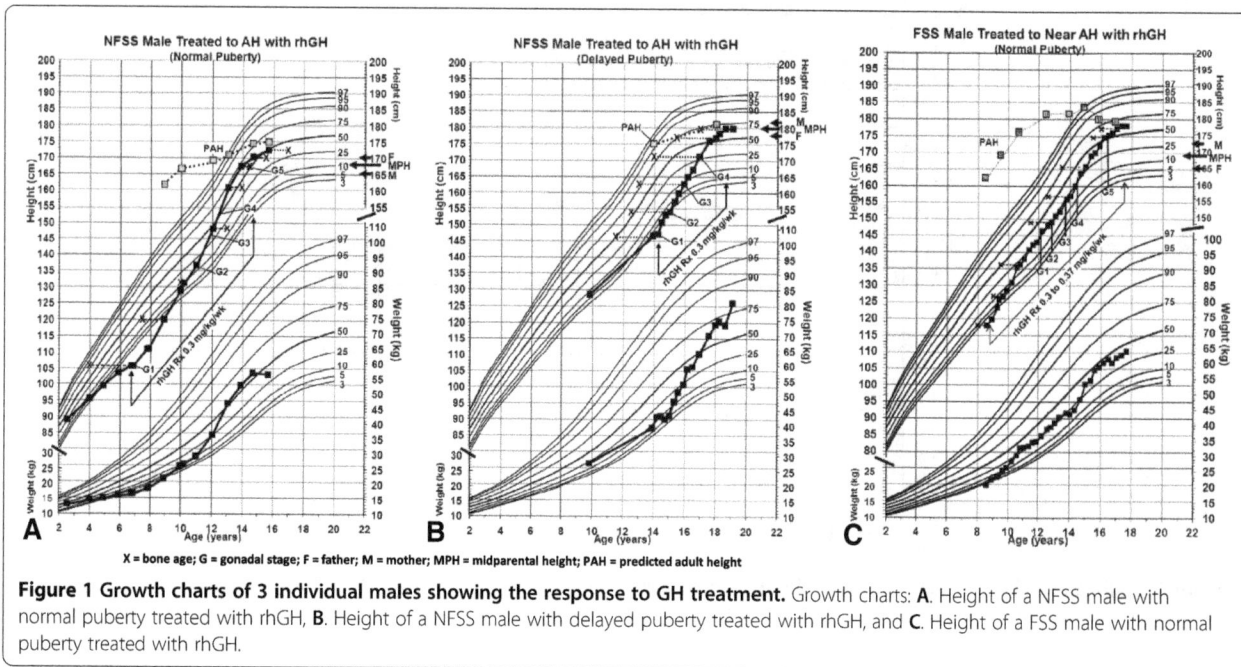

X = bone age; G = gonadal stage; F = father; M = mother; MPH = midparental height; PAH = predicted adult height

Figure 1 Growth charts of 3 individual males showing the response to GH treatment. Growth charts: **A**. Height of a NFSS male with normal puberty treated with rhGH, **B**. Height of a NFSS male with delayed puberty treated with rhGH, and **C**. Height of a FSS male with normal puberty treated with rhGH.

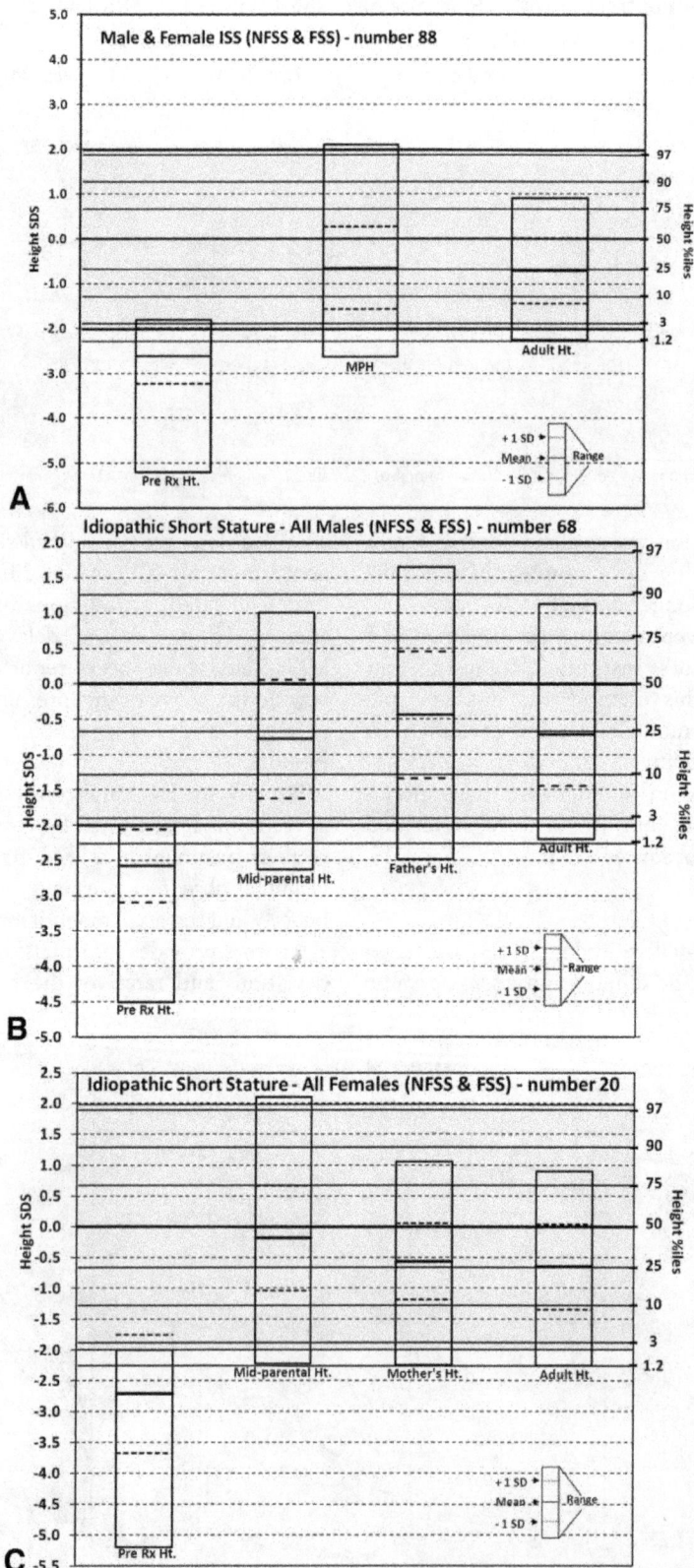

Figure 2 Height SDSs of all subjects, males and females, before and after treatment. Height SDS before and after treatment with rhGH:
A. All ISS males and females, **B**. All ISS males, and **C**. All ISS females. In Table 2 are detailed numbers for means and standard deviations for different measurements to permit comparisons and in Tables 3 and 4 applicable statistics.

treatment, midparental heights, father's or mother's heights and adult heights for different groups. (The individual values for the heights at the beginning of treatment, adult heights, midparental heights, age at the beginning of treatment and when the adult heights were obtained, and means ± standard deviations for different subgroups are given in the additional file 3: Figure S2A, B, C, D and Additional file 4: Figure S3A, B).

In Table 2 are detailed numbers for means and standard deviations for different measurements to permit comparisons and in Tables 3 and 4 applicable statistics.

All the 88 children with ISS (NFSS and FSS), males and females, attained a mean adult height of −0.71 SDS (0.74 SD) (Table 2), all within the normal percentiles – from the 1st to the 80th percentile for males and for females (Figure 2). All of them attained a height within 2 SD except two children with familial short stature, −2.11 and −2.25 SDS (1.2 percentile). The average height of the 88 children was −0.71 SDS (0.74 SD), significantly different than the baseline height of −2.61 SDS (0.62 SD) (p <0.001) (Table 3), equal to the MPH of −0.65 SDS (0.92 SD) (p, 0.638), and the adult height gain (adult height minus baseline height) was +1.9 SDS (0.76 SD) with a range from +0.29 to +4.13 SDS (95% CI, 1.74 to 2.06).

The 68 males (NFSS & FSS) attained a mean height of −0.72 SDS (0.72 SD), (Table 2) higher than the mean at the onset of treatment of −2.58 SDS (0.52 SD) (p <0.001) (Table 3), equal to the MPH of −0.78 SDS (0.84 SD) (p, 0.674), and equal or less than the father's height of −0.44 SDS (0.90 SD) (p ≤ 0.05). The adult height gain was 1.86 SDS (0.69 SD), range 0.29 to 3.92 SDS (95% CI, 1.69 to 2.03).

The 20 females attained an adult height of −0.65 SDS (0.70 SD) (Table 2), significantly higher than the baseline height of −2.71 SDS (0.96 SD) (p <0.001) (Table 3), equal to the MPH of −0.18 SDS (0.85 SD) (p, 0.120) and mother's height of −0.57 SDS (0.62 SD) (p, 0.728). The adult height gain was 2.06 SDS (0.97 SD).

There were no differences between the 68 males and 20 females (Table 3) in regard to baseline height, the SDS for father's and mother's heights, adult height of −0.72 SDS (0.72 SD) for males and for females −0.65 SDS (0.70 SD) or for the adult height gain of 1.86 SDS (0.69 SD) versus 2.06 SDS (0.97 SD) (all p values between 0.40 and 0.72). The only difference between the males and the females was in the MPH of −0.78 SDS (0.84 SD) for the males and −0.18 SDS (0.85 SD) for the females (p, 0.025).

The mean adult height of 171.86 ± 4.82 cm was equal to the target height of 172.76 ± 4.34 cm for the males (p, <0.5 > 0.1). Also for the females the mean adult height of 159.68 ± 4.28 cm was equal to the target height of 162.94 ± 4.53 cm (p, <0.5 > 0.1).

Analysis of the subgroups
NFSS

The results obtained are shown in Table 2, applicable statistics in Table 3 and illustrations or graphs in Figure 2. The mean adult height attained by the 47 males was −0.54 SDS (0.64 SD), significantly higher than the baseline height −2.57 SDS (0.41 SD), (p <0.0001), equal to the MPH of −0.44 SDS (0.73 SD) (p, 0.489) and less than the father's height of −0.18 SDS (0.76 SD) (p, 0.019). The latter statistically different, but it would appear to be of no clinical significance (2.36 cm difference). The adult height of the 20 children with normal puberty, −0.60 SDS (0.67 SD) was equal to the father's height −0.22 SDS (0.89 SD) (p, 0.156). In the 27 children with delayed puberty the adult height of −0.49 SDS (0.61 SD) was near or equal to the father's height of −0.15 SDS (0.64 SD) (p, 0.056).

In the 16 female children with NFSS, the adult height was −0.62 SDS (0.70 SD), higher than the baseline height of −2.74 SDS (0.96 SD) (p < 0.001), less than the MPH of +0.15 SDS (0.85 SD) (p, 0.011), and equal to the mother's height of −0.35 SDS (0.62 SD) (p, 0.269).

The adult height gain for the 47 males with NFSS was 2.04 SDS (0.64 SD), range 0.94 to 3.92 SDS, equal to the adult height gain for the 16 females, 2.12 SDS (0.97 SD) (range 0.99 to 4.13 SDS) (p, 0.969).

FSS

The results obtained in the 21 males and 4 females with FSS are shown in Table 2, applicable statistics in Table 3 and illustrations in Figure 2.

The adult height attained by the 21 males was −1.14 SDS (0.72 SD), significantly higher than the baseline height of −2.59 SDS (0.71 SD) (p <0.001), equal to the MPH of −1.52 SDS (0.51 SD) (p, 0.64), equal to the father's height of −0.99 SDS (0.92 SD) (p, 0.587), and the adult height gain was +1.45 SDS (0.62 SD), range +0.29 to 2.40 SDS (95% CI, 1.17 to 1.73).

The number of females with FSS was only 4 and the values may not accurately represent the values of a larger group. The adult height was −0.78 SDS (1.07 SD), higher than the baseline height of −2.59 SDS, equal or higher than the MPH −1.49 SDS, and equal or higher than mother's height of −1.43 SDS (0.97 SD). The adult height gain was 1.81 SDS (0.80 SD), range 0.66 to 2.82 SDS.

Comparison between NFSS and FSS

The values are in Table 2, statistics in Table 4 and illustrations in Figure 2.

For the 47 males with NFSS and 21 with FSS, there was no difference in the baseline height of −2.57 SDS (0.41 SD) versus −2.59 SDS (0.71 SD) (p, 0.922). The adult height of −0.54 SDS (0.64 SD), 173.1 cm, of the NFSS males was higher than the adult height of males in

Table 2 All ISS (NFSS and FSS) SDS

Males & Females mean SDS (SD)	Treated with GH		
Number	**88**		
Baseline Height (Base H)	−2.61 (0.62)		
MPH	−0.65 (0.92)		
AH (or Near)	−0.71 (0.74)		
AH Gain SDS (AH − Base H)	+1.90 (0.76)		

Males mean SDS (SD)	Total	Normal puberty	Delayed puberty	NP to DP
Number	**68**	**32**	**36**	*p value*
Base H	−2.58 (0.52)	−2.58 (0.63)	−2.58 (0.38)	NS 0.977
MPH	−0.78 (0.84)	−0.94 (0.86)	−0.63 (0.79)	NS 0.141
Fa H.	−0.44 (0.90)	−0.49 (0.96)	−0.39 (0.84)	NS 0.653
AH (or Near)	−0.72 (0.72)	−0.82 (0.77)	−0.64 (0.66)	NS 0.319
AH Gain SDS (AH − Base H)	+1.86 (0.69)	+1.76 (0.67)	+1.94 (0.69)	NS 0.280

Females mean SDS (SD)	Total	Normal puberty	Delayed puberty	NP to DP
Number	**20**	**17**	**3**	*p value*
Base H	−2.71 (0.96)	−2.75 (0.93)	−2.48 (0.44)	NS 0.484
MPH	−0.18 (0.85)	−0.23 (1.08)	+0.09 (0.62)	NS 0.851
Mo H.	−0.57 (0.62)	−0.60 (0.80)	−0.39 (0.94)	NS 0.953
AH (or Near)	−0.65 (0.70)	−0.77 (0.72)	−0.02 (0.82)	NS 0.300
AH Gain SDS (AH − Base H)	+2.06 (0.97)	+1.98 (0.87)	+2.50 (1.23)	NS 0.647

Males with Non-familial Short Stature (NFSS)

Mean SDS (SD)	Total	Normal puberty	Delayed puberty	NP to DP
Number	**47**	**20**	**27**	*p value*
Base H	−2.57 (0.41)	−2.53 (0.47)	−2.60 (0.34)	NS 0.601
MPH	−0.44 (0.73)	−0.58 (0.80)	−0.32 (0.65)	NS 0.262
Fa H	−0.18 (0.76)	−0.22 (0.89)	−0.15 (0.64)	NS 0.758
AH (or Near)	−0.54 (0.64)	−0.60 (0.67)	−0.49 (0.61)	NS 0.603
AH Gain SDS (AH − Base H)	+2.04 (0.64)	+1.94 (0.60)	+2.11 (0.66)	NS 0.372

Males with Familial Short Stature (FSS)

Number	21	12	9	*p value*
Base H	−2.59 (0.71)	−2.65 (0.83)	−2.51 (0.49)	NS 0.669
MPH	−1.52 (0.51)	−1.54 (0.57)	−1.49 (0.43)	NS 0.835
Fa H	−0.99 (0.92)	−0.94 (0.90)	−1.06 (0.95)	NS 0.779
AH (or Near)	−1.14 (0.72)	−1.19 (0.79)	−1.07 (0.62)	NS 0.729
AH Gain SDS (AH − Base H)	+1.45 (0.62)	+1.46 (0.68)	+1.44 (0.52)	NS 0.949

Females with Non-familial Short Stature (NFSS)

				NP to DP
Number	**16**	**13**	**3**	*p value*
Base H	−2.74 (0.96)	−2.80 (1.04)	−2.48 (0.44)	NS 0.484
MPH	+0.15 (0.85)	+0.16 (0.90)	+0.09 (0.62)	NS 0.851
Mo H	−0.35 (0.62)	−0.34 (0.52)	−0.39 (0.94)	NS 0.953
AH (or Near)	−0.62 (0.70)	−0.77 (0.57)	−0.02 (0.82)	NS 0.300
AH Gain SDS (AH − Base H)	+2.12 (0.97)	+2.03 (0.88)	+2.50 (1.23)	NS 0.647

Table 2 All ISS (NFSS and FSS) SDS *(Continued)*

Females with Familial Short Stature (FSS)			
Number	4	4	0
Base H	−2.59 (0.33)	−2.59 (0.33)	
MPH	−1.49 (0.45)	−1.49 (0.45)	
Mo H	−1.43 (0.97)	−1.43 (0.97)	
AH (or Near)	−0.78 (1.07)	−0.78 (1.07)	
AH Gain SDS (AH − Base H)	1.81 (0.80)	1.81 (0.80)	

FSS of −1.14 SDS (0.72 SD) 169.1 cm (p, 0.003). Also the MPH, the father's height and the gain in height were higher in the NFSS than in the FSS, Table 4, with all the p values of less than 0.002. The adult height gain for the 47 NFSS was 2.04 SDS (0.64 SD), range 0.94 to 3.92 SDS, higher that the 1.45 SDS (0.62 SD), range 0.29 to 2.40 SDS, for the 21 FSS children (p, 0.001).

Similar results were obtained when the males and females were grouped, Table 4. There was no difference in the baseline heights, −2.62 SDS (0.60 SD) and −2.59 SDS (0.66 AD), (p, >0.5), for the 63 males and females with NFSS and 25 with FSS. The adult height of −0.56 SDS (0.65 SD) and adult height gain of +2.06 SDS (0.74 SD) for the 63, 47 males and 16 females, with NFSS were higher than the adult height of −1.08 SDS (0.8 SD) and adult height gain of 1.51 SDS (0.66 SD) for the 25, 21 males and 4 females, with FSS (p < 0.01 and <0.001, respectively).

The adult height gain indicates the response to treatment and ranged from 0.29 to 3.92 SDS. The variability in the response to treatment with GH in ISS is well known. This variability was seen in NFSS and FSS. Of interest, however, was that the response to treatment was less in FSS (0.29 to 2.4 SDS) than in NFSS (0.94 to 3.9 SDS).

For the females the number with FSS is small, 4, the result are probably not an accurate reflection of the group and statistics could be doubtful (false results). Nevertheless, comparisons with the 16 females with NFSS were made. The baseline height for the NFSS was equal to the FSS (p, 0.556). The MPH was higher in the NFSS +0.15 SDS (0.85 SD) than in the FSS, −1.49 SDS (0.45) (p, 0.001). There was no difference in the mother's heights, adult heights (159.9 cm vs 158.9 cm) or adult height gain (Table 4, all p values from 0.147 to 0.992).

Variability of the Response to Treatment with Growth Hormone
We definitely observed the variability in response. The AH gain of all the 88 children (males and females) was +1.9 SDS (0.76 SD) with a range for +0.29 to +4.13 SDS, quite a range, (95% CI 1.71 to 2.06). AH was −0.71 SDS (0.74 SD), that would give a range, ± 2 SD, of −2.19 SD to −0.77 SD (page 12). Range of Ahs could be seen in Additional file 3: Figure S2a, b, c, and Additional file 4: Figure S3a and b.

For the 68 males (non-familial and familial short stature), the AH gain was 1.86 SDS (0.69 SD) with a range of +0.29 to 3.92 SDS (95% CI, 1.69 to 2.03). The AH was −0.72 SDS (0.72 SD) giving a range of ± 2 SD of −2.16 to +0.72 SDS.

The AH gain for the 47 males with NFSS was 2.04 SDS (0.64 SD) with a range of 0.94 to 3.92 SDS. The AH gain for the 21 males with FSS was 1.45 SDS (0.62 SD) with a range of 0.29 to 2.40 SDS (p = 0.001).

The AH was −0.54 SDS (0.64 SD), for a range ± 2 SD of −1.82 to +0.74 SDS for the 47 males with NFSS. For the 21 males with FSS the AH was −1.14 SDS (0.72 SD) for a range of ± 2 SD of −2.58 to +0.3 SDS (p = 0.003).

The effect of puberty
The comparison of the values for different measures obtained for all the children with normal puberty and delayed puberty, males 68 and 20 females, in all the subgroups, NFSS and FSS, males and females are shown in Table 2. There was no difference in any of the values for the baseline height, MPH, father's height, mother's height, adult height, and gain in height, for any of the subgroups, for normal and delayed puberty cohorts; all the p values were more than 0.05. There was a difference, however, between NFSS and FSS for normal and delayed puberty.

The effect of age at start of treatment and duration of treatment
In the study of Rekers-Mombarg, et al. [48] comprising 132 children with ISS, the children declined gradually in growth from a length of −0.8 SDS in boys and −1.3 SDS in girls at birth, to a height of −2.7 SDS at 16 years in boys and 13 years in girls, and increasing to a mean of −1.5 SDS in boys and −1.6 SDS in girls. The gain in SDS from childhood height to adult height (adult height gain) varied from 0.1 SDS (1.22 SD) at 3 years to 0.1 SDS (0.60 SD) at 14 years, and to 1.2 for boys at 16 years and 1.1 for girls at 13 years.

It became of interest to know if the changes that we observed in adult height and adult height gain of our treated subjects were somewhat related to age and not to treatment, even though we did not see differences in

Table 3 Comparisons SDS (SD) – Probability

		Mean SDS (SD)			Mean SDS (SD)	p value
All ISS Males & Females (#88)	AH	-0.71 (0.74)	>	Base H	-2.61 (0.62)	<0.0001
	AH	-0.71 (0.74)	=	MPH	-0.65 (0.92)	NS 0.638
Males						
All Males (#68)	AH	-0.72 (0.72)	>	Base H	-2.58 (0.52)	<0.0001
	AH	-0.72 (0.72)	=	MPH	-0.78 (0.84)	NS 0.674
	AH	-0.72 (0.72)	≤	Fa H	-0.44 (0.90)	0.050
Normal puberty (NP) (#32)	AH	-0.82 (0.77)	=	Fa H	-0.49 (0.96)	NS 0.148
Delayed puberty (DP) (#36)	AH	-0.64 (0.66)	=	Fa H	-0.39 (0.84)	NS 0.184
Males NFSS (#47)	AH	-0.54 (0.64)	>	Base H	-2.57 (0.41)	<0.0001
	AH	-0.54 (0.64)	=	MPH	-0.44 (0.73)	NS 0.489
	AH	-0.54 (0.64)	<	Fa H	-0.18 (0.76)	0.019
NP (#20)	AH	-0.60 (0.67)	=	Fa H	-0.22 (0.89)	NS 0.156
DP (#27)	AH	-0.49 (0.61)	≤	Fa H	-0.15 (0.64)	NS 0.057
Males FSS (#21)	AH	-1.14 (0.72)	>	Base H	-2.59 (0.71)	<0.0001
	AH	-1.14 (0.72)	=	MPH	-1.52 (0.51)	NS 0.064
	AH	-1.14 (0.72)	=	Fa H	-0.99 (0.92)	NS 0.587
NP (#12)	AH	-1.19 (0.79)	=	Fa H	-0.99 (0.92)	NS 0.502
	AH	-1.19 (0.79)	=	MPH	-1.52 (0.51)	NS 0.244
DP (#9)	AH	-1.07 (0.62)	=	Fa H	-1.06 (0.95)	NS 0.984
	AH	-1.07 (0.62)	=	MPH	-1.49 (0.43)	NS 0.140
Females						
All Females ISS (#20)	AH	-0.65 (0.70)	>	Base H	-2.71 (0.96)	<0.0001
	AH	-0.65 (0.70)	=	MPH	-0.18 (0.85)	NS 0.120
	AH	-0.65 (0.70)	=	Mo H	-0.57 (0.62)	NS 0.728
Females NFSS (#16)	AH	-0.62 (0.70)	<	MPH	+0.15 (0.85)	0.011
	AH	-0.62 (0.70)	=	Mo H	-0.35 (0.62)	NS 0.269
NP (#13)	AH	-0.77 (0.57)	<	MPH	+0.16 (0.90)	0.006
	AH	-0.77 (0.57)	=	Mo H	-0.34 (0.52)	NS 0.067
Males versus Females						
All Males vs Females		Males [#68]			Females [#20]	p value
	Base H	-2.58 (0.52)	=	Base H	-2.71 (0.96)	NS 0.554
	MPH	-0.78 (0.84)	<	MPH	-0.18 (0.85)	0.025
	Fa H	-0.44 (0.90)	=	Mo H	-0.57 (0.62)	NS 0.568
	AH	-0.72 (0.72)	=	AH	-0.65 (0.70)	NS 0.725
	AH Gain	+1.86 (0.69)	=	Gain	+2.06 (0.97)	NS 0.405
NFSS Males vs Females		Males [#47]			Females [#16]	p value
	Base H	-2.57 (0.41)	=	Base H	-2.74 (0.96)	NS 0.485
	MPH	-0.44 (0.73)	<	MPH	+0.15 (0.85)	0.044
	Fa H	-0.18 (0.76)	=	Mo H	-0.35 (0.62)	NS 0.398
	AH	-0.54 (0.64)	=	AH	-0.62 (0.70)	NS 0.239
	AH Gain	+2.04 (0.64)	=	Gain	+2.12 (0.97)	NS 0.969

Abbreviations: *AH* adult height, *Base H* baseline height, *MPH* midparental height, *Fa H* father's height; *Mo H* Mother's height, *AH Gain* adult height gain, *NS* not significant.

Table 4 Comparisons of NFSS versus FSS – SDS (SD) – Probability

		Mean SDS (SD)			Mean SDS (SD)	p value
Males		**NFSS (#47)**			**FSS (#21)**	
NFSS vs FSS	Base H	−2.57 (0.41)	=	Base H	−2.59 (0.71)	NS 0.922
	MPH	−0.44 (0.73)	>	MPH	−1.52 (0.51)	<0.0001
	Fa H	−0.18 (0.76)	>	Fa H	−0.99 (0.92)	0.002
	AH	−0.54 (0.64)	>	AH	−1.14 (0.72)	0.003
	AH Gain	+2.04 (0.64)	>	Gain	+1.45 (0.62)	0.001
Males & Females		**NFSS (#63)**			**FSS (#25)**	
	Base H	−2.62 (0.60)	=	Base H	−2.59 (0.66)	NS 0.829
	AH	−0.56 (0.65)	>	AH	−1.08 (0.80)	0.008
	AH Gain	2.06 (0.74)	>	Gain	1.51 (0.66)	0.002

our children with normal puberty (usually younger) and those with delayed puberty (usually older). The effect of age on adult height and adult height gain in males with NFSS and FSS (for whom we had adequate numbers) is shown in Table 5. There was a significant difference in the age of children with NFSS with normal puberty (8.6 (2.7 SD) years) and delayed puberty (14.4 (1.0 SD) years) ($p < 0.001$), but there was no difference in the adult height or adult height gain (p >0.6 and >0.3, respectively).

Similarly, there was a significant difference in the age of children with FSS with normal puberty (10.3 (2.47 SD) years) and delayed puberty (14.1 (1.31 SD) years) ($p < 0.001$), but no difference in the adult height and adult height gain (p, 0.729 and 0.949, respectively).

In the 13 young females with NFSS, the adult height and adult height gain was the same as in young males with NFSS.

We correlated AH gain and age at the start of treatment and AH gain and duration of treatment in our 47 NFSS males and 21 FSS males, and there was no significant correlation (correlations shown in supplemental graphs in Additional file 5: Figure S4.

The gain in height is very variable for individuals and averages are not accurate or useful to predict the benefit that an individual will obtain. Based on the averages, Table 5, a male with delayed puberty and NFSS with treatment for 3.5 years could gain 2.11 SDS (16 cm in the USA). The gain in height depends on the pubertal growth, benefit of growth hormone, and bone age. In the aforementioned case, Table 5, depending on the age, bone age, progress of bone age, pubertal growth, and growth hormone response, the gain in height could range from 1.3 SDS to 3.9 SDS (10 to 29 cm). The only way that we could inform the subjects of the benefit that he or she could obtain, is the way that we do it now. Based on the height and the bone age, the predicted adult height is obtained. The subject can be informed that based on our experience, growth hormone should be of benefit to him or her, to improve the adult height.

The benefit could be 5 cm, 7.5, 10 cm or more but cannot be predicted exactly, because it depends on the response to treatment, progress of bone age, and years of treatment. Then the provider and the subject decide whether treatment is continued to attain the maximum height or ended when he or she is satisfied with the height.

Analysis of intent to treat to adult height
Children were observed for a period of time prior to treatment, so that their growth rates could be assessed. In a retrospective review we could know the children who were lost to follow up and, consequently, analyze their growth rates prior to and during treatment.

Growth rates determined for less than 6 months were not included. The growth rates in centimeters per year and the change in the height SDS, prior to treatment, on treatment prior to puberty, and on treatment during the first two years of puberty were not different for treated children lost to follow-up and for those treated to adult height, (p >0.05) (Figure 3 and Table 6). Thus, there was no bias on the reported effect of GH on children treated to adult height.

Safety and IGF-1 levels
Complaints of myalgia or arthralgia of the legs early in the treatment, which promptly subsided without adjustment of the GH dose, were very rare. Two of the 123 children had a low serum TSH and free T_4 (subclinical hypothyroidism) and were treated with levothyroxine, which was discontinued after cessation of treatment.

There were no other side effects.

Concerns have been raised on the possibility of side effects in the future from high levels of IGF-1 because of its mitogenic effect [16,59]. Therefore, it became of interest to know the levels of IGF-1 with treatment. The levels of IGF-1 prior to treatment, during treatment for different stages of puberty, and after treatment are illustrated in Figure 4 and Table 7. Except for a few, all the

Table 5 Effect of Age on Treated Children with ISS

Mean (SD) [min to max]	Number	Treatment start age (yrs)	Stop age (yrs)	Baseline height SDS (SD)	Adult height SDS (SD)	Adult height gain SDS (SD)
Males – NFSS						
Normal puberty	20	8.6 (2.76) [5.0 to 13.4]	16.4 (0.97) [14.7 to 18.3]	−2.53 (0.47) [−3.76 to −1.98]	−0.60 (0.67) [−1.73 to 0.81]	1.94 (0.60) [0.94 to 3.01]
Delayed puberty	27	14.4 (1.10) [12.4 to 16.3]	17.9 (0.84) [16.0 to 19.4]	−2.60 (0.34) [−3.37 to −2.00]	−0.49 (0.61) [−1.36 to 1.13]	2.11 (0.66) [1.30 to 3.91]
		p <0.001		p, 0.601	p, 0.603	p, 0.372
Males – FSS						
Normal puberty	12	10.3 (2.47) [4.7 to 13.7]	16.9 (0.77) [15.7 to 18.1]	−2.65 (0.83) [−4.51 to −1.98]	−1.19 (0.79) [−2.20 to 0.22]	1.46 (0.68) [0.29 to 2.40]
Delayed puberty	9	14.1 (1.31) [11.6 to 15.9]	17.6 (0.65) [16.9 to 18.7]	−2.51 (0.49) [−3.26 to −1.96]	−1.07 (0.62) [−2.20 to 0.24]	1.44 (0.52) [0.86 to 2.20]
		p <0.001		p, 0.669	p, 0.729	p, 0.949
Females – NFSS						
Normal puberty	13	11.4 (1.21) [9.6 to 13.3]	15.5 (0.81) [13.5 to 16.7]	−2.80 (1.04) [−5.20 to −1.81]	−0.77 (0.57) [−1.84 to 0.09]	2.03 (0.88) [1.04 to 4.13]

Abbreviations: min minimum, max maximum.

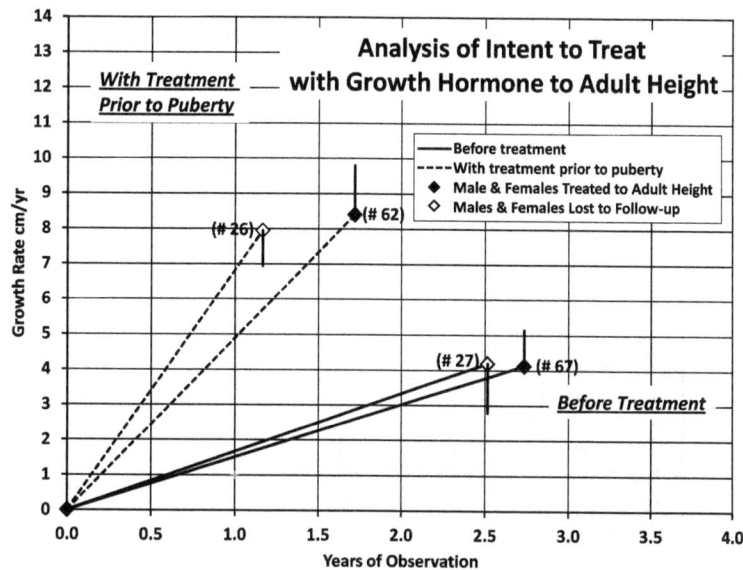

Figure 3 (Analysis of intent to treat).

Table 6 Analysis of Intent to Treat to Adult Height Treatment Response with rhGH

	Number	Years observation (Mean SDS ± SD)	Growth rate cm/yr (Mean SDS ± SD)	Δ Height SDS (Mean SDS ± SD)
Males pretreatment				
Lost to follow-up	22	2.46 ± 1.87	4.29 ± 1.42	−0.31 ± 0.48
Treated to AH	50	2.42 ± 1.37	4.00 ± 1.02	−0.33 ± 0.54
			p, 0.426	p, 0.902
On treatment with rhGH				
Before puberty				
Lost to follow - up	21	1.20 ± 1.02	7.92 ± 0.94	0.53 ± 0.41
Treated to AH	41	1.83 ± 1.51	8.31 ± 1.44	0.71 ± 0.57
			p, 0.207	p, 0.179
During puberty				
Lost to follow - up	7	1.34 ± 0.75	9.09 ± 2.24	0.50 ± 0.28
Treated to AH	50	2.05 ± 1.04	8.31 ± 1.74	0.72 ± 0.48
			p, 0.404	p, 0.116
Females pretreatment				
Lost to follow-up	5	2.76 ± 1.54	3.78 ± 1.40	−0.56 ± 0.49
Treated to AH	17	3.71 ± 2.34	4.56 ± 0.71	−0.50 ± 0.37
			p, 0.293	p, 0.810
On treatment with rhGH				
Before puberty				
Lost to follow - up	5	1.01 ± 0.25	8.06 ± 1.36	0.48 ± 0.32
Treated to AH	10	1.20 ± 0.51	8.94 ± 0.92	0.58 ± 0.27
			p, 0.241	p, 0.593
During puberty				
Lost to follow - up	2	1.02 ± 0.03	9.34 ± 2.07	0.72 ± 0.58
Treated to AH	20	1.94 ± 0.97	7.30 ± 1.77	1.05 ± 0.45
			p, 0.382	p, 0.559

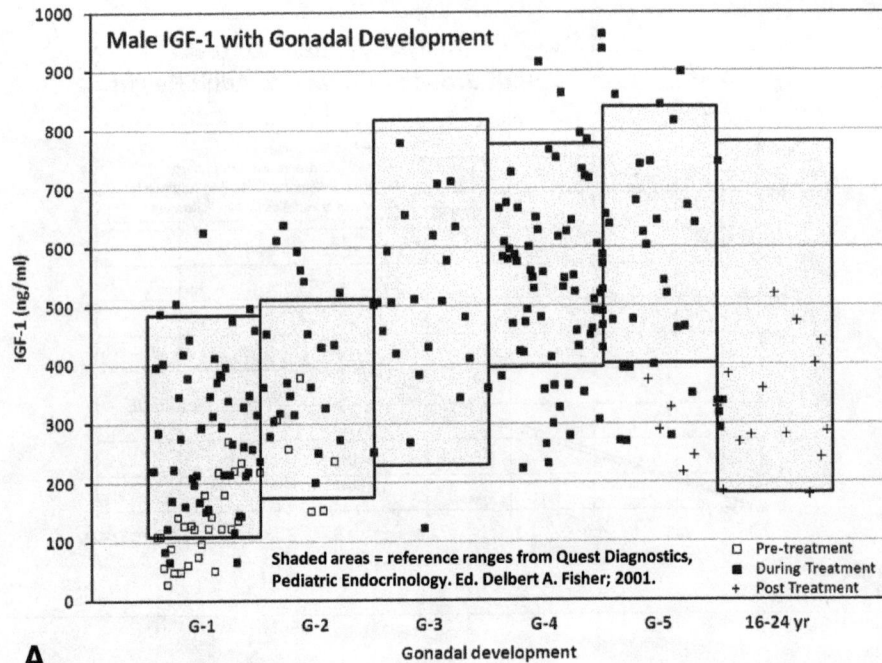

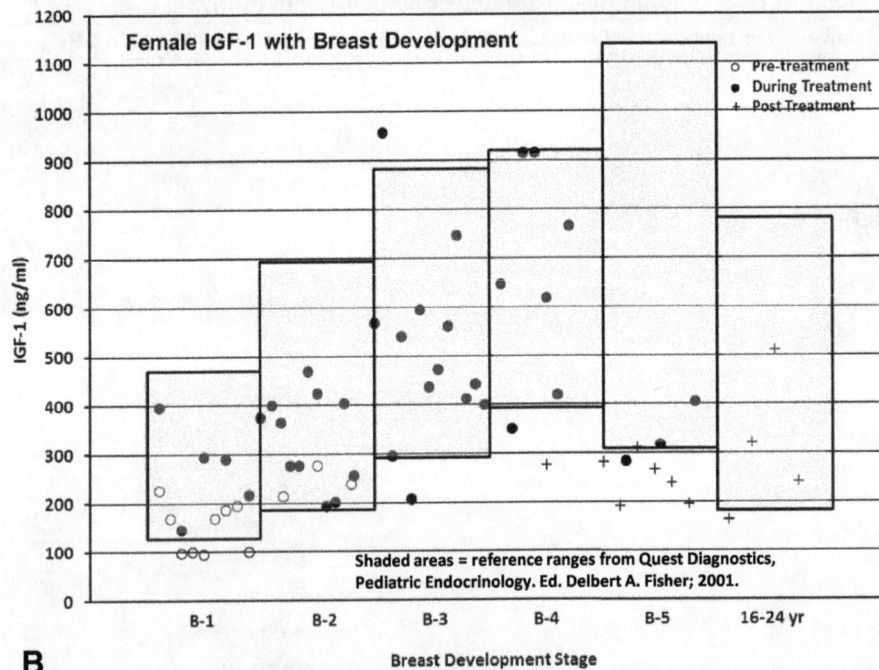

Figure 4 IGF-1 levels pretreatment, during GH treatment & post treatment. Serum levels of IGF-1 before, during and after treatment with rhGH: **A**. relative to gonadal stage in males and **B**. relative to breast developmental stage in females.

values were within the range expected for the pubertal stage. Only 8.4% of the values (20 out of 237) (19 out of 198, 9.6% for the males and 2.5%, 1 out of 39, for the females) exceeded the normal range at one time during the treatment. These values are less than those reported in patients with growth hormone deficiency treated with

0.24 mg/kg/week. Seventeen percent of the values were higher than 2 SD after 2 years of treatment [60].

Benefit obtained by treatment

One of the limitations of our study is the lack of controls. Fortunately, there are, presently, a number of randomized

Table 7 IGF-1

Males	Gonadal stage					
	1	2	3	4	5	Adult
Reference ranges* in ng/ml	109 to 485	174 to 512	230 to 818	396 776	402-839	182 to 780
Pre treatment						
Number	27	7				
Mean	128	250				
SD	64	81				
Minimum	27	151				
Maximum	270	178				
Treated						
Number	53	25	20	68	28	4
Mean	190	415	496	548	575	321
SD	127	130	162	165	184	22
Minimum	64	200	122	224	269	292
Maximum	625	637	777	961	897	338
Post treatment						
Number				1	2	16
Mean				374	286	321
SD					57	101
Minimum					245	178
Maximum					326	520
Females	Breast stage					
Reference ranges in ng/ml	128 to 470	186 to 695	292 to 883	394 920	308-1138	182 to 780
Pre treatment	1	2	3	4	5	Adult
Number	9	3				
Mean	167	243				
SD	80	32				
Minimum	95	214				
Maximum	331	277				
Treated						
Number	6	10	13	7	3	
Mean	287	327	510	662	336	
SD	95	98	192	222	63	
Minimum	146	194	207	352	284	
Maximum	397	470	959	916	406	
Post treatment						
Number				2	5	5
Mean				440	244	300
SD				233	52	130
Minimum				276	192	164
Maximum				605	311	511

*Reference ranges from Quest Diagnostics, Pediatric Endocrinology. Ed. Delbert A. Fisher; 2001.

and nonrandomized controlled studies that would permit assessment of the benefit, by comparisons of the adult height attained and AH gain in our treated children with those of historical untreated controls.

The adult height and adult height gain (AH minus Baseline height) are measurements that the investigators obtain and should be more accurate than comparisons based on attainments of PAH or MPH (see later). MPH was not used to calculate benefit of treatment.

The adult height gain corrects for baseline differences in the different studies in treated subjects and controls, provides information on the benefit of treatment, and permits comparison of groups not matched for baseline heights.

The comparison of adult heights provides also information on the benefit, and when the baselines heights are not different or the AHs are corrected for baseline heights differences, yields the same results as the adult height gain.

The reports on SDS permit comparisons of different populations and calculation of the benefit in centimeters based on the centimeters for SD of adults in a particular population. In this presentation we used 6.75 cm for males and 6.14 cm for females for SD of adult height, the numbers from the US National Health Statistics of 1977. The benefit in centimeters would be different in different populations depending on the centimeters for SD of adults.

1. *Adult height and adult height gain of treated children in our study versus published untreated controls.*

In Figure 5 the adult height of 305 untreated controls, mean SDS and 95% CI, from 9 (3 randomized and 6 nonrandomized) controlled studies, and the adult height, mean SDS and 95% CI, of our 88 treated children are illustrated.

In Figure 6 are similar comparisons for the adult height gain (mean SDS and 95% CI) for the controls and for our treated subjects. The numbers for the different studies for the baseline, adult height and adult height gain of controls and our treated subjects are in Table 8.

A glance at the Figures 5 and 6 clearly shows that there is a significant benefit from treatment.

The benefit from treatment for the adult height for our children (–0.71 SDS) versus the AH (–2.16 SDS) of the controls of the 9 studies, Table 8, was + 1.45 SDS with a range of +1.17 SDS to +1.69 SDS (an average of 9.8 cm for males with a range of 7.9 to 11.4 cm and an average of 8.9 cm for females with a range of 7.2 to 10.3 cm).

The analysis of the adult height gain, Table 8, showed somewhat similar results. The gain of controls in the 9 studies was, on the average, +0.49 SDS (with a range of 0.18 to 0.8 SDS). In our treated children the gain was on the average +1.90 SDS for a difference with controls of +1.41 SDS, range +1.1 to +1.72 SDS (9.5 cm for males with a range of 7.4 to 11.6 cm and 8.6 cm for females, with a range of 6.7 to 10.5 cm).

The average baseline height of the 9 published studies, Table 8, was –2.66 SDS, not different than in our study –2.61 (±0.62) SDS. The baseline of 5 of the 9 studies was not different than ours p >0.1 or >0.5; in two it was higher and in two lower.

In the study of Rekers-Mombarg et al. [48] on the height outcomes of untreated children with ISS, the adult height of 48 NFSS boys of –1.74 SDS (0.91 SD) was 8.3 cm (95% CI, 7.1 to 9.5 cm), less than their target height. The adult height of our 47 treated NFSS boys of –0.54 SDS (0.64 SD) was equal to the target height, suggesting that our treated boys gained 8.3 cm. Actually, the adult height of our 47 NFSS boys of –0.54 SDS (0.64 SD) (95% CI, –0.35 to –0.73) was 1.2 SDS, 8.1 cm (6.8 to 9.3 cm) higher than the adult height of the untreated boys, indicating the benefit obtained by treatment. This benefit of 8.1 cm (6.8 to 9.3 cm) is similar to

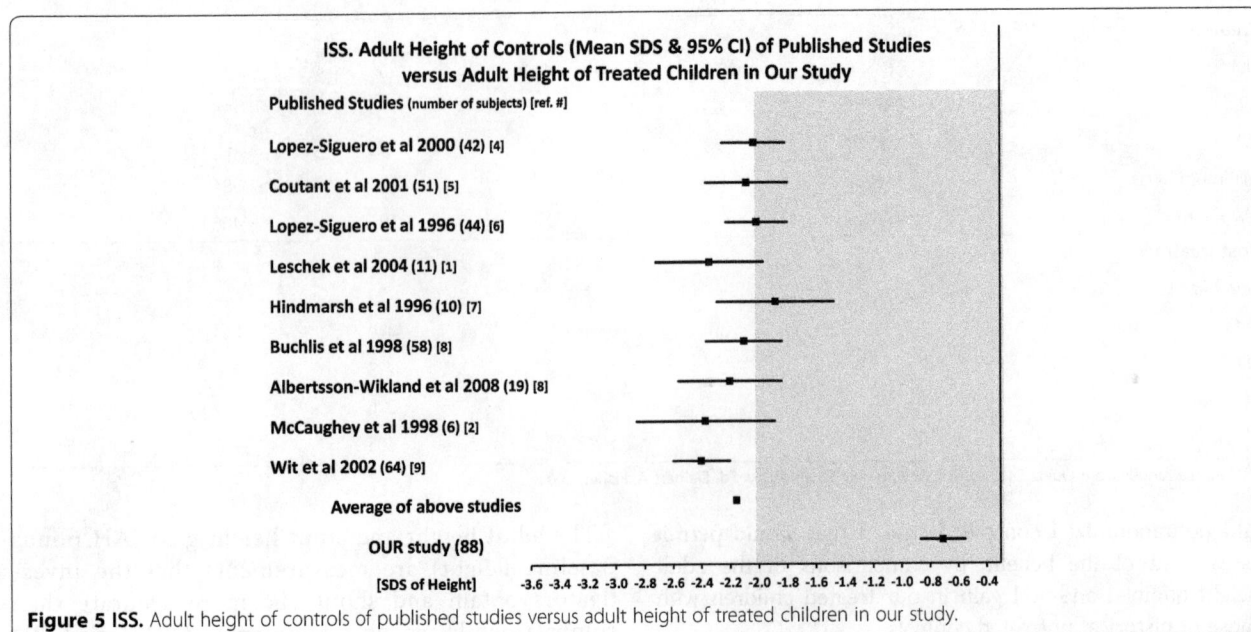

Figure 5 ISS. Adult height of controls of published studies versus adult height of treated children in our study.

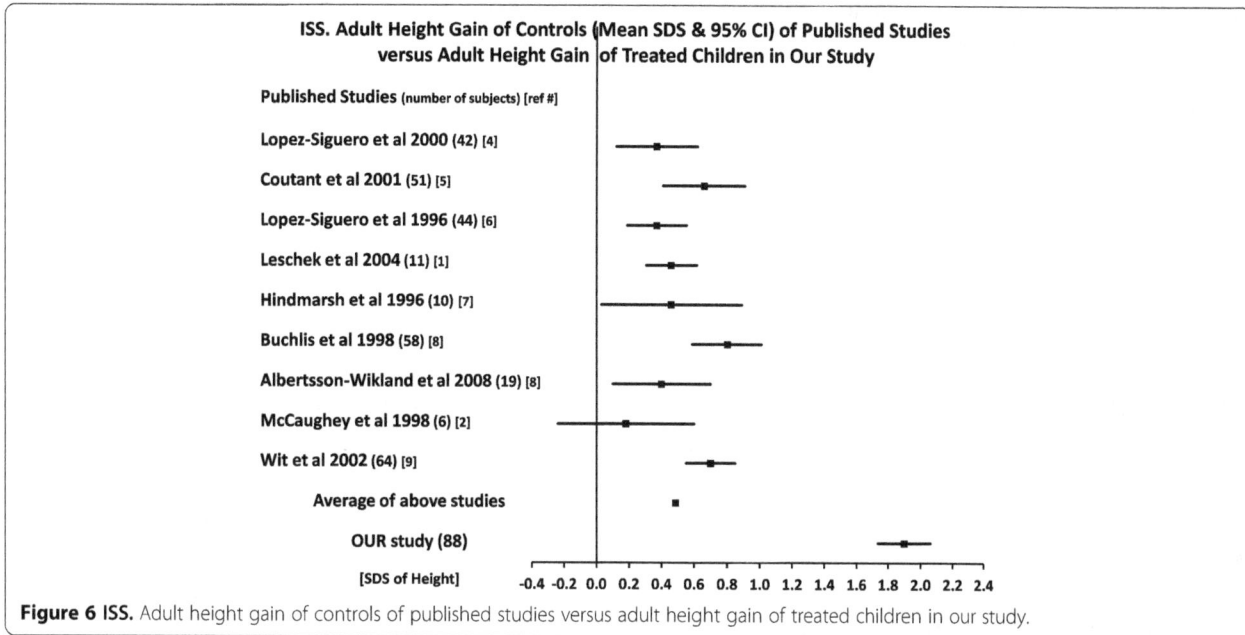

ISS. Adult Height Gain of Controls (Mean SDS & 95% CI) of Published Studies versus Adult Height Gain of Treated Children in Our Study

Figure 6 ISS. Adult height gain of controls of published studies versus adult height gain of treated children in our study.

the benefit found by comparison with other studies and adds confidence in the results of our comparisons.

2. Comparisons of our results with published Adult Heights of controls and treated children.

Table 9 shows the benefit of different doses of growth hormone on the adult height. In published studies the benefit obtained in adult height was usually less than 4 cm over controls with doses of less than 0.3 mg/kg/week. And it was more than 5 cm (6.8, 7.4, 7.5) with doses of 0.3 or more mg/kg/week.

In our study, the benefit with a dose of 0.32 (±0.03 SD) mg/kg/week was 9.8 cm for males and 8.9 cm for females, about 5 cm to 6 cm more than the 4 cm in published studies treated with less than 0.3 mg/kg/week, but, in the range, only 1.5 or 1.35 cm more than in those treated with 0.3 or more mg/kg/week.

3. Comparisons of NFSS and FSS, treated and controls.

There have been only 2 studies comparing NFSS and FSS, the one by Wit et al. [9] and by Albertsson-Wikland et al. [3], Table 10.

The benefit in adult height gain (that corrects for differences in baseline heights) of our treated children were higher than the adult height gain of the controls in the published studies by 1.26 SDS and 1.56 SDS for the NFSS (8.5 and 10.5 cm for males and 7.7 and 9.5 cm for females) and 1.21 SDS and 1.6 SDS for the FSS (8.1 to 10.8 cm for males and 7.4 to 9.8 cm for females); an equal benefit for children with NFSS and FSS.

Even though the benefit with treatment was the same for children with NFSS and FSS, our 25 children with FSS were significantly lower in adult height and adult height gain than our 63 children with NFSS, Table 11; adult height of −1.08 SDS in FSS versus −0.56 SDS in NFSS (p <0.01) and adult height gain 1.51 in FSS versus 2.06 in NFSS (p < 0.001).

Of interest is that the results in the only two studies that have been published are similar, Table 11. The adult height gain of the untreated controls and of the treated subjects were significantly less in the children with FSS than in NFSS (p <0.05). In other words, the adult height gain of treated children with NFSS was higher than in FSS, but also higher was the adult height gain of the NFSS than the FSS controls, so the benefit was the same. This was also the conclusion of Dahlgren J [12] in his analysis of these 2 studies.

This observation seems to be consistent in the three different studies and has implications for interpretation of results with treatment, in studies where the number of children with FSS in the controls and treated subjects is not known, and in the selection of controls for non-randomized or randomized studies.

4. Other Comparisons.

The reported impression, by review of published studies, is that the benefit of treatment of children with ISS is less than in other conditions for which GH has been licensed [20,21,61].

Our results compare well with those obtained in GH treated children in other conditions for which GH has

Table 8 Baseline, Adult height, & Adult height Gain of controls (Mean SDS & 95% CI) in Published studies and of Treated Children in Our Study

Published study [Ref. #]	Number	Baseline Mean SDS	(95% CI)	Adult height Mean SDS	(95% CI)	Adult height gain Mean SDS	(95% CI)
Lopez-Siguero et al. [4]	42	−2.40	−2.52 − −2.28	−2.03	−2.25 − −1.81	0.37	0.37 − 0.80
Coutant et al. [5]	51	−2.74	−2.92 − −2.56	−2.08	−2.36 − −1.80	0.66	0.66 − 0.89
Lopez-Siguero et al. [6]	44	−2.38	−2.50 − −2.26	−2.01	−2.22 − −1.80	0.37	0.37 − 0.60
Leschek et al.* [1]	11	−2.80	−3.20 − −2.40	−2.34	−2.72 − −1.96	0.46	0.46 − 0.23
Hindmarsh et al. [7]	10	−2.34	−2.78 − −1.90	−1.88	−2.29 − −1.47	0.46	0.46 − 0.60
Buchlis et al. [8]	58	−2.90	−3.08 − −2.72	−2.10	−2.36 − −1.84	0.80	0.80 − 0.80
Albertsson-Wikland et al.* [3]	19	−2.76	−2.95 − −2.57	−2.20	−2.56 − −1.84	0.40	0.40 − 0.62
McCaughey et al.* [2]	6	−2.55	−2.89 − −2.21	−2.37	−2.85 − −1.89	0.18	0.18 − 0.40
Wit et al. [9]	64	−3.10	−3.22 − −2.98	−2.40	−2.60 − −2.20	0.70	0.70 − 0.60
Total	**305**						
Mean	**34**	**−2.66**		**−2.16**		**0.49**	
Minimum	**6**	**−3.00**		**−2.40**		**0.18**	
Maximum	**64**	**−2.34**		**−1.88**		**0.80**	
Our study (treated)	*88*	*−2.61*	*−2.74 − −2.48*	*−0.71*	*−0.87 − −0.55*	*1.90*	*1.74 − 2.06*
Difference				*cm*		*cm*	

					M	F		M	F
Mean		*+0.05*		*+1.45*	*9.8*	*8.9*	*+1.41*	*9.5*	*8.6*
Minimum		*−0.27*		*+1.17*	*7.9*	*7.1*	*+1.10*	*7.4*	*6.7*
Maximum		*+0.39*		*+1.69*	*11.4*	*10.3*	*+1.72*	*11.6*	*10.5*

*Randomized controlled trials; M = male; F = Female; [#] reference number.

Table 9 Comparison of Our Results with Published Adult Heights of Controls & Treated Children

Published Study [Ref. #]	Number	mg/kg/wk	AH Controls #305 Mean SDS	AH Treated #212 Mean SDS	Difference Mean SDS	Benefit Males cm	Benefit Females cm
Lopez-Siguero et al. [4]	35	0.16 to 0.25	−2.03	−1.31	0.72	4.86	NA
Coutant et al. [5]	32	0.16	−2.08	−2.10	−0.02	−0.13	−0.12
Lopez-Siguero et al. [6]	20	0.16 to 0.25	−2.01	−1.46	0.55	3.71	NA
Leschek et al.* [1]	22	0.22	−2.34	−1.77	0.57	3.84	3.50
Hindmarsh et al. [7]	16	0.16 to 0.28	−1.88	−1.33	0.55	3.71	3.38
Buchlis et al. [8]	36	0.3	−2.10	−1.50	0.60 0.4 M 1.2 F	3.00	6.8
Albertsson-Wikland et al.* [3]	31	0.47	−2.20	−1.50	0.70	5.0	4.30
McCaughey et al.* [2]	8	0.35 0.4 to 0.31	−2.37	−1.14	1.23	NA	7.55
Wit et al. [9]	12	0.32 0.32 to 0.26	−2.40	−1.30	1.10	7.42	6.75
Total number	**212**						
Mean	**23.6**		**−2.16**	**−1.49**	**0.67**	**3.92**	**4.83**
Minimum	**8**		**−2.40**	**−2.10**	**−0.02**	**−0.13**	**−0.12**
Maximum	**36**		**−1.88**	**−1.14**	**1.23**	**7.42**	**7.55**
Our study treated	*88*	*0.32 (0.03)*	*(−2.16) (Historical)*	*−0.71*	*1.45*	*9.8*	*8.9*
Difference							
Mean			*+0.78*	*+0.78*	*5.2*	*4.8*	
Minimum			*+0.43*	*+0.22*	*1.5*	*1.35*	
Maximum			*+1.39*	*+1.47*	*9.9*	*9.0*	

*Randomized controlled trials; M = male; F = Female.

Table 10 Baseline, Adult height, & Adult height gain of controls (Mean SDS & 95% CI) in Published Studies of NFSS & FSS and of Treated Children in Our Study

Published study [Ref. #]	Number	Baseline mean SDS	(95% CI)	Adult height mean SDS	(95% CI)	Adult height gain mean SDS	(95% CI)
NFSS Wit [9]	45	−3.20	−3.35 − −3.05	−2.40	−2.64 − −2.16	0.80	0.62 − 0.98
NFSS Albertsson-Wikland [3]	36	−2.60	−2.87 − −2.33	−2.10	−2.34 − −1.86	0.50	0.23 − 0.77
Our study NFSS (Treated)	**63**	**−2.62**	**−2.77 − −2.47**	**−0.56**	**−0.72 − −0.40**	**2.06**	**1.87 − 2.25**
Difference — Our study to:					*cm*			*cm*
					M	*F*		*M*	*F*
NFSS Wit [9]		+0.58		+1.84	12.4	11.3	+1.26	8.5	7.7
NFSS Albertsson-Wikland [3]		−0.02		+1.54	10.4	9.4	+1.56	10.2	9.5
FSS Wit [9]	10	−2.50	−2.85 − −2.15	−2.20	−2.83 − −1.57	0.30	−0.05 − 0.65
FSS Albertsson-Wikland [3]	10	−2.80	−3.52 − −2.08	−2.90	−3.57 − −2.23	−0.10	−0.79 − 0.59
Our study FSS (Treated)	**25**	**−2.59**	**−2.86 − −2.32**	**−1.08**	**−1.41 − −0.75**	**1.51**	**1.24 − 1.78**
Difference — Our study to:					*cm*			*cm*
					M	*F*		*M*	*F*
FSS Wit [9]		−0.09		+1.12	7.5	6.9	+1.21	8.1	7.4
FSS Albertsson-Wikland [3]		+0.21		+1.82	12.8	11.2	+1.61	10.8	9.9

M = male, F = female.

been approved, growth hormone deficiency (GHD), small for gestational age (SGA), or Turner syndrome.

The adult height of our 88 children with ISS of −0.71 SDS (0.74 SD) is equal to the adult height of −0.7 SDS (1.2 SD) achieved in 121 children (males and females) with GHD treated with 0.3 mg/kg/week, 3 or 6 times a week, reported by Blethem et al. [62].

In a review of four randomized controlled trials (RCTs) comprising 391 children with SGA treated with growth hormone (range of 0.23 to 0.47 mg/kg/week) [63], the adult height exceeded controls by 0.9 SDS. The adult height gain was 1.25 SDS (1.5 SDS in treated minus 0.25 SDS in untreated subjects). There was no difference between the 2 dose regimens. The adult height gain in our study exceeded controls by 1.41 SDS (1.90 SDS minus 0.49 SDS in controls), Table 8.

Our results of an increase of 7.1 to 10.3 cm of adult height in treated females over controls (Table 8) compares favorably with those obtained in Turner syndrome. In 61 patients with Turner syndrome [64], treated with 0.3 to 0.375 mg/kg/week of growth hormone, the final height was approximately seven cm higher (95% CI, of 6 to 8 cm) than in 43 untreated control patients. Despite this increase, the adult height of treated patient with Turner syndrome was still outside the normal range.

Discussion

Our experience with the growth hormone treatment of children with ISS was a positive one, with the normalization of the height and growth during childhood and adolescence after 2 or 3 years of treatment and the attainment of a normal adult height of −0.71

Table 11 NFSS & FSS Adult Height Gain of Controls and Treated Subjects SDS (95% CI)

Published study	No.	GH Dosage mg/kg/wk	Adult height gain of controls untreated Mean SDS (95% CI)	NFSS to FSS Difference SDS p	Adult height gain of treated subjects Mean SDS (95% CI)	NFSS to FSS Difference SDS p
Wit et al. NFSS [9]	36	0.32 to 0.14	0.8 (0.62 to 0.98)	0.5 SDS p <0.01	1.50 (1.23 to 1.77)	0.7 SDS p <0.05
Wit et al. [9] FSS	5	0.32 to 0.27	0.3 (−0.05 to 0.65)		0.80 (0.06 to 1.54)	
Albertsson-Wikland et al. NFSS [3]	48	0.47	0.5 (0.23 to 0.77)	0.6 SDS p <0.05	1.40 (1.17 to 1.63)	0.5 SDS p < 0.05
Albertsson-Wikland et al. [3] FSS	14	0.47	−0.1 (−0.79 to 0.59)		0.90 (0.44 to 1.36)	
			Adult height		*Adult height gain*	
Our Study NFSS (treated)	63	0.32 (0.03)	−0.56 (−0.72 to −0.40)	0.52 SDS p < 0.01	2.06 (1.87 to 2.25)	0.55 SDS p <0.001
Our Study FSS (treated)	25	0.32 (0.03)	−1.08 (−1.41 to −0.75)		1.51 (1.24 to 1.78)	

SDS (0.74 SD) (95% CI −0.87 to −0.55), the main two aims of treatment; an adult height from the first percentile to the 80th percentile for males and for females.

The treatment was safe. There were no significant adverse effects. The IGF-1 values were essentially within the levels expected for the stages of puberty.

All the parents of the children and the children in our study who attained adult heights were pleased with the results, happy for their children to be normal and grateful for the treatment. The most consistent perception of the parents of the benefit was the improvement of self-esteem in their children, and of the children to be happy to be normal and not different. Other benefits perceived were cessation of teasing, bullying and psychological stress.

The reason for the children lost to follow-up, all growing well and benefiting from treatment, is not known. One can speculate that some were content to be within normal range in height, some may have had difficulty with copays, may have moved, did not care to have more injections, even though all reported that the injections were not painful, and so on.

The benefit obtained in our study seems to be better than that reported in a number of previous studies and there must be some reason. Care was taken in the selection of children to be certain they met qualifications, in the measurements, in the analysis of data and compilation of results.

By our observations, there may be two possible reasons, among others; namely the dose of growth hormone used (dose dependent effect), and the effect of including an unknown number of children with FSS in the group in previous studies.

Benefit of GH treatment – Effect of GH dose

Our observations in 88 children clearly show a significant benefit of GH treatment (0.32 ± 0.03 mg/kg/week) when compared to 305 untreated controls in 9 different studies, a benefit based on adult height gain (that corrects for baseline differences) of 9.5 cm (7.4 to 11.6) for males and 8.6 cm (6.7 to 10.5) for females (Table 8).

The benefit in the adult height of our treated subjects over the adult height of published historical controls was 9.8 cm for males and 8.9 cm for females (Table 9). This benefit is higher by 5 or 6 cm than the benefit obtained in subjects treated with 0.16 or 0.16 to 0.28 mg/kg/week of GH, usually of less than 4 cm. The benefit was only 1.35 or 1.5 cm higher than that obtained in other studies using 0.3 mg/kg or more per week.

This dose dependent effect has been reported previously in studies using 0.3 mg/kg or more of GH a week [65]. A dose effect for children with ISS was shown by Wit et al. [66] with a mean adult height gain of 1.85 SDS (similar to ours) and a benefit of 7.2 cm with a dose of 0.37 mg/kg/week. Also in a randomized controlled study by McCaughey et al. [2], 8 girls (6 of them with FSS) treated with GH 0.35 mg/kg/week (range 0.4 to 0.31), were 7.5 cm taller than the controls; and by others: Buchlis et al. [8] 6.8 cm for females, Albertsson-Wikland et al. [3] 8 cm based on adult height gain, Hintz R et al. [12] 9.2 cm higher for boys and 5.7 cm for girls, and Kemp et al. [67] (Genentech registry) 1.7 to 2.0 SDS in AH gain in children treated for 7 years, results similar to ours.

In view of the aforementioned, it is possible that the stated modest benefit of 4 cm with the treatment of ISS is related to the low dose of GH used and to averaging the results without taking in consideration the difference in the benefit from different doses.

In the meta-analysis conducted by Finkelstein et al. [10], there were only four controlled studies reporting adult height, −1.51 SDS. The reported benefit of treatment over controls, on the average was 5.7 cm, range 2.3 to 8.7 cm, a wide range. Two of the studies used dosages of GH of 0.25 and 0.26 mg/kg/week and the other two doses of 0.3 and 0.4 mg/kg/week, which may account for the 8.7 cm benefit.

In the review of Guyda H et al. [68], comprising 413 treated children in 11 studies the average adult height was −1.7 SDS (range −1.1 to −2.4 SDS). Seven of the studies used doses of GH ranging from 0.21 to 0.26 mg/kg/week for an average of 0.24 mg/kg/week. The difference of the adult height range from −1.1 to −2.4 SDS is 1.3 SDS, a large difference, that could be owing to a difference in the GH dose used. In three of the studies using 0.3 mg/kg/week or more the adult height was −1.1, −1.3, and −1.4 SDS. So the difference of adult height from −1.4 to −2.4 SDS was owing mainly to studies using the lower dose of GH.

As a consequence of the averaging, the improved benefit obtained, in SDS or cm, with the higher doses of GH is not reflected in the reports, as is illustrated in Table 9, averaging results of published studies with no benefit (−0.1 cm) with others with a benefit of 7.5 cm.

The effect of the inclusion of children with FSS

By our results, the adult height and adult height gain were significantly higher by 0.6 SDS (4 cm) in the 47 treated males with NFSS than in the 21 with FSS (Table 4), and in our 63 (males and females) with NFSS (0.55 SDS) higher than in the 25 (males and females) with FSS (Tables 4 and 11).

Similar results were obtained in the only 2 studies reporting the results of NFSS and FSS. The adult height gain of the untreated controls and of treated subjects was significantly higher in the children with NFSS than in FSS (Table 11).

This seems to be a consistent finding in different studies and has implications for the interpretation of the results observed in published studies. The inclusion of a high number of children with FSS in the treated cohort will yield lower results. And also, it has implications for the selection of controls in randomized or non-randomized controlled studies, since the number of children with FSS in the treated or control groups may affect the results.

It is difficult to assess how this has affected the results of previous studies, since most or practically all of the published studies included all the children as ISS and did not mention whether they were NFSS or FSS.

It would seem advisable to identify the two groups NFSS and FSS in future trials.

Assessment of Benefit

The assessment of the benefit from treatment with GH is sometimes difficult, even in controlled studies, because the proportion of children with FSS and NFSS, normal and delayed puberty, and at times IUGR, may not be the same in the treated and control groups.

As previously mentioned, to assess the benefit of treatment, comparison of the AH gain (adult height minus the baseline height) and the AH attained of the treated and control groups would seem to be the best method, because they are based on measurements by the investigator.

Also useful would be the comparison between the groups on the attainment of target height. Target heights, however, are often based on self-reported parental heights. In addition, children with FSS may attain heights near or equal to the MPH without treatment, so the inclusion of a different number of children with FSS in the group may influence the attainment of MPH and render the interpretation as benefit of treatment inaccurate. Furthermore, there are a number of reported methods to calculate MPH [47], which may give different results for the benefit when comparing AHs and MPHs. It would also be difficult to compare the benefit of different studies using different methods for calculating MPH.

Calculation of the benefit to children with ISS, treated with GH, based on the difference of AH attained and PAH at the baseline does not appear accurate. The imprecision and inaccuracy of PAH for both sexes have been indicated in a number of reports and only 33% of the variability in achieved AH is predictable. Commonly used methods tend to over-predict AH, especially in young males and in children with delayed bone age, and under-predict if the bone age is not delayed [69]. Also, the individual variability of the tempo of progression of the bone age, either faster or slower than usually expected, as illustrated in Figure 1, affects the accuracy of the PAH. In a randomized controlled trial, girls with ISS treated with GH were 3.5 cm taller than the originally PAH, but 7.5 cm taller than controls when calculated on the basis of AH and AH gain in SDS, a meaningful difference [2].

Other considerations

Recent critical reviews [20,21,61] concluded that to date no study has fulfilled the criteria for high quality and strong recommendations, in part owing to the small number of children in the studies, and felt that additional high quality trials up to the achievement of adult height would be necessary to determine the efficacy, ideal dosage, long term safety of growth hormone therapy and to address health related quality of life and cost issues.

There is agreement with their recommendations. Even though rhGH has proven to be a remarkably safe medication for 27 years at the doses recommended, long surveillance studies have been suggested by many, because of the mitogenic effect of IGF-1.

Regarding the dose, there has been many and probably enough trials with a dose of less than 0.3 mg/kg/week of GH, to know that it is not an adequate dose to induce a meaningful or satisfactory gain. Doses higher than 0.3, whether it be 0.32, 0.35, 0.37 mg/kg/week, or starting with 0.32 with adjustments may give a satisfactory gain, but the studies have been few; so additional studies would be helpful. It may be preferable to calculate the dose on mg/kg/week; calculations based on m^2 of surface area, would provide higher doses per kg at 6 years of age than later because of the nonlinear relationship of m^2 of surface area and weight.

Additional genetic studies may give useful information to explain the variability of response.

In the past 27 years, since rhGH became available in 1985, there have been 3 or 4 randomized studies, up to the achievement of adult height, and, apparently, they did not provide the answers. It may take 8 or more years to get results from more randomized trials. It is hoped that we do not wait for the answer; many children could benefit while we wait.

One of the main problems that has been often addressed in the past is the significant cost, which limits the availability to children who may need it, raises questions about the use of health resources, and a number of ethical considerations [25]. One may question whether studies would seem applicable to solve the problem of cost; participation from the pharmaceutical industry would be required. The high cost of biopharmaceuticals is a problem concerning public health services around the world, is in the public domain[a], and to reduce cost and increase affordable access to treatment may not be as simple as one may think [70-72].

The wholesale acquisition cost (the list price paid by the distributing pharmacies from the supplier), generally, the price put by the manufacturer of the GH was $50,000 per gram in 2007 [73] and apparently $76,000 in 2010 [74]. The cost to the patients (or insurances) for the purchase of GH from the distributing pharmacies, presently, may be as much as $88,000 to $100,000 per gram. This is based on the pharmacy bills given to the family for the purchase of GH[b].

The estimated cost of GH therapy compared with no therapy, in 2006, was $52,634 per inch (2.54 cm) or $99,959 per child reflecting an incremental growth of 1.9 in (4.8 cm) (Lee JM et al.) [22] and by others, in 2011, at $113,000 per inch or more (Durand-Zaleski I et al.) [23], depending on unit cost and height gain. This cost is applicable to any child treated with GH, whether it be growth hormone deficiency, Turner syndrome, intrauterine growth retardation or ISS.

If the price was reasonable, many of the objections to treatment, concerns for use of heath resources, and ethical considerations would subside. Cost influences pediatric endocrinologists in their decision to treat [75], and third party payers (private insurances or health agencies, state or national) in their decision to support treatment [74]. Also, if the price was reasonable, it, probably, would be the right thing to do to help the children to attain an adult height within the range judged to be normal by National Health Standards and by society. It would not harm anybody.

Conclusion

Children with ISS do not attain a normal adult height: adult heights of −2.4 SDS (0.8 SD) to −1.88 SDS (0.57 SD). Growth hormone treatment significantly increases the adult height, but the benefit obtained with doses of less than 0.3 mg/kg/week is modest, usually less than 4 cm.

The benefit obtained seems dose dependent and a benefit of 7, 7.5, and 8 cm have been reported with higher doses of 0.32 to 0.4 mg/kg/week, but the studies are few.

We conducted a retrospective analysis of our experience with children with ISS treated with rhGH, 0.32 ± 0.03 mg/kg/week. The treatment was quite helpful with normalization of the height and growth during childhood and attainment of normal adult heights. Eighty eight (68 males, 20 females) attained an adult height of −0.71 SDS (0.74 SD) (95%CI −0.87 to −0.55), a benefit over 305 untreated historical controls in 9 different studies of 9.5 cm (7.4 to 11.6 cm) for males and 8.6 cm (6.7 to 10.5 cm) for females, with heights from the 1st to the 80th percentile for males and females.

In the analysis of the subgroups the adult height and adult height gain of children with NFSS were significantly higher than of FSS. Similar results were obtained in the only 2 studies previously reported.

No difference was found in the cohorts with normal or delayed puberty in any of the subgroups, except between the NFSS and FSS subgroups. This has implications for the interpretation of the benefit of treatment in studies where the number of children with FSS in the controls or treated subjects is not known. It would seem advisable to identify the two groups, NFSS and FSS, in future trials.

The treatment was safe. There were no significant adverse events. The IGF-1 values were essentially within the levels expected for the stages of puberty.

There have been, probably, enough trials with a dose of less than 0.3 mg/kg/week to know that it is not an adequate dose to induce a meaningful or satisfactory gain. Studies with doses from 0.3 to 0.375 mg/kg/week are few, so additional trials would be helpful.

Additional high quality studies have been suggested to determine the efficacy, ideal dosage, health related quality of life, long term safety of GH therapy, and cost. There is agreement among investigators for these recommendations. In the past 27 years, since rhGH became available in 1985, there have been 3 or 4 randomized studies to adult height, but, apparently, did not provide the answers. It may take 8 or more years to get results from more randomized trials. It is the hope that we do not wait for the answer; many children could benefit while we wait.

Endnotes

[a]The high price of pharmaceuticals is in the public domain. See The Economist (Economist.com), January 4th – 10th, 2014 – Pharmaceutical pricing, arguments over the cost of drugs are growing – page 10 and 45–46 and January 25th – 31st – Protect patients not patents – page 14.

[b]The pharmacy bill for the purchase of 5 pens, each containing 20 mg of rhGH, (100 mg) was $8,800 every month, $88,000 per gram. Another pharmacy bill for the purchase of a pen containing 15 mg/of rhGH was $1,500, $100,000 per gram.

Abbreviations
AH: Adult height; AH gain: Adult height gain; CBC: Complete blood count; CDGP: Constitutional delay of growth and puberty; CI: Confidence interval; DP: Delayed puberty; F: Female; FDA: Food and Drug Administration; FSS: Familial short stature; GH: Growth hormone; GHD: Growth hormone deficiency; GHR: Growth hormone receptor; IGF-1: Insulin like growth factor 1; IGFBP-3: Insulin like growth factor binding protein 3; ISS: Idiopathic short stature; kDa: Kilodalton; M: Male; MPH: Mid-parental height; NFSS: Non-familial short stature; NP: Normal puberty; PAH: Predicted adult height; rbGH: Recombinant bovine growth hormone; rbST: Recombinant bovine somatotropin; RCT: Randomized control trials; rhGH: Recombinant human growth hormone; RIA: Radioimmunometric assay; SD: Standard deviation; SDS: Standard deviation score; SGA: Small for gestational age; T4: Thyroxine; TSH: Thyroid stimulating hormone.

Competing interests
The authors declare that they have no competing interests.

Authors' contributions
JFS contributed to conception and design, treatment of subjects, acquisition, analysis and interpretation of data, drafting and final approval of the manuscript and agrees to be accountable for all aspects of the work. NJT contributed to testing, acquisition, analysis, and interpretation of data, drafting of the manuscript and final approval of the version to be published.

Authors' information

JFS is Professor of Pediatrics at The Ohio State University, College of Medicine and member of the Section of Pediatric Endocrinology, Metabolism and Diabetes at Nationwide Children's Hospital, Columbus, Ohio. NJT is a research associate of the Section of Endocrinology, Metabolism and Diabetes at Nationwide Children's Hospital, Columbus, Ohio.

Acknowledgments

Our appreciation to the biostatisticians, Igor Dvorchik, PhD, & Han Yin, for their review of the statistical analysis and helpful recommendations.

Author details

[1]Nationwide Children's Hospital, The Ohio State University – College of Medicine, 700 Children's Drive, Columbus, OH 43205, USA. [2]Nationwide Children's Hospital, 700 Children's Drive, Columbus, OH 43205, USA.

References

1. Leschek EW, Rose SR, Yanovski JA, Troendle JF, Quigley CA, Chipman JJ, Crowe BJ, Ross JL, Cassorla FG, Blum WF, Cutler GB Jr, Baron J, National Institute of Child Health and Human Development-Eli Lilly & Co, Growth Hormone Collaborative Group: Effect of growth hormone treatment on adult height in peripubertal children with idiopathic short stature: a randomized, double-blind, placebo-controlled trial. *J Clin Endocrinol Metab* 2004, **89**(7):3140–3148.
2. McCaughey ES, Mulligan J, Voss LD, Betts PR: Randomised trial of growth hormone in short normal girls. *Lancet* 1998, **351**(9107):940–944.
3. Albertsson-Wikland K, Aronson AS, Gustafsson J, Hagenäs L, Ivarsson SA, Jonsson B, Kriström B, Marcus C, Nilsson KO, Ritzén EM, Tuvemo T, Westphal O, Aman J: Dose-dependent effect of growth hormone on final height in children with short stature without growth hormone deficiency. *J Clin Endocrinol Metab* 2008, **93**(11):4342–4350.
4. López-Siguero JP, García-Garcia E, Carralero I, Martínez-Aedo MJ: Adult height in children with idiopathic short stature treated with growth hormone. *J Pediatr Endocrinol Metab* 2000, **13**(9):1595–1602.
5. Coutant R, Rouleau S, Despert F, Magontier N, Loisel D, Limal JM: Growth and adult height in GH-treated children with nonacquired GH deficiency and idiopathic short stature: the influence of pituitary magnetic resonance imaging findings. *J Clin Endocrinol Metab* 2001, **86**(10):4649–4654.
6. Lopez-Siguero JP, Martínez-Aedo MJ, Moreno-Molina JA: Final height after growth hormone therapy in children with idiopathic short stature and a subnormal growth rate. *Acta Pediatr* 1996, **85**:113–147.
7. Hindmarsh PC, Brook CG: Final height of short normal children treated with growth hormone. *Lancet* 1996, **348**(9019):13–16.
8. Buchlis JG, Irizarry L, Crotzer BC, Shine BJ, Allen L, MacGillivray MH: Comparison of final heights of growth hormone-treated vs. untreated children with idiopathic growth failure. *J Clin Endocrinol Metab* 1998, **83**(4):1075–1079.
9. Wit JM, Rekers-Mombarg LT, Dutch Growth Hormone Advisory Group: Final height gain by GH therapy in children with idiopathic short stature is dose dependent. *J Clin Endocrinol Metab* 2002, **87**(2):604–611.
10. Finkelstein BS, Imperiale TF, Speroff T, Marrero U, Radcliffe DJ, Cuttler L: Effect of growth hormone therapy on height in children with idiopathic short stature: a meta-analysis. *Arch Pediatr Adolesc Med* 2002, **156**(3):230–240.
11. Hintz RL, Attie KM, Baptista J, Roche A: Effect of growth hormone treatment on adult height of children with idiopathic short stature. Genentech Collaborative Group. *N Engl J Med* 1999, **340**(7):502–507.
12. Dahlgren J: Growth outcomes in individuals with idiopathic short stature treated with growth hormone therapy. *Horm Res Paediatr* 2011, **76**(Suppl 3):42–45.
13. Lee PA, Germak J, Gut R, Khutoryansky N, Ross J: Identification of factors associated with good response to growth hormone therapy in children with short stature: results from the ANSWER Program®. *Int J Pediatr Endocrinol* 2011, **2011**:6. 10.1186/1687-9856-2011-6.
14. Quigley CA, Gill AM, Crowe BJ, Robling K, Chipman JJ, Rose SR, Ross JL, Cassorla FG, Wolka AM, Wit JM, Rekers-Mombarg LT, Cutler GB Jr: Safety of growth hormone treatment in pediatric patients with idiopathic short stature. *J Clin Endocrinol Metab* 2005, **90**(9):5188–5196.
15. Sävendahl L, Maes M, Albertsson-Wikland K, Borgström B, Carel JC, Henrard S, Speybroeck N, Thomas M, Zandwijken G, Hokken-Koelega A: Long-term mortality and causes of death in isolated GHD, ISS, and SGA patients treated with recombinant growth hormone during childhood in Belgium, The Netherlands, and Sweden: preliminary report of 3 countries participating in the EU SAGhE study. *J Clin Endocrinol Metab* 2012, **97**(2):E213–E217.
16. Rosenfeld RG, Cohen P, Robison LL, Bercu BB, Clayton P, Hoffman AR, Radovick S, Saenger P, Savage MO, Wit JM: Long-term surveillance of growth hormone therapy. *J Clin Endocrinol Metab* 2012, **97**(1):68–72.
17. Ambler GR, Fairchild J, Wilkinson DJ: Debate: idiopathic short stature should be treated with growth hormone. *J Paediatr Child Health* 2013, **49**(3):165–169.
18. Rosenbloom AL: Idiopathic short stature: conundrums of definition and treatment. *Int J Pediatr Endocrinol* 2009, **2009**:470378. 10.1155/2009/470378. Epub 2009 Mar 12.
19. Voss LD: Growth hormone therapy for the short normal child: who needs it and who wants it? The case against growth hormone therapy. *J Pediatr* 2000, **136**(1):103–106.
20. Kelnar CJ: Growth hormone for short children–whom should we be treating and why? *J R Coll Physicians Edinb* 2012, **42**(1):32–33.
21. Deodati A, Cianfarani S: Impact of growth hormone therapy on adult height of children with idiopathic short stature: systematic review. *BMJ* 2011, **342**:c7157.
22. Lee JM, Davis MM, Clark SJ, Hofer TP, Kemper AR: Estimated cost-effectiveness of growth hormone therapy for idiopathic short stature. *Arch Pediatr Adolesc Med* 2006, **160**(3):263–269.
23. Durand-Zaleski I: Developments in idiopathic short stature: cost versus allocation of resources. *Horm Res Paediatr* 2011, **76**(Suppl 3):33–35.
24. Wit JM, Dunkel L: Developments in Idiopathic Short Stature. *Horm Res Paediatr* 2011, **76**(suppl 3):1–2.
25. Allen DB, Fost N: hGH for short stature: ethical issues raised by expanded access. *J Pediatr* 2004, **144**(5):648–652.
26. Theunissen NC, Kamp GA, Koopman HM, Zwinderman KA, Vogels T, Wit JM: Quality of life and self-esteem in children treated for idiopathic short stature. *J Pediatr* 2002, **140**(5):507–515.
27. Sandberg DE, Bukowski WM, Fung CM, Noll RB: Height and social adjustment: are extremes a cause for concern and action? *Pediatrics* 2004, **114**(3):744–750.
28. Sandberg DE: Psychosocial aspects of short stature and its management: good deeds require good science. *Horm Res Paediatr* 2011, **76**(Suppl 3):37–39.
29. Rosenbloom AL: Pediatric endo-cosmetology and the evolution of growth diagnosis and treatment. *J Pediatr* 2011, **158**(2):187–193.
30. Rekers-Mombarg LT, Busschbach JJ, Massa GG, Dicke J, Wit JM: Quality of life of young adults with idiopathic short stature: effect of growth hormone treatment. Dutch Growth Hormone Working Group. *Acta Paediatr* 1998, **87**(8):865–870.
31. Chaplin JE: Growth-related quality of life. *Horm Res Paediatr* 2011, **76**(Suppl 3):51–52.
32. Noeker M: Psychological functioning in idiopathic short stature. *Horm Res Paediatr* 2011, **76**(Suppl 3):52–56.
33. Rosenfeld RG, Hwa V: Toward a molecular basis for idiopathic short stature. *J Clin Endocrinol Metab* 2004, **89**(3):1066–1067.
34. Kiess W, Kratzsch J, Kruis T, Müller E, Wallborn T, Odeh R, Schlicke M, Klammt J, Pfäffle R: Genetics of human stature: Insight from single gene disorders. *Horm Res Paediatr* 2011, **76**(Suppl 3):11–13.
35. Hess O, Khayat M, Hwa V, Heath KE, Teitler A, Hritan Y, Allon-Shalev S, Tenenbaum-Rakover Y: A novel mutation in IGFALS, c.380T>C (p.L127P), associated with short stature, delayed puberty, osteopenia and hyperinsulinaemia in two siblings: insights into the roles of insulin

growth factor-1 (IGF1). *Clin Endocrinol (Oxf)* 2013, **79**(6):838–844.

36. Rojas-Gil AP, Ziros PG, Diaz L, Kletsas D, Basdra EK, Alexandrides TK, Zadik Z, Frank SJ, Papathanassopoulou V, Beratis NG, Papavassiliou AG, Spiliotis BE: **Growth hormone/JAK-STAT axis signal-transduction defect: a novel treatable cause of growth failure.** *FEBS J* 2006, **273**(15):3454–3466.

37. Pugliese-Pires PN, Fortin JP, Arthur T, Latronico AC, Mendonca BB, Villares SM, Arnhold IJ, Kopin AS, Jorge AA: **Novel inactivating mutations in the GH secretagogue receptor gene in patients with constitutional delay of growth and puberty.** *Eur J Endocrinol* 2011, **165**(2):233–241.

38. van Duyvenvoorde HA, van Setten PA, Walenkamp MJ, van Doorn J, Koenig J, Gauguin L, Oostdijk W, Ruivenkamp CA, Losekoot M, Wade JD, De Meyts P, Karperien M, Noordam C, Wit JM: **Short stature associated with a novel heterozygous mutation in the insulin-like growth factor 1 gene.** *J Clin Endocrinol Metab* 2010, **95**(11):E363–E367.

39. Su PH, Yang SF, Yu JS, Chen SJ, Chen JY: **A polymorphism in the leptin receptor gene at position 223 is associated with growth hormone replacement therapy responsiveness in idiopathic short stature and growth hormone deficiency patients.** *Eur J Med Genet* 2012, **55**(12):682–687.

40. Ayling RM, Ross R, Towner P, Von Laue S, Finidori J, Moutoussamy S, Buchanan CR, Clayton PE, Norman MR: **A dominant-negative mutation of the growth hormone receptor causes familial short stature.** *Nat Genet* 1997, **16**(1):13–14.

41. Trovato L, Prodam F, Genoni G, De Rienzo F, Walker GE, Moia S, Riccomagno S, Bellone S, Bona G: **Involvement of genes related to inflammation and cell cycle in idiopathic short stature.** *Pituitary* 2013, **16**(1):83–90.

42. Vasques GA, Amano N, Docko AJ, Funari MF, Quedas EP, Nishi MY, Arnhold IJ, Hasegawa T, Jorge AA: **Heterozygous Mutations in Natriuretic Peptide Receptor-B (NPR2) Gene as a Cause of Short Stature in Patients Initially Classified as Idiopathic Short Stature.** *J Clin Endocrinol Metab* 2013, **98**(10):E1636–E1644.

43. Rao E, Weiss B, Fukami M, Rump A, Niesler B, Mertz A, Muroya K, Binder G, Kirsch S, Winkelmann M, Nordsiek G, Heinrich U, Breuning MH, Ranke MB, Rosenthal A, Ogata T, Rappold GA: **Pseudoautosomal deletions encompassing a novel homeobox gene cause growth failure in idiopathic short stature and Turner syndrome.** *Nat Genet* 1997, **16**(1):54–63.

44. Dunkel L, Wit JM: **Developments in idiopathic short stature.** *Horm Res Paediatr* 2011, **76**(Suppl 3):1–60.

45. Cohen P, Rogol AD, Deal CL, Saenger P, Reiter EO, Ross JL, Chernausek SD, Savage MO, Wit JM, 2007 ISS Consensus Workshop participants: **Consensus statement on the diagnosis and treatment of children with idiopathic short stature: a summary of the Growth Hormone Research Society, the Lawson Wilkins Pediatric Endocrine Society, and the European Society for Paediatric Endocrinology Workshop.** *J Clin Endocrinol Metab* 2008, **93**(11):4210–4217.

46. Savage MO, Bang P: **The variability of responses to growth hormone therapy in children with short stature.** *Indian J Endocrinol Metab* 2012, **16**(Suppl 2):S178–S184.

47. Wit JM, Clayton PE, Rogol AD, Savage MO, Saenger PH, Cohen P: **Idiopathic short stature: definition, epidemiology, and diagnostic evaluation.** *Growth Horm IGF Res* 2008, **18**(2):89–110.

48. Rekers-Mombarg LT, Wit JM, Massa GG, Ranke MB, Buckler JM, Butenandt O, Chaussain JL, Frisch H, Leiberman E: **Spontaneous growth in idiopathic short stature. European Study Group.** *Arch Dis Child* 1996, **75**(3):175–180.

49. Ranke MB, Grauer ML, Kistner K, Blum WF, Wollmann HA: **Spontaneous adult height in idiopathic short stature.** *Horm Res* 1995, **44**(4):152–157.

50. Ranke MB: **Towards a consensus on the definition of idiopathic short stature.** *Horm Res* 1996, **45**(Suppl 2):64–66.

51. Price DA: **Spontaneous adult height in patients with idiopathic short stature.** *Horm Res* 1996, **45**(Suppl 2):59–63.

52. Poyrazoğlu S, Günöz H, Darendeliler F, Saka N, Bundak R, Baş F: **Constitutional delay of growth and puberty: from presentation to final height.** *J Pediatr Endocrinol Metab* 2005, **18**(2):171–179.

53. LaFranchi S, Hanna CE, Mandel SH: **Constitutional delay of growth: expected versus final adult height.** *Pediatrics* 1991, **87**(1):82–87.

54. Crowne EC, Shalet SM, Wallace WH, Eminson DM, Price DA: **Final height in boys with untreated constitutional delay in growth and puberty.** *Arch Dis Child* 1990, **65**(10):1109–1112.

55. Crowne EC, Shalet SM, Wallace WH, Eminson DM, Price DA: **Final height in girls with untreated constitutional delay in growth and puberty.** *Eur J Pediatr* 1991, **150**(10):708–712.

56. Wit JM: **Definition and subcategorization of idiopathic short stature: between consensus and controversy.** *Horm Res Paediatr* 2011, **76**(Suppl 3):3–6.

57. Brown DC, Butler GE, Kelnar CJ, Wu FC: **A double blind, placebo controlled study of the effects of low dose testosterone undecanoate on the growth of small for age, prepubertal boys.** *Arch Dis Child* 1995, **73**(2):131–135.

58. Kelly BP, Paterson WF, Donaldson MD: **Final height outcome and value of height prediction in boys with constitutional delay in growth and adolescence treated with intramuscular testosterone 125 mg per month for 3 months.** *Clin Endocrinol (Oxf)* 2003, **58**(3):267–272.

59. Kamp GA, Ouwens DM, Hoogerbrugge CM, Zwinderman AH, Maassen JA, Wit JM: **Skin fibroblasts of children with idiopathic short stature show an increased mitogenic response to IGF-I and secrete more IGFBP-3.** *Clin Endocrinol (Oxf)* 2002, **56**(4):439–447.

60. Feigerlová E, Diene G, Oliver I, Gennero I, Salles JP, Arnaud C, Tauber M: **Elevated insulin-like growth factor-I values in children with Prader-Willi syndrome compared with growth hormone (GH) deficiency children over two years of GH treatment.** *J Clin Endocrinol Metab* 2010, **95**(10):4600–4608.

61. Bryant J, Baxter L, Cave CB, Milne R: **Recombinant growth hormone for idiopathic short stature in children and adolescents.** *Cochrane Database Syst Rev* 2007, **3**:CD004440.

62. Blethen SL, Baptista J, Kuntze J, Foley T, LaFranchi S, Johanson A: **Adult height in growth hormone (GH)-deficient children treated with biosynthetic GH. The Genentech Growth Study Group.** *J Clin Endocrinol Metab* 1997, **82**(2):418–420.

63. Maiorana A, Cianfarani S: **Impact of growth hormone therapy on adult height of children born small for gestational age.** *Pediatrics* 2009, **124**(3):e519–e531.

64. Baxter L, Bryant J, Cave CB, Milne R: **Recombinant growth hormone for children and adolescents with Turner syndrome.** *Cochrane Database Syst Rev* 2007, **1**:CD003887.

65. Wit JM, Reiter EO, Ross JL, Saenger PH, Savage MO, Rogol AD, Cohen P: **Idiopathic short stature: management and growth hormone treatment.** *Growth Horm IGF Res* 2008, **18**(2):111–135.

66. Wit JM, Rekers-Mombarg LT, Cutler GB, Crowe B, Beck TJ, Roberts K, Gill A, Chaussain JL, Frisch H, Yturriaga R, Attanasio AF: **Growth hormone (GH) treatment to final height in children with idiopathic short stature: evidence for a dose effect.** *J Pediatr* 2005, **146**(1):45–53.

67. Kemp SF, Kuntze J, Attie KM, Maneatis T, Butler S, Frane J, Lippe B: **Efficacy and safety results of long-term growth hormone treatment of idiopathic short stature.** *J Clin Endocrinol Metab* 2005, **90**(9):5247–5253.

68. Guyda HJ: **Four decades of growth hormone therapy for short children: what have we achieved?** *J Clin Endocrinol Metab* 1999, **84**(12):4307–4316.

69. Wit JM: **Idiopathic short stature: reflections on its definition and spontaneous growth.** *Horm Res* 2007, **67**(Suppl 1):50–57.

70. Kelly CJ, Mir FA: **Biological therapies: how can we afford them?** *BMJ* 2009, **339**:b3276.

71. Mullins CD, DeVries AR, Hsu VD, Meng F, Palumbo FB: **Variability and growth in spending for outpatient specialty pharmaceuticals.** *Health Aff (Millwood)* 2005, **24**(4):1117–1127.

72. Saenger P: **Current status of biosimilar growth hormone.** *Int J Pediatr Endocrinol* 2009, **2009**:370329.

73. Bazalo GR, Joshi AV, Germak J: **Comparison of human growth hormone products' cost in pediatric and adult patients. A budgetary impact model.** *Manag Care* 2007, **16**(9):45–51.

74. Cuttler L, Silvers JB: **Growth hormone and health policy.** *J Clin Endocrinol Metab* 2010, **95**(7):3149–3153. 10.1210/jc.2009-2688 Jul.

75. Hardin DS, Woo J, Butsch R, Huett B: **Current prescribing practices and opinions about growth hormone therapy: results of a nationwide survey of paediatric endocrinologists.** *Clin Endocrinol (Oxf)* 2007, **66**(1):85–94.

8

Molecular diagnostic testing for Klinefelter syndrome and other male sex chromosome aneuploidies

Karl Hager[1*], Kori Jennings[1], Seiyu Hosono[1], Susan Howell[2], Jeffrey R Gruen[3,4,5,6], Scott A Rivkees[3,4,7], Nicole R Tartaglia[2] and Henry M Rinder[8]

Abstract

Background: Male sex chromosome aneuploidies are underdiagnosed despite concomitant physical and behavioral manifestations.

Objective: To develop a non-invasive, rapid and high-throughput molecular diagnostic assay for detection of male sex chromosome aneuploidies, including 47,XXY (Klinefelter), 47,XYY, 48,XXYY and 48,XXXY syndromes.

Methods: The assay utilizes three XYM and four XA markers to interrogate Y:X and X:autosome ratios, respectively. The seven markers were PCR amplified using genomic DNA isolated from a cohort of 323 males with aneuploid (n = 117) and 46,XY (n = 206) karyotypes. The resulting PCR products were subjected to Pyrosequencing, a quantitative DNA sequencing method.

Results: Receiver operator characteristic (ROC) curves were used to establish thresholds for the discrimination of aneuploid from normal samples. The XYM markers permitted the identification of 47,XXY, 48,XXXY and 47,XYY syndromes with 100% sensitivity and specificity in both purified DNA and buccal swab samples. The 48,XXYY karyotype was delineated by XA marker data from 46,XY; an X allele threshold of 43% also permitted detection of 48,XXYY with 100% sensitivity and specificity. Analysis of X chromosome-specific biallelic SNPs demonstrated that 43 of 45 individuals (96%) with 48,XXYY karyotype had two distinct X chromosomes, while 2 (4%) had a duplicate X, providing evidence that 48,XXYY may result from nondisjunction during early mitotic divisions of a 46,XY embryo.

Conclusions: Quantitative Pyrosequencing, with high-throughput potential, can detect male sex chromosome aneuploidies with 100% sensitivity.

Keywords: Pyrosequencing, Sex chromosome aneuploidy, Klinefelter (47,XXY) syndrome, 47,XYY syndrome, 48,XXYY syndrome, 48,XXXY syndrome, Male infertility

Introduction

Klinefelter syndrome (KS, also known as 47,XXY) and 47,XYY syndrome are the two most common sex chromosome aneuploidies in humans with prevalence of approximately 1 in 600–1000 males [1-4]. Individuals with KS are usually tall adolescents and adults who have hypergonadotrophic hypogonadism with small testicles. However, the KS phenotype is highly variable and individuals may not show these physical features to a degree that distinguishes them from the general male population.

Males with 47,XYY are also taller than average, but in contrast to KS, they usually do not have phenotypic characteristics to differentiate them from 46,XY males. Compared to 46,XY males, individuals with KS or 47,XYY syndrome exhibit a greater incidence of behavioral problems, psychiatric disorders and neuropsychological characteristics including developmental delays and difficulties in cognitive, verbal and social skills [5]. Yet individuals with both syndromes often fail to be ascertained. Newborn screening studies estimate that only 25% of all individuals with KS, and 10% of all individuals with 47,XYY are diagnosed during their lifetime [6,7].

* Correspondence: karl.hager@jsgenetics.com
[1]JS Genetics, Inc, 2 Church St. South, B-05, New Haven, CT 06519, USA
Full list of author information is available at the end of the article

Table 1 Statistical values calculated from the percent Y allele signals of the three XYM markers for samples grouped together by karyotype

Karyotype	47, XXY (n = 42)			47, XYY (n = 26)			48, XXXY (n = 4)			48, XXYY (n = 45)			46, XY (n = 206)		
Marker	XYM1	XYM2	XYM3	XYM1	XYM2	XYM3	XYM1	XYM2	XYM3	XYM1	XYM2	XYM3	XYM1	XYM2	XYM3
Average	32.3	33.3	33.7	63.7	62.5	64.6	24.4	26.7	26.0	47.4	48.1	49.3	48.2	49.7	49.3
Median	32.3	33.4	33.7	63.6	62.2	64.7	24.1	26.7	25.7	47.6	48.0	49.4	48.2	49.8	49.2
Std Dev	1.53	2.56	1.39	1.55	1.53	0.83	1.54	0.57	0.90	1.17	2.70	1.15	1.46	1.61	1.55
Maximum	38.9	40.6	39.0	67.8	65.9	66.8	26.4	27.3	27.3	50.6	58.3	51.8	51.9	53.2	53.3
Minimum	30.1	27.9	31.0	61.5	57.8	62.3	23.0	25.9	25.3	45.4	44.2	46.1	43.1	41.1	42.8

More complex male sex chromosome aneuploidies, such as 48,XXYY and 48,XXXY, are less common than KS with prevalences ranging from 1 in 18,000 to 1 in 100,000 or greater [1]. While some phenotypic characteristics of 48,XXYY and 48,XXXY syndromes overlap with KS, the unique and significant differences in physical appearance, cognitive function, social and adaptive skills observed in affected individuals differentiate these aneuploidies from KS [8,9].

The gold standard for detection of chromosome aneuploidies is karyotype analysis, an invasive, time-consuming and labor-intensive process. Yet despite the widespread availability of karyotyping, most males with sex chromosome aneuploidy are never diagnosed during their lifetime [6,7]. Thus, the development of more convenient methods for detection of sex chromosome aneuploidies should facilitate identification of these individuals, allowing them to receive early evaluation and therapeutic intervention as indicated. To address this need, we developed a two-stage Pyrosequencing based assay which measures Y:X and X:autosome chromosome ratios. Using this approach, we demonstrated 100% sensitivity in the identification of males with sex chromosome aneuploidy.

Materials & methods

DNA samples
De-identified karyotype-confirmed DNA samples from individuals with male sex chromosome aneuploidies (n = 117) were obtained from Children's Hospital Colorado and the UC Davis MIND Institute (Dr. Flora Tassone). Additional de-identified karyotype-confirmed DNA samples from subjects with 45,X (n = 1), 46,XX (n = 4), 47,

XXX (n = 11), and 46,XY (n = 206) were provided by the above sources, plus the Yale Cytogenetics Lab (Dr. Peining Li) and the Genetics Diagnostic Lab of Children's Hospital Boston (Dr. Bai-Lin Wu). Before use, the DNA samples were diluted 20-fold with nuclease-free water. The concentration of diluted DNA was determined by real time PCR using the human specific probe WIAF699 as described [10]. Only samples with a concentration of diluted DNA ≥1 ng/μl were used as templates for PCR of the XYM and XA markers (see below).

DNA isolation from buccal swabs
Buccal swabs were obtained from patients of Children's Hospital Colorado after informed consent. DNA was isolated from buccal cells using the Qiagen EZ1 robot and EZ1 DNA tissue kit according to the manufacturer's protocol. Extracted DNA was quantified by real time PCR as above.

Assay design
Pyrosequencing (PSQ) assays were designed to interrogate two types of markers. The first class of markers, designated XYM, consisted of regions of the X and Y chromosomes with nearly identical sequence that differ by a chromosome-specific biallelic single nucleotide polymorphism, such that one allele is present only on the X chromosome and the other allele is located on the Y chromosome. Candidate sequences were identified by examining closely related genes present on both X and Y chromosomes outside of the terminal pseudoautosomal regions (see Table 1 of reference [11] and Table 2 of reference [12]). BLAST [13] searches of the human reference genome sequence were used to confirm a single match to

Table 2 Statistical values calculated from the percent X allele signals of the four XA markers for samples grouped together by karyotype

Karyotype	48, XXYY (n = 45)				46, XY (n = 206)			
Marker	XA1	XA2	XA3	XA4	XA1	XA2	XA3	XA4
Average	56.8	54.1	48.5	50.4	42.3	35.3	33.0	32.0
Median	56.4	54.0	48.9	50.8	42.1	35.1	33.3	31.7
Std Dev	1.74	2.57	2.43	3.47	2.51	2.03	2.99	3.56
Maximum	59.7	59.1	51.1	57.8	60.2	42.6	37.2	51.3
Minimum	52.2	49.5	35.3	43.8	35.5	27.4	0.0	20.8

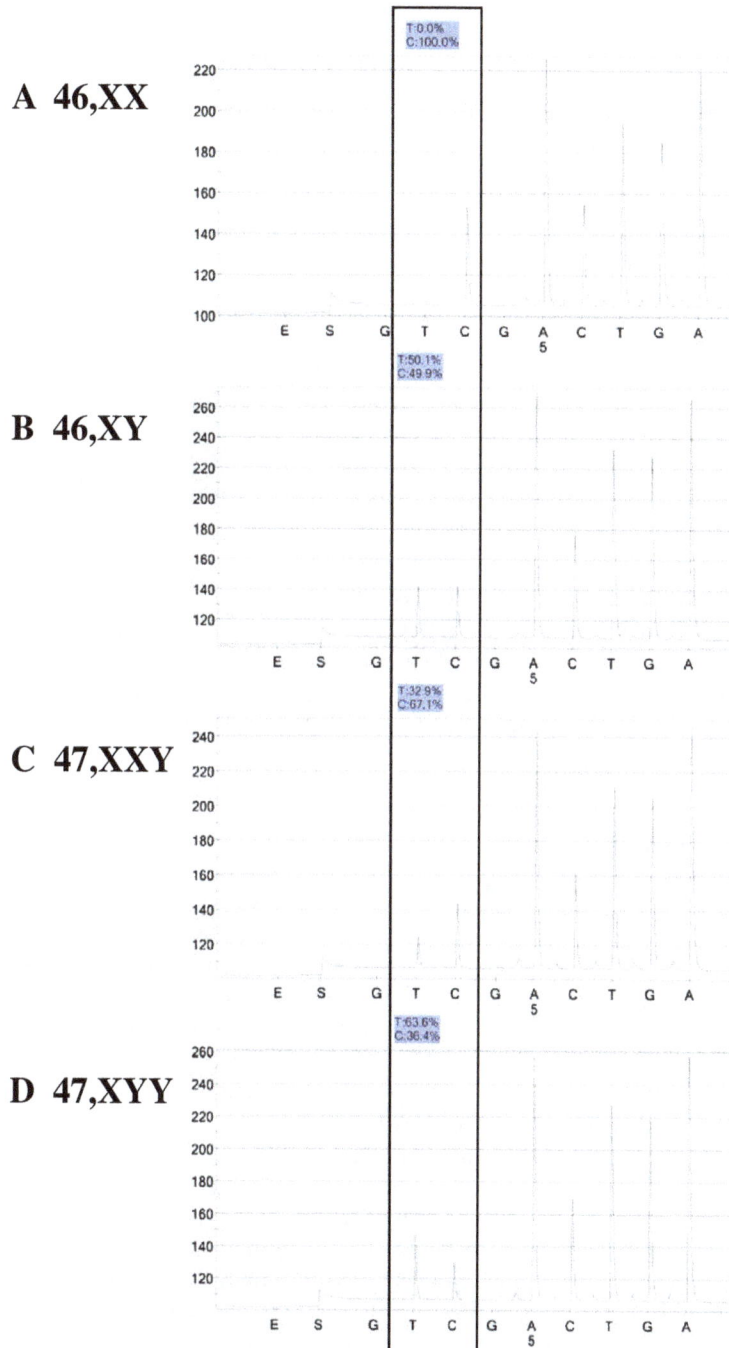

Figure 1 Pyrograms for DNA from a 46,XX female (A), a 46,XY male (B), a 47,XXY KS male (C), and a 47,XYY male (D) using the XYM3 assay. The box encloses the two nucleotide dispensations which define the C/T SNP; the C-allele is derived from the X-chromosome and the T-allele is from the Y-chromosome. The percent of each allele is shown in the shaded box above each pyrogram. The y-axis depicts the intensity of light signal in arbitrary units and the x-axis shows the time of addition of Pyrosequnecing enzymes (E), substrates (S), and each individual nucleotide dispensation (A, C, G, or T).

the X and Y chromosomes for all sequences entered into the PSQ assay design software (version 1.0.6).

The second class of markers, designated XA, represent regions of the X chromosome that are nearly identical with an autosome except for a single chromosome-specific

base. Candidate sequences for assay design were identified by BLAST searching the human genome reference sequence with the set of all X-chromosome transcripts obtained from the ENSEMBL database [14]. High scoring matches where at least 200 bases were >95% identical with one locus on the X-chromosome and one on an autosome were used to generate consensus sequences for assay design by the PSQ software.

PCR and extension primers for high scoring assays were synthesized using standard methods by the W. M. Keck Foundation Biotechnology Resource Lab of Yale University. One of the PCR primers for each assay was labeled at the 5′ end with biotin. For all assays, the extension primer had the same orientation as the forward PCR primer and is complementary to the bio-tinylated template strand generated with the reverse PCR primer.

PCR and pyrosequencing

A minimum of 2.5 ng genomic DNA was used as template in a 25 μl PCR reaction. Each PCR reaction contained 1 X Hotstar buffer (Qiagen), 2.5 mM MgCl$_2$, 200 μM each dNTP, 1 μM each PCR primer, 0.5 U Hotstar Taq Plus (Qiagen). Reactions were performed as follows: initial incubation of 5 min at 95°C; followed by 45 cycles of 30 sec at 95°C, 45 sec at 56°C, and 60 sec at 72 °C; then 5 min at 72 °C and a final hold at 4°C. Upon completion of PCR, the biotinylated template strand was purified using Streptavi-din-Sepharose and the Filter Prep tool (Qiagen) according to the manufacturer's instructions. The resulting single stranded template was annealed to the appropriate exten-sion primer and Pyrosequencing was performed using Pyromark Q96 reagents and PSQ96MA instrument (Qiagen). The allele percentage was calculated by the PSQ software (version 2.1) and exported for analysis by Microsoft Excel.

Results
Principle of assay

The assay measures both Y:X and X:A (X:Autosome) chromosome ratios by Pyrosequencing, a quantitative short-read DNA sequencing technology [15]. For the first step, three XYM loci are PCR amplified with specific primer pairs and the resulting amplicons subjected to Pyrosequencing, yielding the percent of Y-chromosome-specific allele signal for each locus and hence, the ratio of the Y and X chromosomes. Figure 1 shows Pyrosequencing data using the XYM3 marker with DNA from a 46,XX female (A), 46,XY male (B), a 47,XXY individual (C), and a 47,XYY subject (D). The percent Y allele signal has close agreement with the value predicted for each karyotype. The locations of the three XYM markers on the X and Y chromosomes are shown in Figure 2.

In the second step of the assay, Pyrosequencing of the four XA markers determines the X:autosome (X:A) ratio, which permits differentiation between individuals with 46,XY and 48,XXYY karyotypes.

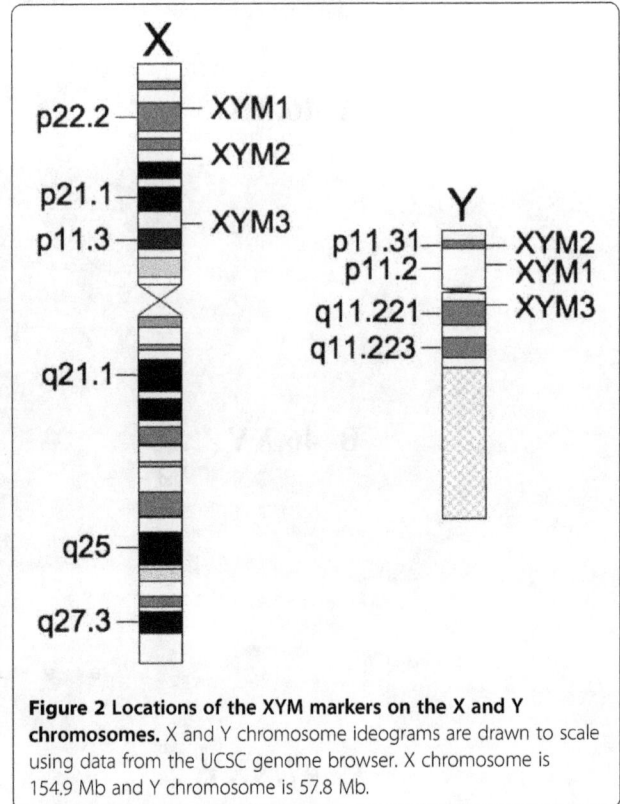

Figure 2 Locations of the XYM markers on the X and Y chromosomes. X and Y chromosome ideograms are drawn to scale using data from the UCSC genome browser. X chromosome is 154.9 Mb and Y chromosome is 57.8 Mb.

Overall performance of XYM markers

To evaluate the ability of the three XYM markers to detect sex chromosome aneuploidies, PCR and Pyrose-quencing were performed on 339 DNA samples from females (n = 16) and males (n = 323), with the technician blinded to each individual's karyotype. Following comple-tion of Pyrosequencing, the karyotype of each sample was matched to the data for all three markers. All samples from phenotypic females, including individuals with a 46,XX karyotype (n = 4) and those with sex chromo-some aneuploidies (45,X, n = 1 and 47,XXX, n = 11), did not display detectable Y allele for any of the three XYM markers (maximum Y allele signal of 1.9%).

Data generated with the three XYM markers were analyzed for the 323 DNA samples from males with karyotype-confirmed sex chromosome aneuploidies (n = 117) or 46,XY (n = 206). Scatter plots of the percent Y allele signal for both the XYM2 and XYM3 markers versus the percent Y allele signal of the XYM1 marker are shown in Figure 3. For all three XYM markers, the data for individuals with the 48,XXXY, 47,XXY, and 47,XYY karyotypes were tightly clustered and distinguish-able from males with a 46,XY karyotype. As expected from the known Y:X chromosome ratio, the percent Y allele signals for the subjects with 48,XXYY karyotype overlapped with those for the 46,XY males. The percent

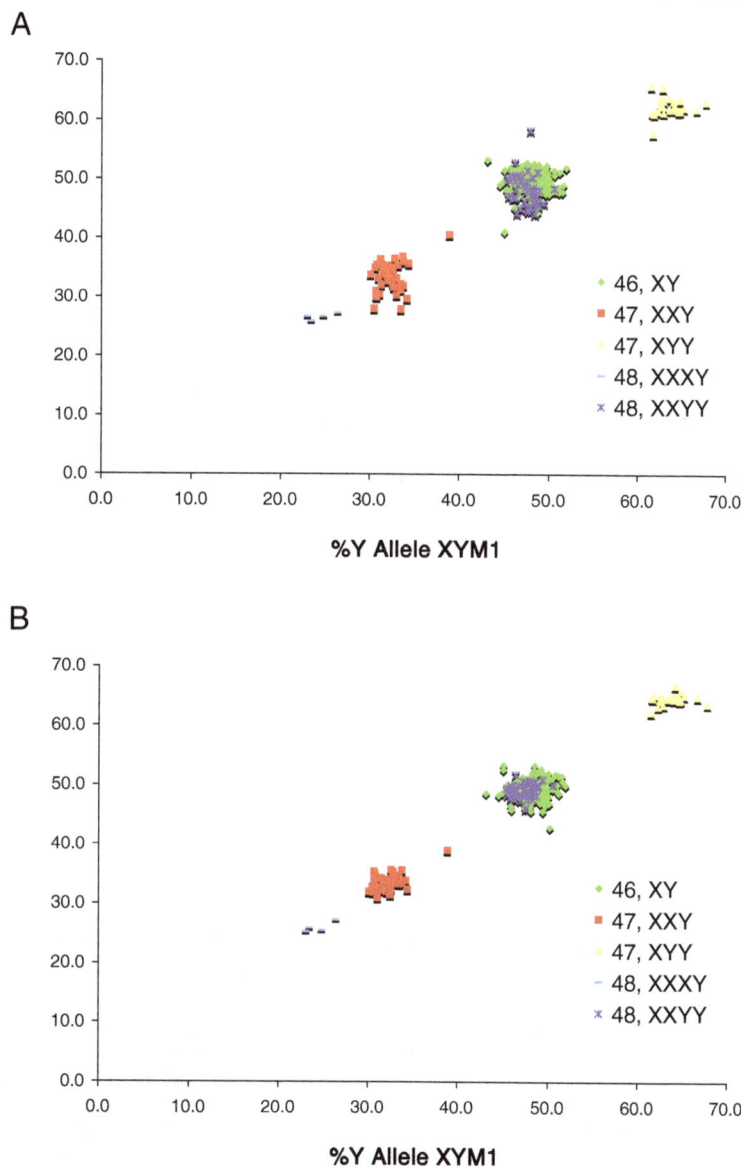

Figure 3 Percent Y allele signal of XYM2 (A) and XYM3 (B) plotted against the percent Y allele signal of XYM1 for 323 DNA samples from male subjects grouped by karyotype. For each marker, the percent Y allele signal is the ratio of signal from the Y-chromosome specific allele divided by the total signal from both the Y- and X-chromosome specific alleles, expressed as a percentage.

Y allele signal for both XYM2 and XYM3 was strongly correlated with XYM1, with correlation coefficients (r^2) of 0.90 and 0.94, respectively. Table 1 summarizes the statistical data calculated for the measured percent Y allele signal of each marker for samples grouped according to karyotype; the average percent Y allele signal for each group was close to the predicted value based on the known karyotype.

Detection of 47,XXY (KS), 48,XXXY and 47,XYY syndromes
To identify 47,XXY, 48,XXXY, or 47,XYY karyotypes, receiver operator characteristic (ROC) curves were

constructed by varying the percent Y allele signal lower and upper thresholds for samples scored as normal 46,XY karyotype (Figure 4). For this analysis, the average percent Y allele signal for the three XYM markers was calculated; the lower threshold was increased from 34% to 48% by 1% increments while sensitivity and false positive rates for detecting 47,XXY (KS) and 48,XXXY karyotypes were calculated. All samples with either 47,XXY or 48,XXXY karyotypes and average percent Y allele signals less than the lower threshold value were classified as true positives. False negative samples had the same karyotypes and the average percent Y allele signal above the threshold. True

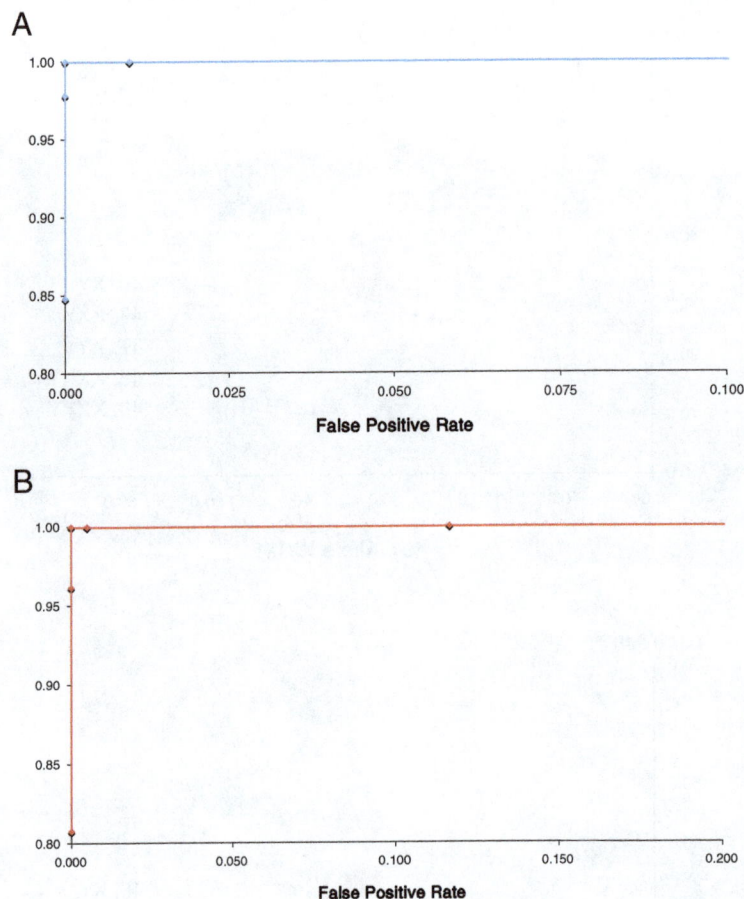

Figure 4 Receiver operator characteristic curves for detection of 47,XXY (KS) and 48,XXXY (A) and 47,XYY syndromes (B). The average of the three XYM marker data points for each sample was calculated and compared to the detection thresholds. The threshold for detecting XXY and XXXY syndromes was varied by 1% increments from 34-48% Y allele signal; that for detecting XYY syndrome was incremented by 1% from 49-63%. The sensitivity (TP/(TP + FN)) and false positive rate (FP/(FP + TN)) were calculated for each value of the appropriate threshold. For XXY and XXXY, true positives (TP) have either a 47,XXY or 48,XXXY karyotype and average Y allele signal less than the threshold; false negatives (FN) have the same karyotypes and average Y allele signal greater than or equal to the threshold. True negatives (TN) for XXY and XXXY are samples with a 46,XY karyotype and average Y allele signal greater than or equal to the threshold; false positives (FP) have a 46,XY karyotype and average Y allele signal below the threshold. For XYY syndrome, true positives have 47,XYY karyotype and average Y allele signal greater than the threshold; false negatives have the same karyotype and average Y allele signal less than or equal to the threshold. True negatives for XYY are samples with a 46, XY karyotype and average Y allele signal less than or equal to the threshold; false positives have a 46,XY karyotype and average Y allele signal above the threshold.

negatives were defined as a 46,XY subject with the average percent Y allele signals greater than the lower limit, while a false positive was defined as having the average percent Y allele signal less than the lower limit.

Conversely for 47,XYY syndrome, the upper threshold was examined from 49% to 63% by 1% increments, and sensitivity and false positive rates were calculated. True positives had 47,XYY karyotype and an average percent Y allele signal above the upper threshold; any 47,XYY sample with the average percent Y allele signal below the upper limit was scored as false negative. True negatives (46,XY) had the average percent Y allele signal less than

or equal to the upper limit; false positives had the average percent Y allele signal above the upper limit.

Examination of the ROC curves indicated that a percent Y allele signal scoring threshold of 43% for 47, XXY and 48,XXXY syndromes and 57% for 47,XYY syndrome yielded 100% sensitivity with a 0% false positive rate. Combining the two thresholds gave a percent Y allele signal range of 43-57% for 46,XY samples. Separate analysis of the individual XYM marker data and the median of the three XYM values generated ROC curves which overlapped the curve generated with the average XYM values; thresholds of 43% and 57%

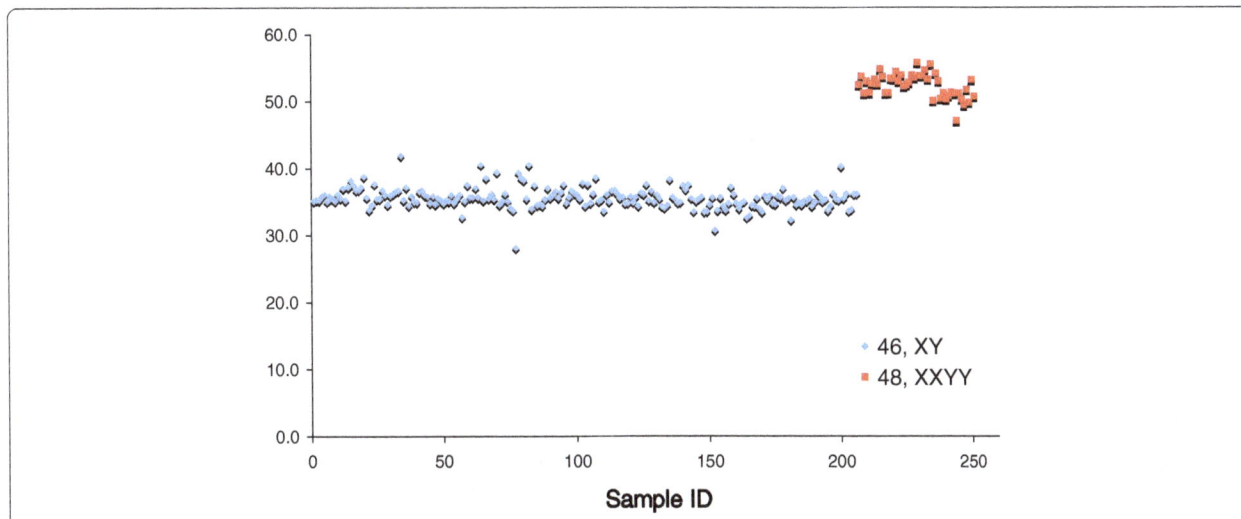

Figure 5 Average percent X allele signal of four XA markers versus sample ID for male samples with 46,XY and 48,XXYY karyotypes. The average percent X allele signal is the average for all four markers of the ratio of signal from the X-chromosome specific allele divided by the total signal from both the X-chromosome and autosome specific alleles, expressed as a percentage.

allow the detection of KS and 47,XYY syndrome with 100% sensitivity and specificity using the data from either each individual marker or the median value.

Detection of 48,XXYY syndrome

As noted above, the percent Y allele signals from 48, XXYY individuals (n = 45) and 46,XY males (n = 206) showed nearly complete overlap (Figure 3 and Table 1). To distinguish these karyotypes, four XA markers were

amplified by PCR and the resulting products examined by Pyrosequencing. Figure 5 is a plot of the average percent X allele for the four XA markers graphed versus the sample ID. The average percent X allele signal differed for the samples with 48,XXYY and 46,XY karyotypes and was close to the expected values of 50% and 33.3%, respectively, based on the known chromosome ratios (Table 2). ROC analysis (Figure 6) performed by comparing the average percent X allele for the four XA markers with a threshold varying

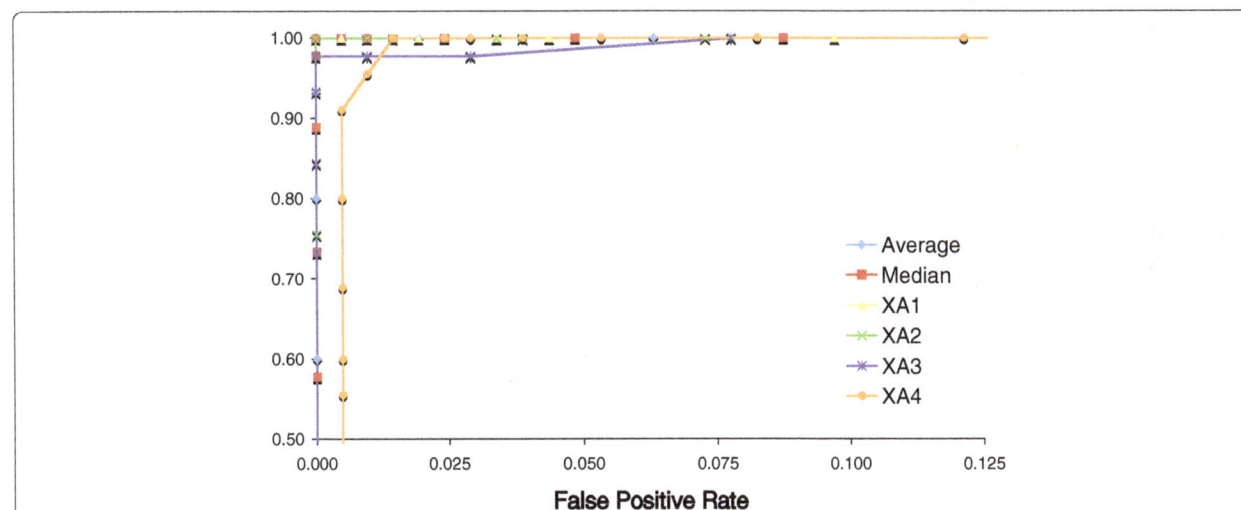

Figure 6 Receiver operator characteristic curves for detection of 48,XXYY syndrome. The average and median of the four XA marker data points for each sample was calculated: either the average, median or individual marker data was compared to the threshold for detecting 48,XXYY syndrome. The threshold was varied by 1% increments from 33-52% X allele signal. The sensitivity (TP/(TP + FN)) and false positive rate (FP/(FP + TN)) were calculated for each value of the appropriate threshold. True positives (TP) have a 48,XXYY karyotype and X allele signal greater than the threshold; false negatives (FN) have the same karyotype and X allele signal less than or equal to the threshold. True negatives (TN) have a 46,XY karyotype and X allele signal less than or equal to the threshold; false positives (FP) have a 46,XY karyotype and X allele signal above the threshold.

Table 3 Statistical values calculated from the average percent allele signals of the XYM and XA marker sets for buccal swab samples grouped together by karyotype

Karytoype Marker Set	47, XXY (n = 8)		47, XYY (n = 3)		46, XY (n = 5)		48, XXYY (n = 13)	
	Average Y Allele XYM	Average X Allele XA	Average Y Allele XYM	Average X Allele XA	Average Y Allele XYM	Average X Allele XA	Average Y Allele XYM	Average X Allele XA
Average	35.1	52.1	65.2	36.3	50.6	38.1	50.1	52.3
Median	35.0	51.5	65.1	36.1	50.7	37.7	50.3	52.1
Std Dev	0.9	1.7	0.2	0.9	0.8	1.3	1.0	1.9
Maximum	36.8	54.3	65.4	37.3	51.6	39.5	52.1	56.3
Minimum	34.0	50.2	65.0	35.6	49.6	36.6	48.0	49.7

from 33-52% in 1% increments indicated that a threshold of 43% gave 100% detection of 48,XXYY karyotype with a 0% false positive rate.

As a confirmatory approach to distinguish males with 48,XXYY and 46,XY karyotypes, 18 X-linked markers were PCR amplified and the amplicons subjected to Pyrosequencing using DNA from all 48,XXYY males. The relative allele strength for each of the X-chromosome specific markers was scored as homozygous, heterozygous, or out-of-range as described for a Turner Syndrome assay [16]. Of the 45 individuals with the 48,XXYY karyotype, 43 demonstrated definitive evidence for the presence of two distinct X-chromosomes, with the number of heterozygous markers ranging from 4 to 12 out of 18 total. Thus, most 48,XXYY individuals either inherit one X-chromosome from each parent or inherit two distinct X chromosomes as a result of nondisjunction in maternal meiosis I. The remaining two individuals were homozygous for all 18 markers, and therefore, appear to have inherited both X chromosomes from their mother due to nondisjuction in maternal meiosis II or as a result of nondisjunction of a 46, XY embryo in early mitotic cell divisions. Thus, for the latter group, only signal from the XA markers distinguished them from 46,XY individuals.

Analysis of Coriell samples with a 47,XXY karyotype
In an additional test of the sex chromosome aneuploidy assay, three XYM markers were measured on DNA obtained from immortalized lymphocyte cultures of 16 individuals with a 47,XXY karyotype (Coriell Institute of Medical Research). For 15 of 16 individuals, the percent Y allele signal for all three markers clustered tightly around the expected 33.3%. One individual had percent Y allele signals between 53.6 and 59% and is known to have a complex mosaic karyotype: 47,XXY [17].ish X (DXZ1x2).ish Y (SRYx1)/47, XYY [28].ish X (DXZ1x1).ish Y (SRYx2)/46,XY [5].ish X (DXZ1x1).ish Y (SRYx1), with prominent contributions from both 47,XXY and 47,XYY cell populations. Based on the mosaic estimate, this subject is expected to have percent Y allele signals near 50%.

Analysis of buccal swab samples
As a final test for assay performance, buccal swabs were obtained from 29 males with known karyotypes. Buccal cell DNA was extracted and all seven markers amplified by PCR. Following Pyrosequencing, the data from all 29 samples were classified using the previously described threshold values for the XYM and XA markers. Table 3 presents the aggregate statistical data for the average allele signal of the buccal swab samples grouped by karyotype. Buccal swab samples demonstrated 100% sensitivity and specificity for detection of male sex chromosome aneuploidies.

Discussion
We report the development of a rapid, high-throughput Pyrosequencing assay for detecting sex chromosome aneuploidies in males. The assay initially interrogates three XYM markers, yielding the percent Y allele signal which is directly related to the Y:X chromosome ratio. Next, to distinguish 46,XY and 48,XXYY karyotypes, the assay utilizes four XA markers to determine the X:A ratio. Using this approach, our assay identifies males with 47,XXY, 47,XYY, 48,XXXY and 48,XXYY karyotypes at 100% sensitivity and specificity (Table 4).

Previous studies of the parental origin of the sex chromosomes in males with 48,XXYY are limited to a total of eight individuals [17-21]. These studies

Table 4 Sensitivity and false positive rate for detection of sex chromosome aneuploidies in males

Karyotype	Total Samples	Sensitivity	False Positive Rate
47,XXY (KS)	65	100%	0%
47,XYY	29	100%	0%
48,XXXY	4	100%	0%
48,XXYY	58	100%	0%

Combination of results for DNAs isolated from buccal swabs (n = 29) or obtained from Colorado Children's Hospital, UC Davis MIND Institute, Children's Hospital Boston, Yale University and Coriell Institute (n = 338). One Coriell sample was omitted from this table due to its complicated mosaic karyotype: 47,XXY [17].ish X (DXZ1x2).ish Y (SRYx1)/47,XYY [28].ish X (DXZ1x1).ish Y (SRYx2)/46,XY [5].ish X (DXZ1x1).ish Y (SRYx1).

concluded that the extra sex chromosomes are paternally derived, resulting from two sequential nondisjunction events in meiosis I and II of spermatogenesis. Our data for 96% of subjects with 48,XXYY (n = 43) are consistent with this mechanism since the DNA samples demonstrated heterozygosity for between 4 and 12 of a total 18 X-linked biallelic SNP markers. However, the data cannot rule out an alternative mechanism whereby the additional X chromosome is maternally derived from nondisjunction in meiosis I of oogenesis and the supernumerary Y is due to nondisjunction in meiosis II of spermatogenesis. Only detailed molecular genetic analysis of the parents of 48,XXYY males can ascertain the relative contribution of these two mechanisms; still, the statistical likelihood of an X aneuploid oocyte being fertilized by a Y aneuploid sperm is quite low. The remaining 4% of subjects with 48,XXYY (n = 2) were shown to have identical X chromosomes due to complete homozygosity of the 18 X-linked markers and thus likely result from nondisjunction during early mitotic divisions of a 46,XY embryo. Alternatively, but less likely, this subset of individuals may result from nondisjunction in meiosis II of both maternal and paternal gametes. The current study has a large enough population (n = 45) to detect this novel mechanism for the chromosomal origin of the supernumerary sex chromosomes in 48,XXYY males.

Our Pyrosequencing based assay is robust and readily interpretable allowing the reliable detection of male sex chromosome aneuploidies with 100% sensitivity and specificity. This particular methodology serves as a rapid, high-throughput screen, and the accuracy of detection for KS and other sex chromosome aneuploidies translates to an extremely low likelihood of discrepant karyotypic analysis if utilized for confirmation. The assay may be completed in 8–10 hrs. which is considerably faster than the time required for either fluorescent in situ hybridization (FISH) or karyotype analysis. Individuals with KS may present clinically at many points during their lifetime [1], and yet, because of variable and often subtle phenotype, they are not recognized and in most cases, never diagnosed [22]. The current assay provides a non-invasive molecular test applicable for rapid diagnosis, thus allowing for earlier assessments and interventions in all facets of therapy for KS, 47,XYY, 48, XXYY and 48,XXXY, including androgen replacement and cognitive and behavioral treatments [23].

For male children suspected of KS or another sex chromosome aneuploidy, the ability to make the diagnosis using DNA isolated from buccal swabs is an advantage over invasive, often traumatic, blood testing. Diagnosis during infancy/childhood, especially for KS, allows for early interventional speech/language therapy and educational planning, as well as promotion of physical activity to inhibit the development of dyspraxia. Endocrine monitoring and early management can be instituted to eventually support puberty, preserve fertility, and determine the timing of androgen replacement [23]. With respect to 47,XYY syndrome, rapid and efficient detection similarly permits initiation of appropriate cognitive and behavioral therapy. Current trials of pharmaceuticals for general developmental disorders in male children that overlap with KS and other supernumerary X chromosome syndromes may also benefit from diagnostic specificity for these relevant aneuploidies.

Even making the delayed diagnosis of KS or other sex chromosome aneuploidies in adulthood offers specific treatment goals for their related complications. KS is one of the most frequent causes of male infertility [24]. For adult males being evaluated for failure to conceive, making this diagnosis earlier offers specific and better options to preserve fertility [25], and this rapid methodology may decrease the stress and anxiety associated with waiting for the diagnosis of KS (or other sex chromosome aneuploidy) by karyotyping. As with male children, making the diagnosis of KS in adulthood is also important for instituting specific endocrine therapies to prevent gynecomastia and osteopenia [23].

The clinical application of this sensitive and specific Pyrosequencing based assay will enable the rapid, efficient and high-throughput detection of sex chromosome aneuploidies in males and allow for early, appropriate assessment and therapeutic interventions for individuals with these common but under-diagnosed genetic conditions.

Competing interests

Karl Hager, Kori Jennings & Seiyu Hosono are employees of JS Genetics, Inc.. Karl Hager, Seiyu Hosono, Jeffrey R. Gruen, Scott A. Rivkees, and Henry M. Rinder hold equity interest in JS Genetics, Inc.. Susan Howell and Nicole R. Tartaglia have no competing interests.

Author details

[1]JS Genetics, Inc, 2 Church St. South, B-05, New Haven, CT 06519, USA. [2]Children's Hospital Colorado, Aurora, CO 80045, USA. [3]Yale Child Health Research Center, Yale University School of Medicine, New Haven, CT 06520, USA. [4]Department of Pediatrics, Yale University School of Medicine, New Haven, CT 06520, USA. [5]Department of Genetics, Yale University School of Medicine, New Haven, CT 06520, USA. [6]Investigative Medicine Program, Yale University School of Medicine, New Haven, CT 06520, USA. [7]Department of Pediatrics, University of Florida, Gainesville, FL 32610, USA. [8]Department of Laboratory Medicine, Yale University, New Haven, CT 06510, USA.

Authors' contributions

KH contributed to study design, developed the hypothesis, analyzed data, and wrote the manuscript; KJ analyzed data and contributed to writing of the manuscript; SH contributed to study design and writing of the manuscript; SH contributed to study design, writing of the manuscript, and collection of patient samples; JG contributed to study design and writing of the manuscript; SR contributed to study design and writing of the manuscript; NT contributed to study design, writing of the manuscript, and collection of patient samples; HR developed the hypothesis, analyzed data, and contributed to study design and writing the manuscript. All authors read and approved the final manuscript.

References

1. Visootsak J, Graham JM: **Klinefelter syndrome and other sex chromosome aneuploidies.** *Orphanet J Rare Diseases* 2006, 1:42.

2. RLNussbaumRRMclnessHFWillard2007Clinical Cytogenetics: Disorders of the Autosomes and the Sex Chromosomes In Thompson & Thompson Genetics in Medicine, Seventh EditionSaunders ElsevierPhiladelphia105107Nussbaum RL, McIness RR, Willard HF: **Clinical Cytogenetics: Disorders of the Autosomes and the Sex Chromosomes.** In *Thompson & Thompson Genetics in Medicine*, Seventh Edition. Philadelphia: Saunders Elsevier; 2007:105–107.

3. Tuttelman F, Gromoll J: **Novel genetic aspects of Klinefelter's syndrome.** *Molec Human Reprod* 2010, 16:386–395.

4. Coffee B, Keith K, Albizua I, Malone T, Mowrey J, Sherman SL, Warren ST: **Incidence of fragile X syndrome by newborn screening for methylated FMR1 DNA.** *Am J Hum Genet* 2009, 85:503–514.

5. Ross JL, Zeger MPD, Kushner H, Zinn AR, Roeltgen DP: **An extra X or Y chromosome: contrasting the cognitive and motor phenotypes in childhood in boys with 47, XYY syndrome or 47, XXY Klinefelter syndrome.** *Dev Disabil Res Rev* 2009, 15:309–317.

6. Bojesen A, Juul S, Gravholt CH: **Prenatal and postnatal prevalence of Klinefelter syndrome: a national registry study.** *J Clin Endocrinol Metab* 2003, 88:622–626.

7. Stockholm K, Juul S, Gravholt CH: **Diagnosis and mortality in 47,XYY persons: a registry study.** *Orphanet J Rare Dis* 2010, 5:15.

8. Tartaglia N, Howell S, Ayari N, D'Epagnier C, Zeitler P: **48,XXYY, 48,XXXY and 49,XXXXY syndromes: Not just variants of Klinefelter syndrome.** *Acta Paediatr* 2011, 100:851–860.

9. Tartaglia N, Davis S, Hench A, Nimishakav S, Beauregard R, Reynolds A, Fenton L, Albrecht L, Ross J, Visootsak J, Hansen R, Hagerman R: **A new look at XXYY syndrome: medical and psychological features.** *Am J Med Genet A* 2008, 146A:1509–1522.

10. Hosono S, Faruqi AF, Dean FB, Du Y, Sun Z, Wu X, Du J, Kingsmore SF, Egholm M, Lasken RS: **Unbiased whole-genome amplification directly from clinical samples.** *Genome Res* 2003, 13:954–964.

11. Ross MT, Grafham DV, Coffey AJ, Scherer S, McLay K, Muzny D, Platzer M, Howell GR, Burrows C, Bird CP, Frankish A, Lovell FL, Howe KL, Ashurst JL, Fulton RS, Sudbrak R, Wen G, Jones MC, Hurles ME, Andrews TD, Scott CE, Searle S, Ramser J, Whittaker A, Deadman R, Carter NP, Hunt SE, Chen R, Cree A, Gunaratne P, Havlak P, Hodgson A, Metzker ML, Richards S, Scott G, Steffen D, Sodergren E, Wheeler DA, Worley KC, Ainscough R, Ambrose KD, Ansari-Lari MA, Aradhya S, Ashwell RI, Babbage AK, Bagguley CL, Ballabio A, Banerjee R, Barker GE, Barlow KF, Barrett IP, Bates KN, Beare DM, Beasley H, Beasley O, Beck A, Bethel G, Blechschmidt K, Brady N, Bray-Allen S, Bridgeman AM, Brown AJ, Brown MJ, Bonnin D, Bruford EA, Buhay C, Burch P, Burford D, Burgess J, Burrill W, Burton J, Bye JM, Carder C, Carrel L, Chako J, Chapman JC, Chavez D, Chen E, Chen G, Chen Y, Chen Z, Chinault C, Ciccodicola A, Clark SY, Clarke G, Clee CM, Clegg S, Clerc-Blankenburg K, Clifford K, Cobley V, Cole CG, Conquer JS, Corby N, Connor RE, David R, Davies J, Davis C, Davis J, Delgado O, Deshazo D, Dhami P, Ding Y, Dinh H, Dodsworth S, Draper H, Dugan-Rocha S, Dunham A, Dunn M, Durbin KJ, Dutta I, Eades T, Ellwood M, Emery-Cohen A, Errington H, Evans KL, Faulkner L, Francis F, Frankland J, Fraser AE, Galgoczy P, Gilbert J, Gill R, Glöckner G, Gregory SG, Gribble S, Griffiths C, Grocock R, Gu Y, Gwilliam R, Hamilton C, Hart EA, Hawes A, Heath PD, Heitmann K, Hennig S, Hernandez J, Hinzmann B, Ho S, Hoffs M, Howden PJ, Huckle EJ, Hume J, Hunt PJ, Hunt AR, Isherwood J, Jacob L, Johnson D, Jones S, de Jong PJ, Joseph SS, Keenan S, Kelly S, Kershaw JK, Khan Z, Kioschis P, Klages S, Knights AJ, Kosiura A, Kovar-Smith C, Laird GK, Langford C, Lawlor S, Leversha M, Lewis L, Liu W, Lloyd C, Lloyd DM, Loulseged H, Loveland JE, Lovell JD, Lozado R, Lu J, Lyne R, Ma J, Maheshwari M, Matthews LH, McDowall J, McLaren S, McMurray A, Meidl P, Meitinger T, Milne S, Miner G, Mistry SL, Morgan M, Morris S, Müller I, Mullikin JC, Nguyen N, Nordsiek G, Nyakatura G, O'Dell CN, Okwuonu G, Palmer S, Pandian R, Parker D, Parrish J, Pasternak S, Patel D, Pearce AV, Pearson DM, Pelan SE, Perez L, Porter KM, Ramsey Y, Reichwald K, Rhodes S, Ridler KA, Schlessinger D, Schueler MG, Sehra HK, Shaw-Smith C, Shen H, Sheridan EM, Shownkeen R, Skuce CD, Smith ML, Sotheran EC, Steingruber HE, Steward CA, Storey R, Swann RM, Swarbreck D, Tabor PE, Taudien S, Taylor T, Teague B, Thomas K, Thorpe A, Timms K, Tracey A, Trevanion S, Tromans AC, d'Urso M, Verduzco D, Villasana D, Waldron L, Wall M, Wang Q,

Warren J, Warry GL, Wei X, West A, Whitehead SL, Whiteley MN, Wilkinson JE, Willey DL, Williams G, Williams L, Williamson A, Williamson H, Wilming L, Woodmansey RL, Wray PW, Yen J, Zhang J, Zhou J, Zoghbi H, Zorilla S, Buck D, Reinhardt R, Poustka A, Rosenthal A, Lehrach H, Meindl A, Minx PJ, Hillier LW, Willard HF, Wilson RK, Waterston RH, Rice CM, Vaudin M, Coulson A, Nelson DL, Weinstock G, Sulston JE, Durbin R, Hubbard T, Gibbs RA, Beck S, Rogers J, Bentley DR: **The DNA sequence of the human X chromosome.** *Nature* 2005, 434:325–337.

12. Skaletsky H, Kuroda-Kawaguchi T, Minx PJ, Cordum HS, Hillier L, Brown LG, Repping S, Pyntikova T, Ali J, Bieri T, Chinwalla A, Delehaunty A, Delehaunty K, Du H, Fewell G, Fulton L, Fulton R, Graves T, Hou SF, Latrielle P, Leonard S, Mardis E, Maupin R, McPherson J, Miner T, Nash W, Nguyen C, Ozersky P, Pepin K, Rock S, Rohlfing T, Scott K, Schultz B, Strong C, Tin-Wollam A, Yang SP, Waterston RH, Wilson RK, Rozen S, Page DC: **The male-specific region of the human Y chromosome is a mosaic of discrete sequence classes.** *Nature* 2003, 423:825–837.

13. Altschul SF, Gish W, Miller W, Myers EW, Lipman DJ: **Basic local alignment search tool.** *J Mol Biol* 1990, 215:403–410.

14. Flicek P, Amode MR, Barrell D, Beal K, Brent S, Chen Y, Clapham P, Coates G, Fairley S, Fitzgerald S, Gordon L, Hendrix M, Hourlier T, Johnson N, Kähäri A, Keefe D, Keenan S, Kinsella R, Kokocinski F, Kulesha E, Larsson P, Longden I, McLaren W, Overduin B, Pritchard B, Riat HS, Rios D, Ritchie GR, Ruffier M, Schuster M, Sobral D, Spudich G, Tang YA, Trevanion S, Vandrovcova J, Vilella AJ, White S, Wilder SP, Zadissa A, Zamora J, Aken BL, Birney E, Cunningham F, Dunham I, Durbin R, Fernández-Suarez XM, Herrero J, Hubbard TJ, Parker A, Proctor G, Vogel J, Searle SM: **Ensembl 2011.** *Nucleic Acids Res* 2011, 39(Database issue):D800–D806.

15. Fakhrai-Rad H, Pourmand N, Ronaghi M: **Pyrosequencing: an accurate detection platform for single nucleotide polymorphisms.** *Hum Mutat* 2002, 19:479–485.

16. Rivkees SA, Hager K, Hosono S, Wise A, Li P, Rinder HM, Gruen JR: **A highly sensitive, high-throughput assay for the detection of Turner syndrome.** *J Clin Endocrinol Metab* 2011, 96:699–705.

17. Lorda-Sanchez I, Binkert F, Hinkel KG, Moser H, Rosenkranz W, Maechler M, Schinzel A: **Uniparental origin of sex chromosome polysomies.** *Hum Hered* 1992, 42:193–197.

18. Leal CA, Belmont JW, Nachtman R, Cantu JM, Medina C: **Parental origin of the extra chromosomes in polysomy X.** *Hum Genet* 1994, 94:423–426.

19. Iitsuka Y, Bock A, Nguyen DD, Samango-Sprouse CA, Simpson JL, Bischoff FZ: **Evidence of skewed X-chromosome inactivation in 47, XXY and 48, XXYY Klinefelter patients.** *Am J Med Genet* 2001, 98:25–31.

20. Hillig U, Hoo JJ: **A case of 48, XXYY–paternal origin of the extra X chromosome.** *Humangenetik* 1974, 25:159–161.

21. Rinaldi A, Archidiacono N, Rocchi M, Filippi G: **Additional pedigree supporting the frequent origin of XXYY from consecutive meiotic non-disjunction in paternal gametogenesis.** *J Med Genet* 1979, 16:225–226.

22. Abramsky L, Chapple J: **47, XXY (Klinefelter syndrome) and 47, XYY: estimated rates and indication for postnatal diagnosis with implications for prenatal counseling.** *Prenat Diagn* 1997, 17:363–368.

23. Radicioni AF, De Marco E, Gianfrilli D, Granato S, Gandini L, Isidori AM, Lenzi A: **Strategies and advantages of early diagnosis in Klinefelter's syndrome.** *Mol Hum Reprod* 2010, 16:434–440.

24. Lanfranco F, Kamischke A, Zitamann M, Nieschlag E: **Klinefelter's syndrome.** *Lancet* 2004, 364:273–283.

25. Ferhi K, Avakian R, Griveau JF, Guille F: **Age as only predictive factor for successful sperm recovery in patients with Klinefelter's syndrome.** *Andrologia* 2009, 41:84–87.

9

Changes in diet and physical activity in adolescents with and without type 1 diabetes over time

Franziska K Bishop*, R Paul Wadwa, Janet Snell-Bergeon, Nhung Nguyen and David M Maahs

Abstract

Background: Diet and physical activity (PA) are fundamental aspects of care in type 1 diabetes, but scant longitudinal data exist on these behaviors in adolescents with type 1 diabetes, especially compared to non-diabetic controls.

Methods: Data in 211 adolescents with type 1 diabetes (baseline age = 15.3 ± 2.2 years, diabetes duration = 8.8 ± 3.1 years, A1c = 9.0 ± 1.5%, 51% male) and 67 non-diabetic (age = 14.9 ± 1.7 years, 52% male) controls were collected at baseline (V1) and again at 2-year follow-up (V2) (mean follow up = 2.2 ± 0.4 years). Diet data (meals/day, snacks/day, and weekly consumption of breakfast, fruit, vegetables and fried foods), and PA were collected using interviewer administered questionnaires. T-tests and chi-squared tests were used for comparisons.

Results: Both adolescents with type 1 diabetes and non-diabetic controls reported increased vegetable (2.8 v. 3.6 and 3.1 v. 3.8 times weekly, respectively, p < 0.0001) and fruit (2.9 v. 3.8, both groups, p < 0.0001) intake (times per week) and increased PA (hours/day; 1.8 v. 2.2, p = 0.005 and 1.5 v. 1.9, p = 0.008, respectively) from V1 to V2. Adolescents with type 1 diabetes reported eating breakfast (3.3 v. 3.8 weekly, p = 0.0002) but also fried foods (1.9 v. 2.3, p = 0.0005) weekly more often from V1 to V2. Adolescents with and without type 1 diabetes met PA recommendations of 60 minutes or more of moderate-to-hard PA daily at both V1 (74% v. 70%, respectively, p = 0.58) and V2 (70% v. 78%, respectively, p = 0.78).

Conclusions: Over 2 years, adolescents with and without type 1 diabetes had a healthier diet with increased fruit and vegetable intake and increased PA. However, neither group met the guidelines of daily breakfast, fruit and vegetable intake. Some diet and PA improvements were seen in adolescents with type 1 diabetes over a 2-year period. Therefore, adolescence could be a beneficial time to target diet and lifestyle interventions to take advantage of this time period when behaviors are being modified.

Keywords: Diet, Physical activity, Type 1 diabetes, Screen time, Adolescents

Background

Diet and physical activity (PA) are fundamental aspects of care in type 1 diabetes, but scant data exist on diet and PA behaviors of adolescents with type 1 diabetes, especially compared to non-diabetic (non-DM) controls [1]. The nutrition guidelines for children with type 1 diabetes are similar to those for the general population with a focus on healthful eating to provide energy intake and nutrients to ensure normal growth and development [2-4]. The USDA Guidelines for Americans 2010 recommends to "build a healthy plate" with half a plate of fruits and vegetables; cut back on foods high in saturated fat, added sugar and salt; choose whole grains and be physically active [5]. The American Academy of Pediatrics (AAP) recommends eating 3 balanced meals/day, eating breakfast daily, and limiting sugary beverages and energy dense foods [6]. The American Diabetes Association (ADA) recommends a diet that includes carbohydrates from fruits, vegetables, and whole grains and limit saturated fat and cholesterol [4].

* Correspondence: Franziska.Bishop@ucdenver.edu
Barbara Davis Center for Childhood Diabetes, University of Colorado Denver, 1775 Aurora Ct, MS F527, 80045 Aurora, CO, USA

The SEARCH for Diabetes in Youth study reported that adolescents with type 1 diabetes do not meet the ADA and AAP dietary recommendations in cross-sectional data [7]. Similarly, youth without diabetes also do not meet the U.S. dietary guidelines [8,9]. Adolescents with and without diabetes do not consume adequate fruit and vegetables and consume too much saturated fat [7,10,11]. However, few studies have compared dietary patterns in adolescents with type 1 diabetes to non-DM controls, and none longitudinally [1].

Youth with type 1 diabetes are encouraged to exercise for health to promote benefits such as weight control, cardiovascular fitness, improved blood pressure, and lipid profile [12]. The ADA recommends moderate-intensity PA for at least 30-60 minutes per day [12] and limiting sedentary activities. Current PA guidelines recommend that all school-age children participate in at least 60 minutes of moderate-to-vigorous intensity daily [13] and the AAP recommends no more than 1-2 hours of screen time per day [14]. Excessive screen time can replace or limit PA and has been linked to obesity, poorer glycemic control, behavioral problems, and impaired academic performance [14,15].

Herein we report diet, PA and screen time patterns in youth with and without type 1 diabetes in the "Determinants of Macrovascular Disease in Adolescents with Type 1 Diabetes" study at baseline and at the 2-year follow-up visit. Our objective is to examine the differences in diet and PA in adolescents with and without type 1 diabetes over 2 years. Diet and PA recommendations are similar for adolescents with and without type 1 diabetes; however, adolescents with type 1 diabetes receive regular care from their diabetes care team and should receive more diet and PA education, support and counseling. Therefore, we hypothesized that adolescents with type 1 diabetes would have improved diet and PA patterns compared to non-DM controls at baseline and over the course of the study period.

Methods
The Determinants of Macrovascular Disease in Adolescents with Type 1 Diabetes study prospectively assessed early cardiovascular disease (CVD) risk factors in youth with and without type 1 diabetes [16-18]. The main specific aim was to assess the prevalence, treatment, and control of established CVD risk factors, including glycemic control, blood pressure, and lipid levels, and their association with vascular function in a cohort of 300 youth with type 1 diabetes, age 12-19 years. Secondly, the study compared the CVD risk profile of the 300 youth with type 1 diabetes with that of 100 non-DM controls of similar age and gender. The study then followed the cohort for 2 years. Enrollment began in 2008 for the baseline visit (V1) and concluded in 2012 for the 2-year follow-up visit (V2). At

V1, participants were ages 12-19 and those with type 1 diabetes were diagnosed by the presence of islet antibodies or by provider clinical diagnosis, had diabetes duration > 5 years at entry into the study, and received care at the Barbara Davis Center for Childhood Diabetes. Non-DM control participants were recruited from campus and community advertisements as well as from friends of the study participants. No siblings of patients with type 1 diabetes were included. Participants were excluded for diabetes of any other type. The study was approved by the Colorado Multiple Institution Review Board and informed consent and assent (for subjects <18 years) was obtained in all participants. All study participants were invited back for V2.

At V1 and V2 all participants had anthropometric and questionnaire data collected. Diet data (meals/day, snacks/day, and weekly consumption of breakfast, fruit, vegetables, sweets/desserts, fried foods, restaurant meals, and sugary beverages), physical activity, and screen time (T.V., video games, and computer) were collected using interviewer-administered questionnaires (Additional file 1). Adolescents were administered the questionnaire alone without parent(s) in the room. Dietary practices consisted of frequency of consumption of the following: restaurant meals (including fast food), sweetened beverages, meals per day, snacks per day, breakfast, fruit, vegetables, fried foods and sweets/desserts. Frequency was coded as times per week. Meals per day and snacks per day were reported as: one, two, three, four or five or more per day. For PA, days per week, hours per day (on days where PA took place) and exercise level (light, moderate and hard; the definition of intensity was explained to participants with examples) were asked. Meeting PA guidelines was defined as 60 minutes or more of moderate-to-hard physical activity daily per U.S and international PA recommendations. For screen time; hours per day on TV, hours per day on computer and hours per day on video/electronic games were asked. For total screen time, TV, computer and video/electric games hours per day were combined. Height was measured by a wall-mounted stadiometer to the nearest 0.1 cm with shoes removed and weight by a Detecto scale to the nearest 0.1 kg. Waist circumference was measured at the navel on bare skin using the Figure Finder Tape Measure by Novel Products, Inc (Rockton, IL), which provides consistent and repeatable 4 oz. of tension and accuracy to 3/32 inch. BMI was calculated and in subjects <20 years of age, BMI z-score and BMI percentile was calculated using the 2000 Centers for Disease Control and Prevention growth chart standards. When calculating BMI-z-score and BMI-percentile at V2, 42 participants were excluded from the analysis due to age cutoffs (>20 years old). HbA1c was measured on the DCA Advantage by Siemens at the Children's Hospital Colorado (Aurora, CO) main clinical lab.

Statistical analysis

Stratified two sample t-tests were used to examine differences across groups for continuous variables, and chi square tests were used to test for differences in categorical data. Change between V1 and V2 in each group was measured using paired t-tests. Only participants that completed both V1 and V2 were included (N = 278). Pearson correlations were performed to calculate correlation coefficients for BMI-z and HbA1c with dietary habits, PA, and screen time for T1D and non-DM. Multivariate analyses were used to determine the effect of sex on dietary habits, PA, and screen time. A p-value less than 0.05 was considered significant. Analyses were performed using SAS version 9.3 (SAS Institute, Cary, NC).

Results

A total of 400 participants completed V1 (type 1 diabetes n = 300, non-DM n = 100) and 278 participants completed V2 (type 1 diabetes n = 211, non-DM n = 67). Data in 211 adolescents with type 1 diabetes (baseline age = 15.3 ± 2.2 years, diabetes duration = 8.8 ± 3.1 years, A1c = 9.0 ± 1.5%, 51% male) and 67 non-DM controls (age = 14.9 ± 1.7 years, 52% male) were collected at V1 and again at V2 (mean follow up = 2.2 ± 0.4 years) and were included for this analysis (Table 1). Age and gender were similar in both groups at V1 and V2, but race-ethnicity differed, and adolescents with type 1 diabetes were slightly older than non-DM controls at V2. Adolescents with type 1 diabetes had higher BMI (p = 0.05) and BMI z-score (p = 0.01) at V1; there were no differences between diabetes status and BMI percentile categories (normal, <85th percentile and overweight or obese, ≥85th percentile) at V1. At V2, BMI z-score was significantly higher in adolescents with type 1 diabetes compared to non-DM controls (p = 0.04). There were no differences in BMI-percentile categories (normal, <85th percentile vs.

overweight or obese, >85th percentile) in adolescents with type 1 diabetes compared to non-DM controls at V2. Waist and hip measurements were similar in both groups at both visits.

Table 2 shows the diet, PA, and screen time data for both groups at V1 and V2 and the change between visits within adolescents with type 1 diabetes and within non-DM controls. Both adolescents with and without type 1 diabetes reported increased vegetable and fruit intake from V1 to V2 and these changes were significant (all p-values <0.0001). Adolescents with type 1 diabetes reported eating breakfast more often from V1 to V2; however, at V2 both adolescents with type 1 diabetes and non-DM controls ate breakfast fewer than 4 times per week (3.8 vs. 3.7, respectively, p = 0.0002). Both adolescents with and without type 1 diabetes consumed 3 meals per day and this frequency was consistent from V1 to V2. Snack consumption was the same in both groups at approximately 2 snacks per day and this did not change from V1 to V2. Surprisingly, at V1 adolescents with type 1 diabetes consumed as many sugary beverages as non-DM controls (2.6 vs. 2.8 per week, respectively, p = 0.32); however, at V2 adolescents with type 1 diabetes consumed less sugary beverages (2.7 vs. 3.2, respectively, p = 0.02). For restaurant meals there was no difference in adolescents with and without type 1 diabetes at V1 or V2; however, adolescents with type 1 diabetes did eat significantly fewer restaurant meals at V2 than V1 (2.1 vs. 1.7, p = .0008). At V1, adolescents with and without type 1 diabetes consumed fried foods at the same frequency per week (1.9 v. 1.8, respectively, p = 0.51). At V2, adolescents with type 1 diabetes reported more fried food consumption (1.9 vs. 2.3, p = 0.0005) while there was no change in consumption for non-DM controls. Overall there was no difference in consumption of sweets/desserts among adolescents with and without type 1 diabetes with both groups consuming

Table 1 Demographics at baseline (V1) and 2-year follow-up (V2)

	Visit 1			Visit 2		
	T1D	Non-DM	p-value	T1D	Non-DM	p-value
Age, years	15.3 ± 2.2	14.9 ± 1.7	0.13	17.5 ± 2.3	16.9 ± 1.9	0.04
Male, %	51%	52%	0.88	NA	NA	–
Race-Ethnicity, % NHW	86%	73%	0.01	NA	NA	–
T1D Duration, years	8.8 ± 3.1	NA	–	11.0 ± 3.2	NA	–
CSII pump, %	62%	NA	–	61%	NA	–
HbA1c, %	9.0 ± 1.5	5.3 ± 0.3	<0.0001	9.1 ± 1.7	5.2 ± 0.2	<0.0001
BMI, kg/m²	22.6 ± 3.7	21.4 ± 4.5	0.05	23.8 ± 3.6	22.8 ± 5.1	0.13
BMI z-score	0.61 ± 0.76	0.22 ± 1.1	0.01	0.55 ± 0.83	0.24 ± 1.05	0.04
Waist, cm	76.5 ± 9.9	74.4 ± 12.1	0.17	81.8 ± 9.3	78.7 ± 13.6	0.08
Hip, cm	94.0 ± 10.2	91.1 ± 11.1	0.06	97.7 ± 7.6	95.0 ± 11.2	0.07

T1D: Type 1 Diabetes.
Non-DM: non-diabetic control.

Table 2 Change between baseline (V1) and 2-year follow-up (V2) within T1D and non-DM

	T1D			Non-DM		
	Visit 1	Visit 2	Change	Visit 1	Visit 2	Change
Diet						
Meals/day	3.0 ± 0.6	2.9 ± 0.6	-0.1 ± 7.5**	3.0 ± 0.7	2.9 ± 0.7	-0.06 ± 0.6
Snacks/day	2.3 ± 1.2	2.3 ± 1.3	-0.05 ± 1.3	2.2 ± 1.0	2.2 ± 1.1	-0.01 ± 1.2
Breakfast[#]	3.3 ± 1.2	3.8 ± 1.6	0.45 ± 1.7**	3.5 ± 1.0	3.7 ± 1.8	0.15 ± 1.7
Vegetables[#]	2.8 ± 1.1*	3.6 ± 1.4	0.87 ± 1.5**	3.1 ± 1.2*	3.8 ± 1.3	0.69 ± 1.3**
Fruit[#]	2.9 ± 1.2	3.8 ± 1.3	0.89 ± 1.4**	2.9 ± 1.3	3.8 ± 1.5	0.85 ± 1.6**
Sugary beverages[#]	2.6 ± 1.4	2.7 ± 1.7*	0.06 ± 2.1	2.8 ± 1.3	3.2 ± 1.7*	0.45 ± 2.2
Restaurant meals[#]	2.1 ± 1.6	1.7 ± 1.0	-0.44 ± 1.9**	2.2 ± 1.6	1.8 ± 1.2	-0.34 ± 2.3
Fried foods[#]	1.9 ± 1.2	2.3 ± 1.3	0.41 ± 1.7**	1.8 ± 1.1	2.1 ± 1.2	0.27 ± 1.6
Sweets/Desserts[#]	2.1 ± 1.3	2.2 ± 1.3	0.11 ± 1.7	2.3 ± 1.3	2.4 ± 1.7	0.18 ± 1.9
Physical activity (PA)						
PA days/week	5.0 ± 1.8	4.8 ± 1.7	-0.29 ± 2.2	4.9 ± 1.7	4.5 ± 1.9	-0.41 ± 2.3
PA hours/day	1.8 ± 1.2*	2.2 ± 1.4	0.35 ± 1.6**	1.5 ± 0.8*	1.9 ± 1.3	0.43 ± 1.2**
PA level[†]	1.9 ± 0.6	2.0 ± 0.5	0.06 ± 0.7	2.0 ± 0.5	2.1 ± 0.6	0.12 ± 0.7
Screen time						
Computer hours[+]	1.5 ± 1.7	2.5 ± 2.5	0.98 ± 2.6**	1.6 ± 1.7	2.2 ± 2.4	0.61 ± 1.9**
TV hours[+]	2.0 ± 1.9	1.9 ± 1.7	-0.12 ± 1.7	1.7 ± 1.6	1.9 ± 1.4	0.14 ± 1.5
Video games hours[+]	0.9 ± 1.3	0.8 ± 1.2	-0.08 ± 1.2	0.8 ± 1.1	0.7 ± 1.2	-0.04 ± 1.1
Total screen time[+]	4.3 ± 3.3	5.1 ± 3.5	0.78 ± 3.3**	4.1 ± 2.8	4.8 ± 3.0	0.7 ± 2.4**
Anthropometric						
BMI z-score	0.6 ± 0.8*	0.5 ± 0.8*	-0.04 ± 0.56	0.2 ± 1.1*	0.2 ± 1.1*	0.04 ± 0.46

T1D: Type 1 Diabetes.
Non-DM: non-diabetic control.
[#]Times per week.
[†]PA level: 1 = mild, 2 = moderate, 3 = hard.
[+]hours per day.
*p < 0.05 comparing T1D and non-DM at visit 1 or visit 2.
**p < 0.05 comparing change between visit 1 and visit 2 within T1D and non-DM.

sweets/desserts twice a week. There were no significant changes in BMI-z score for adolescents with and without type 1 diabetes over time from V1 to V2 (Table 2).

At V1 74% of adolescents with type 1 diabetes met PA recommendations of 60 minutes or more of moderate-to-hard PA daily compared to 70% of non-DM controls (p = 0.58). At V2 the percentage of adolescents with and without type 1 diabetes that met PA recommendations increased to 80% and 78%, respectively, and the difference between groups was not significant (p = 0.78). Additionally, the change within adolescents with type 1 diabetes and within non-DM controls from V1 to V2 was not significant. Both groups performed PA on most days of the week at a moderate-to-hard level for at least 60 minutes on days PA was performed (see Table 2). At V1, adolescents with type 1 diabetes reported more time spent performing PA than non-DM controls (p = 0.02) yet the number of days of PA and level of intensity were the same in both groups. There were no differences reported in days per week PA was performed at V2 between groups,

although both adolescents with and without type 1 diabetes reported an increase in PA time (hours per day on days PA was performed) from V1 to V2 (p = 0.005 and p = 0.008, respectively).

For screen time, TV and video/electronic game hours per day were the same for both adolescents with and without type 1 diabetes at V1 and V2 and there were no changes within each group from V1 to V2. Computer hours per day did increase for adolescents with type 1 diabetes and non-DM controls from V1 to V2 (1.5 vs. 2.5, p < 0.0001 and 1.6 vs. 2.2, p = 0.01, respectively). Total screen time increased to over 4 hours per day for adolescents with and without type 1 diabetes (p = 0.0009 and p = 0.02, respectively) due to the increased computer time reported.

In post-hoc analyses the associations between A1c and BMI-z score and diet, PA, and screen time in adolescents with type 1 diabetes were performed. At V1, there was a positive association with A1c and exercise (hours per day, p = 0.02) in adolescents with type 1 diabetes. At V2, A1c was positively correlated with screen time (TV hours, video game hours, overall screen time, $p = 0.02$, $p = 0.02$, $p = 0.001$, respectively) in adolescents with type 1 diabetes. BMI-z score was negatively correlated with meals per day ($p = 0.001$) and frequency of snacks ($p = 0.04$) at V2 in adolescents with type 1 diabetes.

Discussion

Over 2 years, adolescents with and without type 1 diabetes reported a healthier diet with increased fruit and vegetable intake and increased PA. However, both groups are far from meeting the guidelines of daily fruit and vegetables intake or daily consumption of breakfast. Adolescents with type 1 diabetes also reported increased fried food intake from V1 to V2. This suggests that further attention to dietary recommendations and education are needed for adolescents with type 1 diabetes.

The SEARCH for Diabetes in Youth study also showed poor adherence to dietary guidelines with less than 50% of the cohort meeting ADA recommendations for total fat, fiber, fruits, vegetables and grains [7]. Although the SEARCH for Diabetes in Youth study used detailed food frequency methodology for diet data collection, the SEARCH data and our data similarly demonstrate that adolescents with type 1 diabetes did not meet the dietary guidelines of eating fruits and vegetables daily. Additionally, we were able to compare dietary patterns between adolescents with and without type 1 diabetes over time. Neither group met dietary recommendations despite adolescents with type 1 diabetes receiving dietary education from their diabetes care team.

In cross-sectional data, Nansel et al. reported that children and adolescents consume less than half of the recommended intake of fruit, vegetables, and whole grains and exceed saturated fat intake [19]. In addition, results from the Coronary Artery Calcification in Type 1 Diabetes (CACTI) study demonstrated that young adults with type 1 diabetes consume excess fat and saturated fat [20]. Similarly our data found that adolescents with type 1 diabetes are consuming more fried foods over time. A recent study in adolescents with type 1 diabetes reported that over half of youth with type 1 diabetes consume more cholesterol than recommended by U.S. and international guidelines and this was positively correlated with A1c and calories consumed as fat [21]. Poor dietary habits start in youth and can persist into adulthood, which is of particular concern for adolescents with type 1 diabetes due to their elevated risk of cardiovascular disease.

The majority of adolescents with type 1 diabetes (74%) and non-DM controls (70%) met the PA guidelines of 60 minutes or more of moderate-to-hard PA daily over the 2-year study period. Even though adolescents with type 1 diabetes reported increased PA time on active days compared to non-DM controls at V1, BMI and BMI z-score were higher in adolescents with type 1 diabetes. At V2, BMI z-score continued to be higher in adolescents with type 1 diabetes compared to non-DM controls. The T1D Exchange has recently reported that 39% of 13-19 year olds had a BMI > 85th% for age and sex [22]. The Hvidoere study group reported that adolescents with type 1 diabetes are only physically active for 60 minutes or more 3-4 days per week; therefore, not meeting international PA recommendations for 60 minutes of exercise daily [23] in contrast to our data. Overby et al. reported that only 54% of children and adolescents with type 1 diabetes meet PA recommendations [24]. NHANES data from 1999-2006 in U.S. adolescents aged 12-17 reported that less than 20% of adolescents reported meeting the 2008 Physical Activity Guidelines for Americans [25]. However, our cohort is from Colorado which is one of the healthiest states in the U.S. and ranked lowest for BMI and sedentary activity [26] and therefore may not be representative of the U.S. as a whole. The Youth and Risk Behavior Survey in 2011 reported that 53% of Colorado high school students reported physical activity at least 60 minutes per day on 5 or more days [27]. Additionally 23% of Colorado children are overweight or obese [28] with an obesity ranking of 23rd among the US states [29]. In our study 30% of adolescents with and without type 1 diabetes were overweight or obese. Even though this study's participants meet the PA recommendations they are similarly overweight and obese compared to Colorado as a whole.

There may be sex-specific differences in PA; men with type 1 diabetes from the CACTI study reported increased PA than non-DM men but women with type 1 diabetes reported less PA than non-DM women [30]. The Hvidoere Study also found similar patterns in their adolescent cohort with males with type 1 diabetes being more active than females with type 1 diabetes [23]. These data suggest sex-specific differences in PA in adults and adolescents with type 1 diabetes. The current study found small differences between males and females with type 1 diabetes for time spent in PA at V1 or V2. Males with type 1 diabetes did report higher PA intensity at V2 ($p = 0.047$) than females with type 1 diabetes, and females reported more exercise days per week at V2 ($p = 0.05$) than males, but overall PA time was the same.

Screen time was elevated in both groups well over the 1-2 hour per day guidelines. Excess screen time is associated with many health and wellness issues such as obesity, higher A1c, poor academic performance, and decreased PA. Specifically, Overby et al. showed that children with type 1 diabetes watch an excess of amount of TV (>2 hours per day) and TV viewing was related to overweight children and adolescents with type 1 diabetes [24]. Similarly, the Hvidoere study group also reported that adolescents with type 1 diabetes watch more than 2 hours of TV daily [23]. In our study, adolescents with type 1 diabetes and non-DM adolescents also exceeded the TV viewing or screen time recommendation of less than 2 hours per day, and A1c and screen time were positively associated in adolescents with type 1 diabetes.

Strengths of this study include a non-DM control group and longitudinal data over a 2-year study period. All questionnaires were interviewer-administered and asked without parent(s) in the room to improve accuracy of data (see Additional file 1: Questionnaires). Limitations of these data include self-reported diet, PA and screen time, therefore reporting bias may exist. The questionnaires used for assessing diet, PA and screen time were not validated. Diet, PA and screen time were not variables associated with the specific aims of the study and there was limited time for lifestyle-related questions. For this reason 3-day food and PA records, a standard for dietary and PA assessment were not used. Diet, PA and screen time questions were created to assess dietary, PA and screen time patterns as recommended by national guidelines (such as daily fruit and vegetable intake and daily PA). Frequency of servings of foods (meals, fruits, vegetables and fried foods) vs. percent or amount of foods consumed was asked to limit the impact of increased energy intake as adolescents get older. The diet, PA and screen time questionnaires were designed to assess lifestyle patterns only and not detailed nutrient intake or direct measures of energy expenditure; however, this would not explain differences reported between groups. We looked at percent of participants who met the PA guidelines in order to compare our findings with the literature and further explain the data. All adolescents were asked how often they consumed sugary beverages on a weekly basis. However, the questionnaire did not differentiate sugary beverages consumed to treat hypoglycemia, although interview-administrators told participants with type 1 diabetes to exclude sugary beverages used to treat hypoglycemia.

Only study participants that completed both study visits were included in this analysis. There were no differences in adolescents with type 1 diabetes for age, sex, A1c, BMI, BMI z-score, BMI percentile, or diabetes duration that completed V1 and V2 compared to adolescents with type 1 diabetes that only completed V1. Among non-DM controls, there were no differences in sex, BMI, BMI z-score, and BMI percentile that completed V1 and V2 compared to non-DM adolescents that only completed V1. Non-DM controls that completed V1 and V2 were significantly younger than those who only completed V1 (14.9 vs. 16.3, p = 0.0023). Although significant, the age difference between non-DM controls who completed V1 vs. V1 and V2 was not substantial (15 years old vs. 16 years old) or clinically relevant. Adolescents with type 1 diabetes reported more non-Hispanic White race/ethnicity which would be expected given that the disease prevalence is higher in the non-Hispanic White race/ethnicity. Factors that may have affected study participants completing V2 include the nature of the age range (adolescents and young adults) and the location of the Barbara Davis Center. The Barbara Davis Center may not be very convenient to visit for the general population since it is a part of a large medical campus, while the adolescents with type 1 diabetes are at the center regularly for their routine clinic visits and their study visit was often scheduled the same day. The teenage and young adult age range is known to be a difficult age to recruit and retain as teenagers become more independent and often leave for college, move away from home and become in charge of their medical care.

Conclusions

Adolescents with and without type 1 diabetes have similarly poor dietary habits. Over a 2-year period, adolescents with and without type 1 diabetes reported consuming more fruits and vegetables; however, adolescents with type 1 diabetes do not meet the guidelines of daily fruit, vegetable and breakfast intake. Furthermore, fried food intake increased over the 2 year period for adolescents with type 1 diabetes which is of particular concern due to their elevated risk of cardiovascular disease. Adolescents with type 1 diabetes do meet the PA guidelines yet BMI and BMI z-score are higher in adolescents with type 1 diabetes compared to non-DM controls. Screen time was also elevated over the recommended 2 hours or less per day and total screen time increased over time. Adolescents with type 1 diabetes and non-DM controls have similarly poor dietary patterns, despite adolescents with type 1 diabetes receiving dietary education and support through their diabetes care. Some diet and PA improvements were seen in adolescents with type 1 diabetes over a 2-year period. Therefore, adolescence could be a beneficial time to target diet and lifestyle interventions to take advantage of this time period when behaviors are being modified.

Competing interests
The authors declare that they have no competing interests.

Authors' contributions
FKB coordinated and supervised the data collection, wrote the manuscript and approved the final manuscript for submission. RPW conceptualized and designed the study, researched, contributed to discussion, reviewed and revised the manuscript and approved the final manuscript for submission. JSB reviewed and revised the manuscript and approved the final manuscript for submission. NN analyzed data and reviewed and revised the manuscript and approved the final manuscript for submission. DMM researched, analyzed data, contributed to the discussion and reviewed and revised the manuscript and approved the final manuscript for submission. All authors read and approved the final manuscript.

Acknowledgments

We would like to thank the study participants and their families as well as the staff of the Barbara Davis Center for Childhood Diabetes for making this study possible. Dr. Maahs was supported by a grant from NIDDK (DK075360) and Dr. Wadwa by an early career award from the Juvenile Diabetes Research Foundation (11-2007-694). This project was supported in part by NIH/NCATS Colorado CTSI Grant Number UL1 TR000154. Its contents are the authors' sole responsibility and do not necessarily represent official NIH views. The authors have no conflicts of interest to disclose.

References

1. Rovner AJ, Nansel TR: **Are children with type 1 diabetes consuming a healthful diet?: a review of the current evidence and strategies for dietary change.** *Diabetes Educ* 2009, **35**:97–107.

2. Smart C, Slander-van VE, Waldron S: **Nutritional management in children and adolescents with diabetes.** *Pediatr Diabetes* 2009, **10**(Suppl 12):100–117.

3. Bantle JP, Wylie-Rosett J, Albright AL, Apovian CM, Clark NG, Franz MJ, Hoogwerf BJ, Lichtenstein AH, Mayer-Davis E, Mooradian AD, Wheeler ML: **Nutrition recommendations and interventions for diabetes: a position statement of the American Diabetes Association.** *Diabetes Care* 2008, **31**(Suppl 1):S61–S78.

4. Franz MJ, Bantle JP, Beebe CA, Brunzell JD, Chiasson JL, Garg A, Holzmeister LA, Hoogwerf B, Mayer-Davis E, Mooradian AD, Purnell JQ, Wheeler M: **Evidence-based nutrition principles and recommendations for the treatment and prevention of diabetes and related complications.** *Diabetes Care* 2003, **26**(Suppl 1):S51–S61.

5. USDA: *USDA Guidelines for Americans.* 2010. http://www.cnpp.usda.gov/dietaryguidelines.htm. 1-31-2011.

6. Gidding SS, Dennison BA, Birch LL, Daniels SR, Gillman MW, Lichtenstein AH, Rattay KT, Steinberger J, Stettler N, Van HL: **Dietary recommendations for children and adolescents: a guide for practitioners.** *Pediatrics* 2006, **117**(2):544–559.

7. Mayer-Davis EJ, Nichols M, Liese AD, Bell RA, Dabelea DM, Johansen JM, Pihoker C, Rodriguez BL, Thomas J, Williams D: **Dietary intake among youth with diabetes: the SEARCH for Diabetes in Youth Study.** *J Am Diet Assoc* 2006, **106**:689–697.

8. Krebs-Smith SM, Guenther PM, Subar AF, Sharon LK, Dodd KW: **American do not meet federal dietary recommendations.** *J Nutr* 2010, **140**(10):1832–1838.

9. Kirkpatrick SI, Dodd KW, Reedy J, Krebs-Smith SM: **Income and race/ethnicity are associated with adherence to food-based dietary guidance among US adults and children.** *J Acad Nutr Diet* 2012, **112**:624–635.

10. U.S. Department of Agriculture: *Continuing Survey of Food Intakes by Individuals 1994-96.* 1998.

11. Eaton DK, Kann L, Kinchen S, Shanklin S, Ross J, Hawkins J, Harris WA, Lowry R, McManus T, Chyen D, Lim C, Whittle L, Brener ND, Wechsler H: *Youth Risk Behavior Surveillance - U.S. 2010.* 2010.

12. Silverstein J, Klingensmith G, Copeland K, Plotnick L, Kaufman F, Laffel L, Deeb L, Grey M, Anderson B, Holzmeister LA, Clark N: **Care of children and adolescents with type 1 diabetes: a statement of the American Diabetes Association.** *Diabetes Care* 2005, **28**:186–212.

13. Strong WB, Malina RM, Blimkie CJ, Daniels SR, Dishman RK, Gutin B, Hergenroeder AC, Must A, Nixon PA, Pivarnik JM, Rowland T, Trost S, Trudeau F: **Evidence based physical activity for school-age youth.** *J Pediatr* 2005, **146**:732–737.

14. American Academy of Pediatrics: **Children, adolescents, and television.** *Pediatrics* 2001, **107**:423–426.

15. Margeirsdottir HD, Larsen JR, Brunborg C, Sandvik L, Dahl-Jorgensen K: **Strong association between time watching television and blood glucose control in children and adolescents with type 1 diabetes.** *Diabetes Care* 2007, **30**:1567–1570.

16. Specht BJ, Wadwa RP, Snell-Bergeon JK, Nadeau KJ, Bishop FK, Maahs DM: **Estimated insulin sensitivity and cardiovascular disease risk factors in adolescents with and without type 1 diabetes.** *J Pediatr* 2013, **162**:297–301.

17. Clements SA, Anger MD, Bishop FK, McFann KK, Klingensmith GJ, Maahs DM, Wadwa RP: **Lower A1c among adolescents with lower perceived A1c goal: a cross-sectional survey.** *Int J Pediatr Endocrinol* 2013, **2013**:17.

18. Maahs DM, Prentice N, McFann K, Snell-Bergeon JK, Jalal D, Bishop FK, Aragon B, Wadwa RP: **Age and sex influence cystatin C in adolescents with and without type 1 diabetes.** *Diabetes Care* 2011, **34**:2360–2362.

19. Nansel TR, Haynie DL, Lipsky LM, Laffel LM, Mehta SN: **Multiple indicators of poor diet quality in children and adolescents with type 1 diabetes are associated with higher body mass index percentile but not glycemic control.** *J Acad Nutr Diet* 2012, **112**:1728–1735.

20. Snell-Bergeon JK, Chartier-Logan C, Maahs DM, Ogden LG, Hokanson JE, Kinney GL, Eckel RH, Ehrlich J, Rewers M: **Adults with type 1 diabetes eat a high-fat atherogenic diet that is associated with coronary artery calcium.** *Diabetologia* 2009, **52**:801–809.

21. O'Brecht L, Streisand R, Holmes CS, Mackey ER: **Nutrition intake in early adolescents with type 1 diabetes.** *PES* 2013, Abstract 1522.291.

22. Wood JR, Miller KM, Maahs DM, Beck RW, Dimeglio LA, Libman IM, Quinn M, Tamborlane WV, Woerner SE: **Most youth with type 1 diabetes in the T1D exchange clinic registry do not meet American Diabetes Association or International Society for Pediatric and Adolescent Diabetes Clinical Guidelines.** *Diabetes Care* 2013, **36**:2035–2037.

23. Aman J, Skinner TC, de Beaufort CE, Swift PG, Aanstoot HJ, Cameron F: **Associations between physical activity, sedentary behavior, and glycemic control in a large cohort of adolescents with type 1 diabetes: the Hvidoere Study Group on Childhood Diabetes.** *Pediatr Diabetes* 2009, **10**:234–239.

24. Overby NC, Margeirsdottir HD, Brunborg C, Anderssen SA, Andersen LF, Dahl-Jorgensen K: **Physical activity and overweight in children and adolescents using intensified insulin treatment.** *Pediatr Diabetes* 2009, **10**:135–141.

25. Song M, Carroll DD, Fulton JE: **Meeting the 2008 physical activity guidelines for americans among U.S. youth.** *Am J Prev Med* 2013, **44**:216–222.

26. America's Health Rankings: *United Health Foundation. Colorado 2012*; 2012.

27. Eaton DK, Kann L, Kinchen S, Shanklin S, Flint KH, Hawkins J, Harris WA, Lowry R, McManus T, Chyen D, Whittle L, Lim C, Wechsler H: **Youth risk behavior surveillance - United States, 2011.** *MMWR Surveill Summ* 2012, **61**:1–162.

28. Colorado Department of Public Health and Environment: *Colorado Child Health Survey.* Colorado: Department of Public Health and Environment; 2010.

29. *2007 National Survey of Children's Health.* 2007, www.childhealthdata.org/docs/nsch-docs/childhealthmeasures_03_vs_07_v2_508-pdf.pdf. Online source.

30. Bishop FK, Maahs DM, Snell-Bergeon JK, Ogden LG, Kinney GL, Rewers M: **Lifestyle risk factors for atherosclerosis in adults with type 1 diabetes.** *Diab Vasc Dis Res* 2009, **6**:269–275.

10

Physical, social and societal functioning of children with congenital adrenal hyperplasia (CAH) and their parents, in a Dutch population

Sarita A Sanches[1,2], Therese A Wiegers[1*], Barto J Otten[3] and Hedi L Claahsen-van der Grinten[3]

Abstract

Background: Most research concerning congenital adrenal hyperplasia (CAH) and related conditions caused by primary adrenal insufficiency, such as Addison's or Cushing's disease, has focused on medical aspects rather than on patients' quality of life. Therefore, our objective was to investigate the physical, social and societal functioning of children with CAH and their parents in a Dutch population.

Methods: The study is descriptive and cross-sectional. Self-designed questionnaires, based on questionnaires developed in the Netherlands for different patient groups, were sent to parents of children with CAH between 0 and 18 years old. Participants were recruited through the Dutch patient group for Adrenal Disease (NVACP) and six hospitals in the Netherlands. Three different questionnaires were designed for parents: for children aged 0 - 4, aged 4 - 12 and aged 12 - 18. Additionally, a fourth questionnaire was sent to adolescents with CAH aged 12 - 18. Main outcome measures were experienced burden of the condition, self-management and participation in several areas, such as school and leisure time.

Results: A total of 106 parents returned the questionnaire, 12 regarding pre-school children (0-4 years), 63 regarding primary school children (4-12 years), and 32 regarding secondary school children (12-18 years), combined response rate 69.7%. Also, 24 adolescents returned the questionnaire. Children and adolescents with CAH appear to be capable of self-management at a young age. Experienced burden of the condition is low, although children experience several health related problems on a daily basis. Children participate well in school and leisure time. Few children carry a crisis card or emergency injection with them.

Conclusions: Overall, our research shows that, according to their parents, children with CAH experience few negative effects of the condition and that they participate well in several areas such as school and leisure time. However, improvements can be made concerning the measures parents and children must take to prevent an adrenal crisis.

Keywords: CAH, children, quality of life, social functioning, burden of disease, self-management, participation, Netherlands, parents, comorbidity, preventive measures

Background

Congenital Adrenal Hyperplasia (CAH) is an inherited disorder of the adrenal cortex caused by deficiency of enzymes involved in adrenal steroidogenesis, most often a deficiency of 21-hydroxylase [1-4]. This defect results in an impaired production of cortisol and mostly also of aldosterone and an excessive production of adrenal androgens. The clinical picture depends on the degree of the enzymatic block: the most severe form, the classic CAH (almost always apparent at birth) and the mild non-classic form (mostly diagnosed later in life). In general, CAH has larger implications for females than males. Furthermore, the classical form is subclassified in the salt wasting (SW) and the simple virilising form (SV) [3]. Females with the classic form of CAH are born with ambiguous external genitalia caused by the excessive

* Correspondence: T.Wiegers@nivel.nl
[1]Netherlands institute for health services research (NIVEL), P.O. Box 1568, 3500 BN Utrecht, The Netherlands
Full list of author information is available at the end of the article

amount of androgens already in utero [3,5]. In these cases, surgery is often necessary to correct the external genitalia. Treatment of CAH consists of long-term glucocorticoid and mostly also mineralocorticoid substitution [6]. Increased dosages of glucocorticoids are necessary in case of physical stress to prevent life threatening Addisonian (adrenal) crisis. Overtreatment can lead to growth inhibition, excess weight, and several daily health related problems such as sleepiness and abdominal pain. Undertreatment can lead to symptoms of androgen excess such as signs of early puberty, early growth acceleration and reduced final height. In the Netherlands, the prevalence of CAH is about 1 in 12.000. Every year, 15 to 20 infants are newly diagnosed with the disorder [7]. Since 2000, CAH is part of the neonatal screening programme in the Netherlands to prevent life threatening Adrenal crisis.

Studies focussing on quality of life in patients with adrenal diseases are rare. Only recently some studies have been published about the quality of life of adult patients with Addison's disease. Most of these studies have shown a reduced quality of life, especially in adult patients with comorbidity. Furthermore, a recent study [8] found that the objective and subjective health status in adult CAH patients in the United Kingdom was significantly impaired. However, no research has been carried out to study the quality of life of children with primary adrenal insufficiency.

The aim of our study is to investigate the quality of life of children and adolescents with CAH and their parents by studying physical, social and societal functioning of children with CAH and their parents.

Methods
Subjects
Parents of children with all types of CAH were recruited through the Dutch patient group Adrenal Disease (NVACP). Additionally, several hospitals in the Netherlands were asked to inform their patients about the research. A total of six hospitals participated in the study, five university hospitals and one general hospital.

Assessments
Self designed questionnaires, based on questionnaires developed in the Netherlands for different patient groups, were used to measure the following sub-concepts: social demographics (i.e. sex, age, parents' education, country of origin), characteristics of the condition (i.e. CAH subtype, comorbidity, CAH-medication use), experienced burden of the condition (physical and mental problems, constraints, adrenal crisis), self management (lifestyle, social support, general medication use) and participation in several areas such as school and leisure time. The questions were derived from the Second National Survey of General Practice (DNSGP-2) [9], a Dutch study concerning quality

of life of (adult) patients with Addison's disease, Cushing's disease and CAH [10] and a Dutch study concerning young adults with chronic digestive disorders [11].

Three different questionnaires were developed for parents of different age groups. A questionnaire for parents of children aged 0 - 4, 4 - 12 and 12 - 18. This distinction was based on the Dutch schooling system. Children aged 0 - 4 do not go to school yet, children aged 4 - 12 receive primary education and children aged 12 - 18 receive secondary education. The questionnaires were largely the same, except for some age-specific questions, for instance, about school, work and going out. Adolescents of 12 - 18 years were also invited to fill out a questionnaire themselves [12].

Study design
In this study, quality of life is defined according to the sub-concepts used by Heijmans et al [10] in a Dutch report about the impact of Addison's disease, Cushing's disease and CAH on the daily life of adult patients. The sample of CAH patients in that study was too small to draw conclusions from and children were excluded.

An exploratory design was used to describe the several sub-concepts (see assessments).

Parents and adolescents had the possibility to fill out a paper version or an online version of the questionnaire. For the online version, they received a link to the questionnaire by email. A first reminder was sent after 2-3 weeks. If needed, a second reminder was sent again 2-3 weeks later.

Ethical approval
Ethical approval is not required for this kind of study in the Netherlands.

Analysis
Due to the division in three separate age groups, the number of subjects in each age group was relatively small, which hampered the use of statistical models. Therefore, the results are mainly descriptive. Each concept was described for each group and groups were compared to study possible differences on the various concepts. Six (for age group 0-4) or seven (for both other age groups) questions have been combined in order to create the scale 'Parents' experiences'. Eight questions were combined to create the scale 'Difficulties'. The reliability of these scales is expressed in Cronbach's alpha. Where possible, comparisons were made with data from the second Dutch National Survey of General Practice (DNSGP-2). DNSGP-2 is a Dutch nationwide study, containing representative information on morbidity in the population, use of health services at patient level, health determinants and sociodemographic characteristics [9]. DNSGP-2 contains data about approximately 50.000 children in the Netherlands,

which makes it a very powerful dataset for comparison. All analyses were carried out with Stata 10.

Results
Response
250 invitations were sent to parents of children with CAH with information about the study and 152 parents enrolled and received a questionnaire. Of those questionnaires 106 were returned fully completed (response rate of 69.7%). Twelve questionnaires were returned by parents of children of 0-4 years, 62 for children of 4-12 years and 32 for adolescents 12-18 years of age. Adolescents themselves returned 24 questionnaires.

Sample characteristics
Parent questionnaires
Sample characteristics are listed in Table 1. The groups 0-4 and 4-12 consisted of slightly more boys than girls. This was reversed in the group 12-18. The age distribution within the groups was skewed. Children under the age of 1 year were not represented in the youngest age group. The middle age group was relatively old with 69% of children being over 7 years old. On the other hand, the oldest age group was relatively young with almost 63% of children being under 15 years old. The mean age of children in the group 0-4 was 2.4 years, in the middle age group 8.5 years and in the oldest age group 15.0 years. Most children (75%) had the salt wasting type of CAH, only 5% of children had the nonclassic type of CAH. In all age groups, boys were more often diagnosed as salt wasters than girls (boys ≥ 80% SW, girls 50-75% SW). The time from the first symptoms until the

definitive diagnosis was shorter for younger children than for older children. Furthermore, younger children experienced fewer health related problems before the time of diagnosis than older children.

Adolescent questionnaires
Sample characteristics are listed in Table 2. 24 questionnaires were returned (62.5% girls). 79% indicated to have reached puberty. 79.2% had salt wasting CAH, 8.3% SV CAH and 1 person (4.2%) had the nonclassic form of CAH. 33% of adolescents reported to experience no daily health related problems, 17% experienced one, 13% two, 4% three, and 33% more than four daily health related problems.

Health related problems at diagnosis
Health related problems often mentioned by parents in all age groups are weight loss, severe somnolence, accelerated growth/development, inability to retain fluids and lack of appetite. About 31% of the children had CAH related complications in the neonatal period. Genital anomalies occurred most often, dehydration due to loss of salt was second. Girls in the younger age groups more often underwent reconstructive surgery than in the older group. One parent of a child aged 0-4 years was dissatisfied with the results of the operation, whereas all other parents of operated children (n = 24) were satisfied with the results of the operation.

Current health related problems and comorbidity
Table 3 shows the number of daily health related problems and the incidence of chronic conditions beside CAH such as asthma or eczema in the sample from the parent questionnaires compared to data from DNSGP-2. Although chronic conditions in addition to CAH were

Table 1 Sample characteristics and characteristics of the condition from parent questionnaires

	0-4 year		4-12 year		12-18 year		Total	
	n	(%)	n	(%)	n	(%)	n	(%)
Total	12	(100)	62	(100)	32	(100)	106	(100)
Sex								
Male	7	(58)	34	(55)	15	(47)	56	(53)
Female	5	(42)	28	(45)	17	(53)	50	(47)
CAH subtype								
Salt wasting form	9	(75)	50	(81)	21	(66)	80	(75)
Simple virilizing form	3	(25)	9	(14)	8	(25)	20	(19)
Non-classical form	0	-	3	(5)	2	(6)	5	(5)
Unknown	0	-	0	-	1	(3)	1	(1)
Diagnosis								
Within 1 week after birth	11	(92)	45	(73)	12	(38)	68	(64)
Health related problems before diagnosis								
Yes	6	(50)	42	(68)	24	(75)	72	(70)
Complications at birth								
Yes	5	(42)	19	(31)	9	(28)	33	(31)
Reconstructive surgery (girls)	n = 5		n = 28		n = 17		n = 50	
Yes	3	(60)	15	(54)	6	(35)	24	(48)

Table 2 Sample characteristics and characteristics of the condition from adolescent questionnaires

	Adolescents	
	n	(%)
Total	24	(100)
Sex		
Male	9	(37.5)
Female	14	(62.5)
Age		
12 - 15	14	(62.5)
15 - 18	9	(37.5)
Reached puberty		
Yes	19	(79)
No	5	(21)
CAH subtype		
Salt wasting form	19	(79)
Simple virilizing form	2	(8)
Non-classical form	1	(4)
Unknown	2	(8)
Number of daily health-related problems		
0	8	(33)
1	4	(17)
2	3	(13)
3	1	(4)
≥ 4	8	(33)

rare in the study population, 71% of the children experienced daily health related problems in the two weeks preceding the questionnaire. The daily health related problems that occurred most often in children with CAH were excessive sweating, mood swings, lack of energy, excitability, fever, sleepiness, crying and pain in the legs and abdomen. However, in all age groups, children with CAH seem to have less daily health related problems than their peers in DNSGP-2 but this finding was not tested for significance. Only children aged 4-12 seem to have more daily health related problems than the other age groups and than children from DNSGP-2.

Experienced burden of the condition

Only 8% of the parents reported that their children experienced constraints in daily life as a result of CAH (Table 4). According to the parents, an adrenal crisis was experienced by 33% of the children. Most parents (83%) indicated that they did not fear the occurrence of an adrenal crisis. About 30% of children aged 4-18 have been absent of school due to CAH in the past year. The percentage of parents feeling their actions can influence the course of the condition declines when the age of the children increases. In total, 96% of the parents indicated to be satisfied with the overall health of their children. All adolescents were satisfied with their own health and 84% of them have no problem with controlling the condition (not shown in Table).

Two scales have been constructed about parents' experiences (Table 5). The scale 'Experiences parents' contains items about parents' experience with the condition of their child (including their own ability to control the condition). The average score on this scale in all three age groups is slightly higher than 3, which indicates that parents are inclined to a more positive feeling. The scale 'Difficulties' contains items about the reasons why parents find it difficult to keep the condition of their child under control, including an item about their fear of an adrenal crisis. The average score on this scale is below

Table 3 Comorbidity and number of daily health-related problems (according to parents) in children with CAH and control children from DNSGP-2

	0-4 CAH	0-4 DNSGP-2	4-12 CAH	5-12 DNSGP-2	12-18 CAH	13-18 DNSGP-2	total CAH	total DNSGP-2
chronic conditions *								
0	0.0	71.8	0.0	70.6	0.0	65.4	0.0	69.3
1	83.0	24.0	72.6	21.7	78.0	23.7	77.9	23.1
≥ 2	17.0	4.2	27.4	7.7	22.0	10.9	22.1	7.6
Total	100.0	100.0	100.0	100.0	100.0	100.0	100.0	100.0
N	12	766	62	1494	32	874	106	3134
Number of daily health-related problems								
0	42.0	17.0	26.0	20.6	31.0	8.7	33.0	15.4
1	16.6	20.9	6.0	21.9	16.0	16.4	12.9	19.7
2	8.0	19.3	18.0	16.9	19.0	15.2	15.0	17.1
3	16.6	14.9	10.0	12.5	12.0	14.3	12.9	13.9
≥ 4	16.6	27.9	40.0	28.1	22.0	45.4	26.2	33.8
Total	100.0	100.0	100.0	100.0	100.0	100.0	100.0	100.0
N	12	766	62	1494	32	874	106	3134

* chronic conditions, including CAH
Age boundaries differ slightly between CAH groups and DNSGP-2 groups.

Table 4 Experienced burden of the condition (by parents)

	0-4 year		4-12 year		12-18 year		Total	
	n	(%)	n	(%)	n	(%)	n	(%)
Total	12	(100)	62	(100)	32	(100)	106	(100)
Constraints in daily life ((totally) agree)	0	-	6	(10)	2	(6)	8	(8)
Adrenal crisis experienced (yes)	3	(25)	20	(32)	12	(38)	35	(33)
Fear for adrenal crisis ((totally) agree)	3	(25)	15	(24)	0	-	18	(17)
School absence due to CAH (yes)	n/a	-	19	(31)	9	(28)	28	(30)
Influence on condition ((totally) agree)	9	(75)	38	(61)	19	(59)	66	(62)
General health (good/very good/excellent)	12	(100)	60	(97)	30	(94)	102	(96)

n/a = not applicable

3 for all age groups. This means that on average, parents do not find it difficult to keep the condition of their child under control. The same holds true for the adolescents who have a mean score of 2.03 on the 'Difficulties' scale (not in Table).

Management

About 6% of children older than 4 years do not use medication daily (Table 6). On the other hand, 82% of children use two or more different medicines for CAH, most often Hydrocortisone and Fludrocortisone. Approximately 88% of the parents report that a proper balance in medication use is achieved. Medication is administered at a set time by 83% of the parents. The percentage of parents that administer medication at fixed times declines when children get older. Of the adolescents, 17% (n = 4) indicate not to use any CAH related medication (not in Table). All of the children and adolescents that do not use medication (or, in case of the adolescents, say they do not use medication) have the classic form of CAH.

Medication is most often raised in response to flu, fever, physical injury, and illness in general (Table 6). Parents of children younger than 12 years often mentioned

inoculation or drawing blood as a reason to increase the medication whereas parents of children older than 12 years often mentioned exams as a reason to increase the medication.

Self-management

Almost 63% of children aged 4-12 take their medicines independently or with some support of their parents and 56% of children aged 12-18 take their medication independently, according to their parents. 63% of the adolescents indicate that they take their medication independently from their parents and 38% of those adolescents receive help from a parent or other family member. The mean age at which children start to self-administer medication is 7.6 years (CI: 6.81 - 8.48). Approximately 67% of parents of children aged 12-18 years check whether the medication has been taken correctly. Approximately 75% of the adolescents take their medication according to the instructions of their physician.

Preventive measures

The measures that children and their parents take to prevent an adrenal crisis were also investigated. Only 7 of 106 children were able to inject themselves glucocorticoids intramuscularly in case of an adrenal crisis. On

Table 5 Parents' experience with the condition

	0-4 year	4-12 year	12-18 year
Scale 'Experiences parents'			
Average scale score (95% CI)	3.50 (3.06-3.94)	3.08 (2.92-3.25)	3.22 (2.94-3.50)
Cronbach's alpha	0.76	0.71	0.72
Number of items (range)	6 (1-5)	7 (1-5)	7 (1-5)
1————————— 3 —————————5 Negative neutral positive			
Scale 'Difficulties'			
Average scale score (95% CI)	2.18 (1.80-2.55)	2.27 (2.12-2.42)	1.82 (1.61-2.03)
Cronbach's alpha	0.78	0.73	0.85
Number of items (range)	8 (1-5)	8 (1-5)	8 (1-5)
1————————— 3 —————————5 Less diff. neutral more diff.			

Table 6 Self management and Participation (according to parents)

	0-4 year		4-12 year		12-18 year		Total	
	n	(%)	n	(%)	n	(%)	n	(%)
Total	12	(100)	62	(100)	32	(100)	106	(100)
Self management								
Daily medication use								
0 CAH med.	0	-	4	(6)	2	(6)	6	(6)
1 CAH med.	0	-	7	(11)	6	(19)	13	(12)
2 CAH meds.	9	(75)	29	(47)	11	(34)	49	(46)
3 CAH meds.	3	(25)	22	(36)	13	(41)	38	(36)
Medication at fixed time	11	(92)	53	(85)	24	(75)	88	(83)
Increased medication in past 12 months?								
0 times	0	-	3	(5)	5	(16)	8	(7.5)
1-10 times	11	(92)	43	(69)	19	(59)	73	(69)
> 10 times	1	(8)	11	(18)	5	(16)	17	(16)
Unknown	0	-	5	(8)	3	(9)	8	(7.5)
Participation								
Contact with school because of problems	n/a	-	22	(35)	8	(25)	30	(32)
Child exercises as much as peers without CAH	n/a	-	41	(66)	22	(69)	63	(67)
Child engages in a sport	n/a	-	46	(74)	31	(97)	77	(82)

n/a = not applicable

average 59% of all children carry an SOS bracelet or badge, children aged 4-12 more often (66%) than older (59%) or younger (25%) children. More than half of the adolescents carry an SOS bracelet or badge. However, only 17% carry a crisis card or emergency injection. According to parents, 31% of children aged 12-18 always carry a crisis card or emergency injection with them. For the younger age groups, parents most often carry a crisis card or emergency injection with them. Most parents of children with CAH state that their children's friends are aware of the fact that their child has a chronic medical condition.

Participation

As shown in Table 4 in the past 12 months, 30% of children have been absent from school for CAH related reasons. The average duration of school absence was approximately 7 days. 32% of the parents had contact with school because of school problems in the past 12 months. The reasons for contact varied from providing information and education to teachers to problems with bullying, behavioural problems and problems caused by comorbidity such as autism or dyslexia. With regard to physical exercise, 67% of the parents indicate that their child exercises just as much as peers without CAH (Table 6). Furthermore, 82% of children engage in a sport, often mentioned are horse riding, swimming, soccer and tennis. About 84% of parents of children older than 4 years indicate that their children have one or more hobbies. Playing outdoors, and playing computer games are often mentioned among children aged 4-12

and playing outdoors, meeting with friends, playing computer games and playing a musical instrument are often mentioned among children aged 12-18. About 28% of children older than 12 have a part time job next to school. On average they work 5.8 (+/-1.26) hours a week. According to their parents, none of these children experience problems at work as a consequence of CAH.

To evaluate the degree of protectiveness or even over-protectiveness that parents may display towards their children, some questions were asked only to parents of children of certain age groups. Firstly, parents of children aged 0-4 were asked if they make use of child care facilities and 75% indicated to do so. A playgroup or day nursery was mentioned most often. Secondly, parents of children aged 4-12 were asked whether their child sometimes spends the night away from home, for example, with family or friends. About 85% of parents reported that this sometimes occurred.

None of the adolescents indicated to experience impediments like concentration problems, physical discomfort or pain. When asked how they would rate their own level of functioning in daily life, all adolescents reported to be satisfied, with answers varying from good (35%) to very good (30%) and excellent (35%).

Finally, parents of children aged 12-18 were asked if their children go out by themselves or whether they go on holiday independent of their parents. Less than half of the children (41%) go out by themselves and 69% has occasionally been on holiday independent of their parents. Unfortunately, for these participation questions we have no comparative data available from the general population.

Discussion

In this study, we evaluated the physical, social and societal functioning of children with CAH and their parents. Previous research has focused mainly on adult patients with Addison's disease and CAH so to our knowledge this study is the first describing health state and quality of life of children with CAH and their parents.

In general, our results show that children with CAH experience few negative CAH related effects and that they participate well in several areas such as school and leisure time. Adolescents are confident about the management of their condition and their participation in daily life. Parents do not seem to be exceptionally protective of their children and are capable of leaving the care of their child to others.

Depending on the tools used mixed results are found but previous studies in Norway [13,14], Germany [15,16] and the United Kingdom [8,17] have shown impaired quality of life in adult patients with Addison's disease and CAH. Particularly, reduced energy, vitality and general health perception were reported. The parents of children with CAH in our population, however, did not report any of these problems. Instead, most parents indicated they were satisfied with the general health of their child with CAH. Comorbidity was present in most adult CAH patients studied by Erichsen [13]. In contrast, in our population comorbidity was scarce. That may explain the absence of impaired quality of life in our group children. Recently, Arlt et al. described the health status of adult CAH patients in the United Kingdom [8] and showed that a minority of adult CAH patients in the United Kingdom are under endocrine specialist care and that androgen levels are often poorly controlled whereas children with CAH are managed using established guidelines. This may be another important factor in explaining the higher quality of life in children compared to adults. Our results show some discrepancy between the answers of parents of adolescents and adolescents themselves with regard to medication intake. 17% of adolescents indicate not to use any CAH related medication compared to only 6% indicated by their parents. This may be explained by the assumption that parents may not be aware of the fact that their child has stopped taking medication.

Our results show that as children grow older, parents become less afraid of an adrenal crisis. This is probably because parents get more familiar with the disease. When children grow older, the responsibility for the management shifts from parent to child, as is the case in all chronic conditions and healthy children. This transfer of responsibility and control is often difficult for parents as their role in managing the disease decreases [18]. We found that the increasing importance of self-management seems to pose few problems for children with CAH since

they are partly capable of self-management already at a young age. However, measures to prevent adrenal crisis can be improved. Although CAH patients have to carry a card or SOS bracelet that indicates the use of glucocorticoids in case an emergency occurs, our results show that many children don't do so It is important to stress the necessity of such preventive measures.

A limitation of our study is a lack of a reference group of healthy children for all variables. Furthermore, we used questionnaires adapted from a previous Dutch study [16] that hinders comparisons to other studies.

Because group sizes were relatively small detailed statistical models could not be used.

Conclusions

In conclusion, our study shows that quality of life is not reduced in children with CAH and their parents. The children do experience several daily health related problems but these do not hamper them in their daily activities and participation in society. Parents themselves do not experience a lot of fear about the occurrence of an adrenal crisis and feel that they can influence the condition of their child. However, measures for prevention of adrenal crisis could be improved.

Acknowledgements
The authors wish to thank the Dutch Society for Addison and Cushing patients (NVACP), especially Alida Noordzij, Esther Groenhuijzen and Martijn van der Lee, the specialists and hospitals and all parents of children with CAH for their cooperation in this study. This study was made possible through financial support from the Dutch patient group for Addison, Cushing and CAH patients (NVACP) and fonds Nuts/Ohra.

Author details
[1]Netherlands institute for health services research (NIVEL), P.O. Box 1568, 3500 BN Utrecht, The Netherlands. [2]VU Medical Centre, department of Rehabilitation Medicine, room PK -1 Y 158, De Boelelaan 1118, 1081 HZ, The Netherlands. [3]Department of Paediatric Endocrinology, Radboud University Nijmegen Medical Centre, P O Box 9101, 6500 HB Nijmegen, The Netherlands.

Authors' contributions
SS and TW designed the questionnaires and conducted the study. SS drafted the manuscript and performed the statistical analysis. TW helped to draft the manuscript. HC and BO participated in the design of the questionnaires, participation of patients and revised the manuscript. All authors read and approved the final manuscript.

Competing interests
There are no potential conflicts of interest with respect to financial or personal relationships.

References
1. Trakakis E, Loghis C, Kassanos D: Congenital Adrenal Hyperplasia Because of 21-Hydroxylase Deficiency. A Genetic Disorder of interest to Obstetrics and Gynecologists. Obstet Gynecol Surv 2009, 64:177-187.
2. Claahsen- van der Grinten HL: Van gen naar ziekte; het adrenogenitaal syndroom en het CYP21A2-gen (From gene to disease: adrenogenital

syndrome and the CYP21A2 gene). *Nederlands tijdschrift voor geneeskunde* 2007, **151**(Suppl 21):1174-1177.

3. Grosse SD, Van Vliet G: **How many deaths can be prevented by newborn screening for Congenital Adrenal Hyperplasia?** *Horm Res* 2007, **67**:284-291.

4. Bachelot A, Chakthoura Z, Rouxel A, Dulon J, Touraine P: **Classical Forms of Congenital Adrenal Hyperplasia due to 21-Hydroxylase Deficiency in Adults.** *Horm Res* 2008, **69**:203-211.

5. Malouf MA, Inman AG, Carr AG, Franco J, Brooks LM: **Health-related quality of life, mental health and psychotherapeutic considerations for women diagnosed with a disorder of sexual development: Congenital Adrenal Hyperplasia.** *Int J Ped Endocrinol* 2010, **2010**:253465.

6. Speiser PW, Azziz R, Baskin LS, Ghizzoni L, Hensle TW, Merke DP, Meyer-Bahlburg HFL, Miller WL, Montori VM, Oberfield SE, Ritzen M, White PC: **Congenital Adrenal Hyperplasia Due to Steroid 21-Hydroxylase Deficiency: An Endocrine Society Clinical Practice Guideline.** *J Clin Endocrinol Metab* 2010, **95**(Suppl 9):4133-4160.

7. RIVM: *Informatieblad in het kader van het landelijke neonatale screeningsprogramma (Information leaflet of the national neonatal screening program)* Bilthoven; 2006.

8. Arlt W, Willis DS, Wild SH, Krone N, Doherty EJ, Hahner S, Han TS, Carroll PV, Conway GS, Rees DA, Stimson RH, Walker BR, Connell JMC, Ross RJ, the United Kingdom Congenital Adrenal Hyperplasia Adult Study Executive (CaHASE): **Health status of adults with congenital adrenal hyperplasia: A cohort study of 203 patients.** *J Clin Endocrinol Metab* 2010, **95**(Suppl 11):5110-5121.

9. Westert GP, Schellevis FG, de Bakker DH, Groenewegen PP, Bensing JM, van der Zee J: **Monitoring health inequalities through general practice: the Second Dutch National Survey of General Practice.** *Eur J Public Health* 2005, **15**(Suppl 1):59-65.

10. Heijmans MJWM, Rijken M: *De impact van de ziekte van Addison, AGS of het syndroom van Cushing op het dagelijks leven en de zorg: een onderzoek vanuit patiëntenperspectief (The impact of Addison's disease, CAH and Cushing's syndrome on daily life and healthcare: a study from the patient's perspective.)* Utrecht: NIVEL; 2006.

11. Calsbeek H: *The social position of adolescents and young adults with chronic digestive disorders* Utrecht: NIVEL; 2003.

12. Sanches S, Wiegers T: *Het fysiek, sociaal en maatschappelijk functioneren van kinderen met AGS (en hun ouders) (The physical, social and societal functioning of children with CAH (and their parents)* Utrecht: NIVEL; 2010.

13. Erichsen MM, Løvås K, Skinningsrud B, Wolff AB, Undlien DE, Svartberg J, Fougner KJ, Berg TJ, Bollerslev J, Mella B, Carlson JA, Erlich H, Husebye ES: **Clinical, immunological, and genetic features of autoimmune primary adrenal insufficiency: Observations from a Norwegian registry.** *J Clin Endocrinol Metab* 2009, **94**:4882-4890.

14. Løvås K, Loge JH, Husebye ES: **Subjective health status in Norwegian Patients with Addison's disease.** *Clin Endocrinol (Oxf)* 2002, **56**:581-588.

15. Bleicken B, Hahner S, Loeffler M, Ventz M, Allolio B, Quinkler M: **Impaired subjective health status in chronic adrenal insufficiency: impact of different glucocorticoid replacement regimens.** *Eur J Endocrinol* 2008, **159**:811-817.

16. Hahner S, Loeffler M, Fassnacht M, Weisman D, Koschker AC, Quinkler M, Decker O, Arlt W, Allolio B: **Impaired subjective health status in 256 patients with adrenal insufficiency based on cross sectional analysis.** *J Clin Endocrinol Metab* 2007, **92**:3912-3922.

17. Gurnell EM, Hunt PJ, Curran SE, Conway CL, Pullenayegum EM, Huppert FA, Compston JE, Herbert J, Chatterjee VK: **Longterm DHEA replacement in primary adrenal insufficiency: a randomized, controlled trial.** *J Clin Endocrinol Metab* 2008, **93**:400-409.

18. Witchel SF: **The medical home concept and Congenital Adrenal Hyperplasia: a comfortable habitat!** *Int J Ped Endocrinol* 2010, **2010**:561526.

11

Efficacy of Leuprolide Acetate 1-Month Depot for Central Precocious Puberty (CPP): Growth Outcomes During a Prospective, Longitudinal Study

Peter A Lee[1,2]*, E Kirk Neely[3], John Fuqua[2], Di Yang[4], Lois M Larsen[4], Cynthia Mattia-Goldberg[4] and Kristof Chwalisz[4]

Abstract

Introduction: Gonadotropin-releasing hormone analogs (GnRHa) are the treatment of choice for CPP. We investigated growth in GnRHa-naïve subjects, treated with leuprolide acetate 1-month depot for CPP.

Methods: This prospective, open-label study had a long-term, observational, follow-up period. Forty-nine females and 6 males were enrolled. Leuprolide acetate depot was administered intramuscularly every 28 days. Height and growth rate during and after treatment until adulthood were measured.

Results: Among 30 of 49 females having an adult height (AH) measurement, 29 had target heights available (mean = 163.8 cm) and 27 had pretreatment predicted adult heights (PAHs; mean = 157.4 cm). After treatment, the mean AH at mean age 21.8 years [range 13.7-26.7 years] was 162.5 cm, a mean height gain over baseline PAH of 4.0 cm. The mean height standard deviation score was -0.1 at AH.

Conclusions: Treatment of CPP with leuprolide acetate 1-month depot had beneficial effects on growth rate and preservation of AH.

Introduction

Central precocious puberty (CPP) commonly refers to the development of pubertal sex characteristics as a consequence of the premature activation of the hypothalamic-pituitary-gonadal (HPG) axis before the age of 8 years in girls and 9 years in boys. The pathogenesis of CPP includes early activation of pulsatile release of gonadotropin-releasing hormone (GnRH), leading to an increase in secretion of gonadotropins and gonadal steroids. Central precocious puberty occurs much more frequently among females than males (greater than 20:1 ratio) [1].

The treatment goals for children with CPP include hormonal suppression, regression or cessation of

development of pubertal characteristics and the prevention of short stature in adulthood. Patients with CPP are at risk of short stature in adulthood because of disproportionately advanced skeletal maturation in relation to growth acceleration, resulting in early epiphyseal fusion that limits growth potential [2].

Analogs of GnRH (GnRHa) have been the standard of care for the treatment of children with CPP for more than 20 years [2], with the usage of the depot form reported in 1989 [3]. However, despite the widespread use of GnRHa in the treatment of CPP, the factors that impact adult height outcomes after GnRHa therapy in children with CPP are poorly understood [4-13].

The few previous studies that have examined outcomes during and after treatment with leuprolide acetate have utilized variable treatment doses, and generally small numbers of patients [14-16]. The objectives of this longitudinal, prospective study were to evaluate the

* Correspondence: plee@psu.edu
[1]The Milton S. Hershey Medical Center, College of Medicine, Pennsylvania State University, Hershey, PA 17033, USA
Full list of author information is available at the end of the article

suppression of hormonal and clinical sexual characteristics and to examine the long-term impact of baseline and during-treatment factors on the growth pattern and adult height after treatment with leuprolide acetate 1-month depot in females with CPP. In this report, we describe the auxological outcomes of the study and analyze the effect of multiple baseline and during-treatment factors that potentially affect height outcomes in females. Though males were included in the study, firm conclusions regarding height outcomes cannot be drawn due to the small sample size. However, brief descriptive results have been included herein. A separate article reports the hormonal and reproductive outcomes of the study [17].

Patients and Methods

Patients

Patients were females with Tanner breast stage ≥ 2 before 8 years of age whose chronological age (CA) was less than 9 years. Males with Tanner genitalia stage ≥ 2 before 9 years of age whose CA was less than 10 years were also included. All had a baseline GnRH-stimulated LH level ≥ 10 IU/L. This level was chosen to ensure that all enrolled patients clearly had CPP, even though it was realized that some patients with CPP would be excluded. Additional inclusion criteria were bone age (BA) advancement ≥ 1 year over CA by the Fels Method [18], and treatment naïve to GnRHa. Institutional review board approval was obtained at each site, and written informed consent was provided by patients' parents or legal guardians prior to screening or any study related procedures.

Study Design

This was a prospective, longitudinal, multicenter study that consisted of an open-label treatment period and a long-term post-treatment follow-up period. The study was conducted from 1991 to 2009 at nine U.S. centers. The primary outcomes of treatment in the study were the assessment of clinical sexual characteristics evaluated by Tanner staging and the decrease in serum gonadotropin and sex steroid concentrations to prepubertal levels. During the long-term follow-up into adulthood, the outcomes were adult height (based on stadiometer measurement or self-reported by questionnaire as adults) and information reported concerning reproductive system function.

Leuprolide acetate 1-month depot was started at a dose of 300 µg/kg (minimum starting dose of 7.5 mg) administered intramuscularly (IM) every 28 days. Incremental dose adjustments of 3.75 mg were made at each clinic visit, if necessary, based on the results of the previous GnRH stimulation test and hormonal parameters. GnRH stimulation tests for LH were performed by using a standard method (Factrel 100 µg IV bolus) in all patients. LH concentrations were measured by using DELFIA™ with a lower limit of quantitation of 0.15 IU/L.

Treatment period visits occurred at weeks 4, 8, 12, 24, 36, 48, and then every 6 months until study drug discontinuation. Study procedures included a physical examination with measurement of height and weight, assessment of Tanner stage, GnRH stimulation testing, and blood collection for gonadotropin and sex steroid levels. Bone radiographs were taken at baseline, week 24, week 48, and every 12 months thereafter. Radiographs were sent to a central reader (Wright State University School of Medicine, Lifespan Health Research Center, Kettering, OH) for determination of BA using the Fels Method [18]. Levels of gonadotropins and estradiol were determined by dissociation-enhanced lanthanide fluorescence immunoassay and radioimmunoassay, respectively (University of Pittsburgh Children's Hospital; Pittsburgh, PA). Target height was calculated by mid parental height plus or minus 6.5 cm for males and females, respectively; target height range was calculated by target height ± 8.5 cm. Predicted adult heights (PAH) were calculated by dividing a subject's height by the average percent of mature height associated with a given BA. The average percents of mature height were derived from tables for accelerated boys and girls prepared by Bayley and Pinneau [19]. Study drug was discontinued at the appropriate age for puberty at the discretion of the investigator.

After study drug withdrawal, patients entered into an optional follow-up period, with study visits occurring every 6 months until physical and laboratory measurements reached pubertal levels, and then annually until age 21 years. Follow-up study visits included a physical examination with measurement of height and weight, Tanner staging, basal levels of gonadotropins and sex steroids after evidence of pubertal response was observed with stimulated levels, menstrual and sexual history, and bone radiographs of the left hand and wrist. Adult height data were collected at adulthood (after age 18), during an office visit or by a patient-reported questionnaire (n = 19). For patients who were missing adulthood height data, adult height was established if the final height obtained during follow-up was associated with a growth velocity of <1 cm/year or a BA ≥ 14 years in females (n = 11) or ≥ 15 years in males.

Statistics

Mean incremental growth rate was calculated as the ratio of the change in height to the change in CA at approximately six month intervals (1 month = 28 days to match dosing interval) during the treatment period and through the first year of the follow-up period, and at approximately one year intervals thereafter. Baseline growth rate was calculated as the growth rate during the year prior to the start of the treatment period.

The ratio of the change in BA during each one year interval to the change in CA during the one year interval was computed. Mean height and mean height standard deviation score (HtSDS) were calculated at each visit during the treatment and the follow-up periods and at adult height.

Pearson's correlation coefficients were calculated between baseline characteristics (CA, BA, BA-CA, time to treatment from onset of CPP, basal and peak LH, basal and peak FSH, growth rate, height SDS and target height), during-treatment variables (duration of treatment, average growth rate, the mean ratio of change in BA to change in CA, mean basal and peak LH, and mean basal and peak FSH), and end of treatment variables (CA, BA, BA-CA, growth rate, and height SDS) and gain over baseline PAH, height gain over end of treatment height, and at adult height. Dependent variables that were statistically significantly correlated at α = 0.05 level with each auxological outcome were entered into a stepwise multiple regression analysis to determine the best predictors (statistically significant at α = 0.05 level) of each auxological outcome.

Results
Female Patients
This study consisted of a mean ± SD treatment period of 3.9 ± 2.0 years and a post-treatment follow-up period of 3.5 ± 2.2 years [17]. The study enrolled both females and males, however, too few males (n = 5) were enrolled to draw conclusions, and, therefore, were not included in the primary analysis presented in this report. Forty-nine females were enrolled in the treatment period and 35 of them participated in the long-term follow-up period (Figure 1). No premature discontinuations (n = 9) were related to lack of efficacy. All patients were naïve to treatment with GnRHa. Patient demographics and baseline characteristics for the female study population are summarized in Table 1. Overall, 61.2% of patients were Caucasian. At baseline, the mean age was 7.3 years and BA was advanced over CA by an average 3.0 years. Overall, the mean time since diagnosis of CPP was 0.3 years in the study population. All subjects had peak stimulated LH suppressed to <1.75 IU/L during treatment with leuprolide acetate 1-month depot, with 5 subjects requiring an increased dosage to obtain or retain suppression over the course of treatment. After discontinuation from study drug, the mean ± SD time to first menses was 1.5 ± 0.5 years (range of 0.5-2.5 years). The gonadotropin and sex steroid data are discussed in detail in a separate paper.

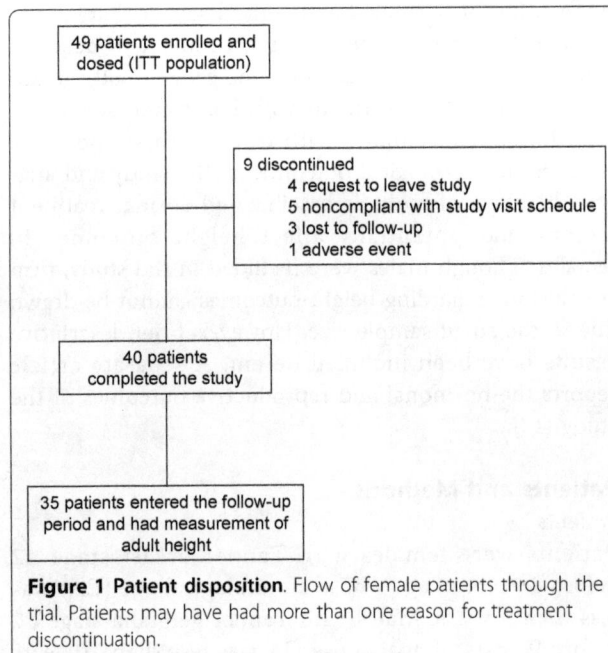

Figure 1 Patient disposition. Flow of female patients through the trial. Patients may have had more than one reason for treatment discontinuation.

Growth During Treatment
The mean incremental growth rate was greatly reduced from 10.6 cm/year at baseline to approximately 5-6 cm/year during the first 72 weeks of therapy and then 4-4.5 cm/year from week 72 to week 192 (Figure 2). These mean growth rates during treatment were generally comparable to normal growth rates in prepubertal girls.

Post-treatment Growth
During the last 6 months of treatment, among patients who were enrolled into the follow-up period of the study, the mean incremental growth rate was 4.0 cm/year. Following withdrawal of study drug, mean incremental growth rate increased to 4.4 cm/year (Figure 2) at the 24 week follow-up visit, showing a small growth spurt, before gradually decreasing to 0.4 cm/year by follow-up week 192.

Bone Age and Predicted Height
Prior to the initiation of treatment, mean BA advance over CA was 3 years. Treatment with leuprolide acetate 1-month depot rapidly controlled the advance in BA, with mean ΔBA/ΔCA of 0.7 after the first year of treatment, and not more than 0.6 in during the next 3 years of treatment (Figure 3).

Adult Height and Height Gain
Among the 30 females with adult height data, 29 females had a mean target height of 163.8 cm at baseline, and 27 subjects had a mean PAH of 157.4 cm at baseline. Of the 30 females with adult height data, 22 were measured with stadiometer, and 8 were self-reported. The mean adult height was 162.5 cm, which represents a mean height gain over baseline PAH of

Table 1 Pretreatment subject demographics and baseline characteristics

Characteristic	Female Patients N = 49
Race, n (%)	
Caucasian	30 (61.2)
African American	11 (22.4)
Asian	0
Hispanic	8 (16.3)
Age, years	
Mean (SD)	7.3 (1.9)
Range	1.2-9.4
Weight, kg	
Mean (SD)	33.6 (9.72)
Range	13.0-52.2
Height, cm	
Mean (SD)	131.6 (14.97)
Range	84.6-154.7
Height Standardized Score	
Mean (SD)	1.5 (1.29)
Range	-1.4-3.4
Tanner Stage, n (%)	
Breast/Genitalia I	1 (2.0)[a]
II	9 (18.4)
III	25 (51.0)
IV	13 (26.5)
V	1 (2.0)
Growth Velocity, cm/yr	
Mean (SD)	10.7 (3.40)
Range	5.5-21.2
BA, years	
Mean (SD)	10.2 (2.13)
Range	2.5-12.1
BA - CA, years	
Mean (SD)	3.0 (0.80)
Range	1.3-4.5
History of Menstrual Bleeding, n (%)	
No	36 (75)
Yes	12 (25)

[a]A one year old patient was enrolled in the trial with breast Tanner stage I based on qualifying peak stimulated LH (84.7 IU/L) and E_2 (90 pg/mL).

4.0 cm. (Figure 4). In addition, mean height SDS was -0.1 at adult height, indicating that these patients essentially reached the mean height of the normal population by adulthood (Figure 5). Among the 29 females with menarche status at baseline and adult height, subjects who were premenarchal (n = 22) or post-menarchal (n = 7) had similar mean ± SD adult height outcomes (162.8 ± 6.77 cm vs 162.0 ± 1.6 cm, respectively).

Analysis of Factors Potentially Predictive of Height Outcomes

Univariate analyses were performed to identify factors that were strongly correlated with adult height, height gain over baseline PAH, and height gain after treatment (Tables 2, 3, and 4). After stepwise multiple linear regression of the factors that were significantly correlated in the univariate analysis, there were significant positive associations of average growth rate during treatment (p = 0.0002) and height SDS at baseline (p < 0.0001) with adult height (Table 2). For height gain over baseline PAH, BA minus CA at baseline (p = 0.0028) and time to treatment from onset of CPP (p = 0.0245) were found to be significantly positively and negatively associated, respectively (Table 3). Finally, for height gain after treatment, significant negative associations were found for BA at baseline (p < 0.0001) and duration of treatment (p = 0.0002, Table 4).

Male Patients

While auxological outcome analyses are not presented herein, the descriptive data on growth during treatment, post-treatment growth, and bone age and predicted height are presented below. A total of 6 males were enrolled in the treatment period, and 5 males participated in the long-term follow-up period. At baseline, the mean age of the 6 males was 7.5 years and on average, BA was advanced over CA by 3.2 years. Treatment with leuprolide acetate 1-month depot rapidly controlled the advancement in BA, with mean ΔBA/ΔCA of 1.2 after the first year of treatment. Mean growth rate during treatment was reduced from 9.6 cm/year at baseline to 4.5-9 cm/year during the first 72 weeks and 4.5-6 cm/year from week 72 through week 192, respectively. The mean incremental growth rate was 2.0 cm/year at the end of treatment; however, following withdrawal of study drug, the rate increased to 4.5 cm/year at the 24-week follow-up visit. The mean final adult height (n = 3) during follow-up was 4.7 cm less than the PAH at baseline. None of the male patients had final adult heights recorded at adulthood (after age 18).

Discussion

The results of this prospective, longitudinal study show that leuprolide acetate 1-month depot effectively suppressed the advanced growth rate and rate of bone maturation in females with CPP who were naïve to treatment with GnRHa, similar to the effects observed in previous studies [20-24]. After discontinuation of study drug, a small increase in growth rate was observed during the first year post-treatment, suggesting the occurrence of a limited pubertal growth spurt. Furthermore, on average, patients in this study population

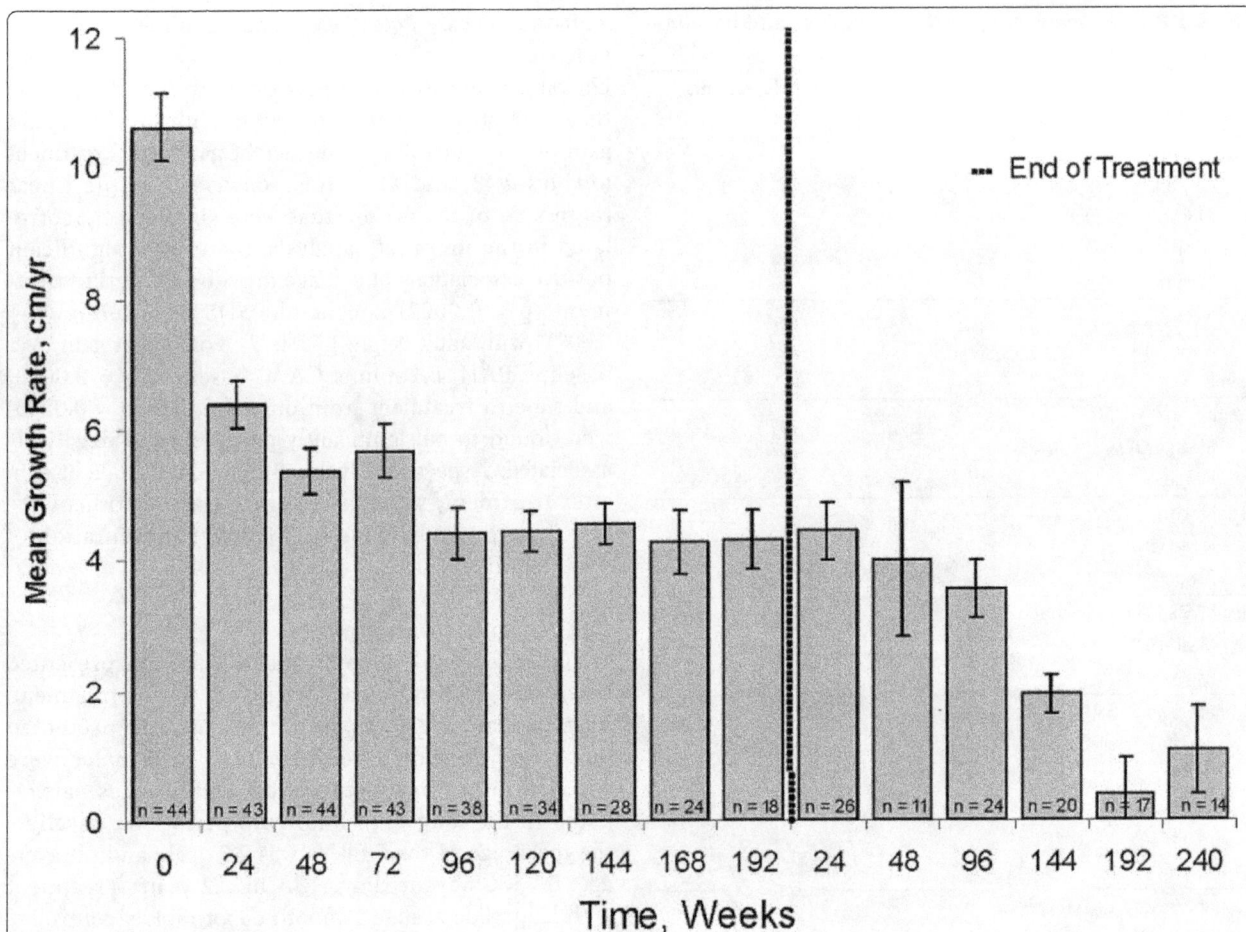

Figure 2 Mean ± SE growth rates for females. Incremental growth rates were calculated every 6 months. The baseline growth rate was defined as the growth rate for 1 year prior to the start of study drug. Numbers reflect available results.

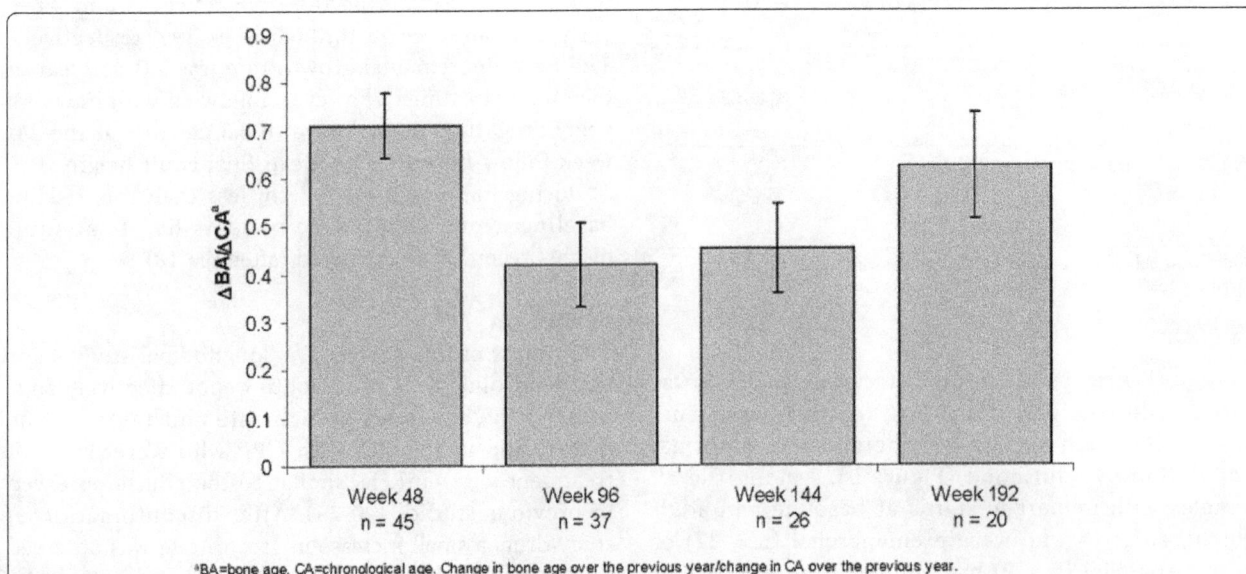

[a]BA=bone age, CA=chronological age. Change in bone age over the previous year/change in CA over the previous year.

Figure 3 Change in bone age to change in chronological age during each year of treatment for females. The ratio of the change in BA from the previous visit to the change in CA from the previous visit was calculated at approximately one year intervals. Numbers reflect available results

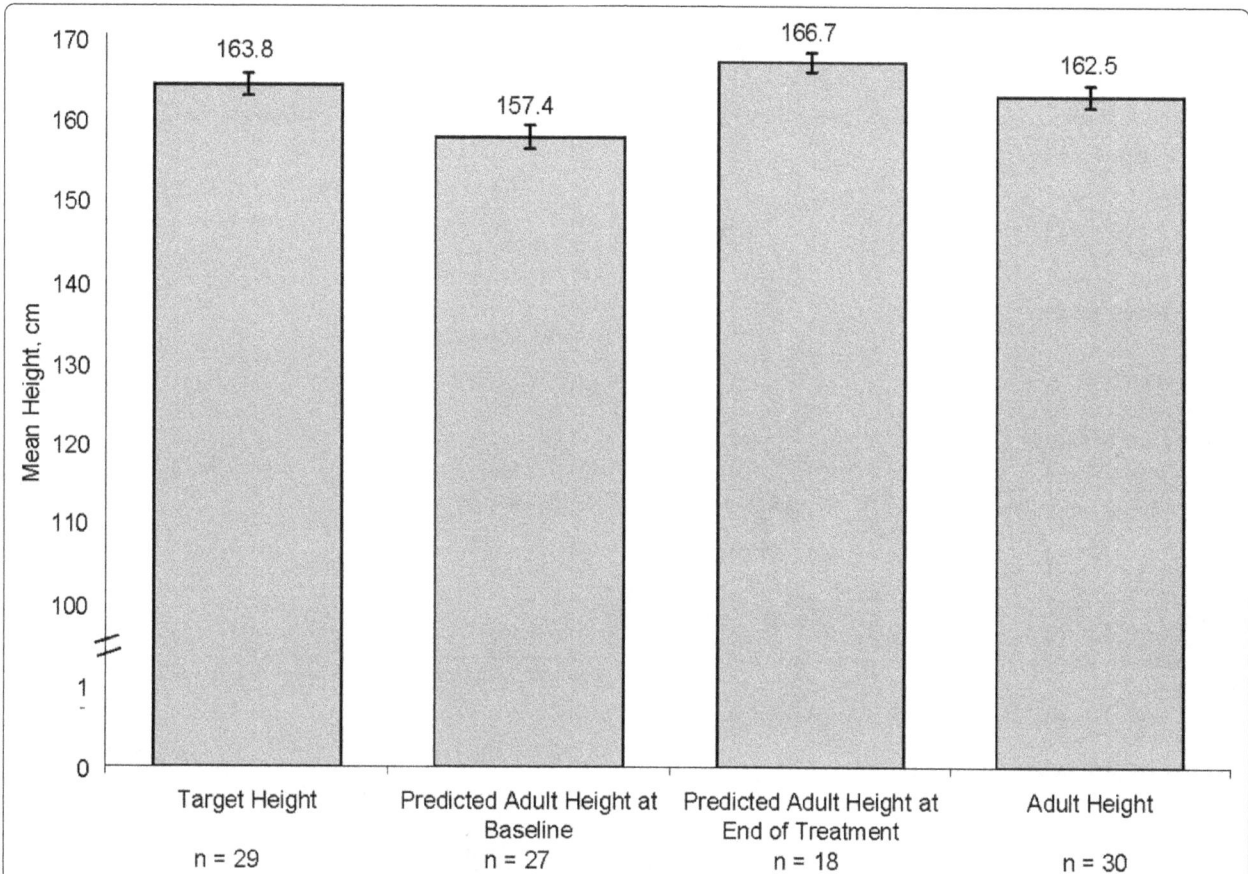

Figure 4 Height outcomes for females during the study. Adult height includes data from patients whose height was collected at adulthood after age 18. For patients who were missing adulthood height data, adult height was established when their growth velocity was <1 cm/year or bone age was ≥14 years during the follow-up period.

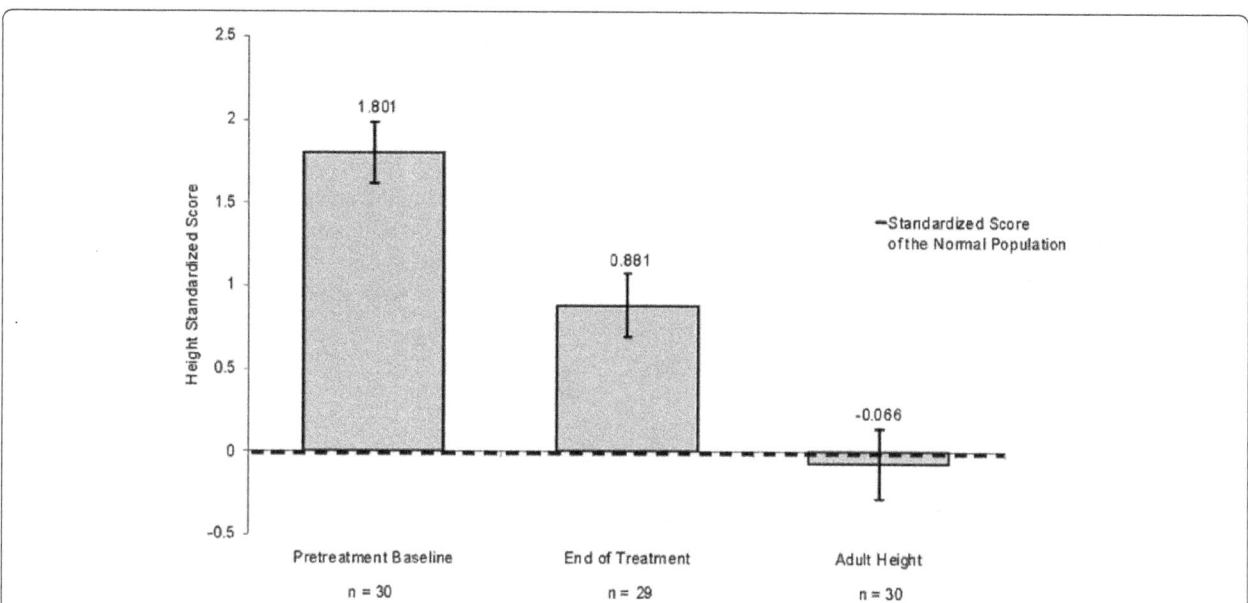

Figure 5 Height standardized scores for females during the study. The pretreatment baseline is the mean standardized height score of patients before initiation of leuprolide acetate therapy. The height at the end of treatment refers to the mean standardized height score for patients at the end of the treatment period. Adult height includes standardized scores for those patients whose height was collected at adulthood after age 18. For those without adult height available, adult height was established when their growth velocity was <1 cm/year or bone age was ≥14 years during the follow-up period.

Table 2 Analysis of factors significantly associated with adult height in females

Adult Height[a]		
Univariate Analysis	Correlation Coefficient	P-value
At the start of therapy		
CA (yr)	-0.37	0.0348
BA (yr)	-0.38	0.0306
Peak FSH	0.35	0.0466
Growth rate	0.39	0.0336
Height SDS	0.82	<.0001
Target height	0.53	0.0019
During therapy		
Averaged growth rate	0.62	0.0001
At the end of therapy		
Height SDS	0.82	<.0001
Multiple Linear Regression	**Beta Coefficient**	**P-value**	**R^2**
Average growth rate during treatment	3.05	0.0002	
Height SDS at baseline	5.11	<0.0001	0.82

[a]Adult height was established when the height was associated with a growth velocity of <1 cm/year or a bone age ≥14 years in females

Table 4 Analysis of factors significantly associated with height gain after treatment

Height Gain After Treatment[b]		
Univariate Analysis	Correlation Coefficient	P-value
At the start of therapy		
CA (yr)	-0.58	0.0005
BA (yr)	-0.73	<.0001
BA minus CA	-0.62	0.0001
Peak FSH	0.38	0.0344
Growth rate	0.44	0.0151
During therapy		
Duration of the treatment	0.39	0.0292
Averaged growth rate	0.58	0.0006
ΔBA/ΔCA	0.54	0.0015
Basal FSH	-0.36	0.0447
At the end of therapy		
BA	-0.63	0.0001
Multiple Linear Regression	**Beta Coefficient**	**P-value**	**R^2**
BA at baseline	-3.08	<0.0001	
Duration of treatment	-1.87	0.0002	0.72

[a]Final adult height minus height at the end of treatment

reached adult height of the standard normal population after treatment with leuprolide acetate 1-month depot.

Using the Bayley-Pinneau method at baseline to predict the adult height of our study population, adult heights were on average 4.0 cm greater than PAH at onset of treatment with leuprolide acetate among female patients. This is consistent with previous studies using depot GnRHa for CPP, which have demonstrated that females between the ages of 6-8 years have a moderate height increase that ranges from 4.5 cm to 7.2 cm

Table 3 Analysis of factors significantly associated with gain over predicted adult height

Gain Over Baseline Predicted Adult Height[a]		
Univariate Analysis	Correlation Coefficient	P-value
At the start of therapy		
CA (yr)	-0.43	0.0221
BA minus CA	0.53	0.004
Time to treatment from onset of CPP (yr)	-0.39	0.0395
During therapy		
Duration of the treatment	0.52	0.0048
At the end of therapy		
CA	0.40	0.0369
Multiple Linear Regression	**Beta Coefficient**	**P-value**	**R^2**
BA-CA at baseline	3.37	0.0028	
Time to Treatment from onset of CPP (yr)	-3.84	0.0245	0.41

[a]Adult height minus predicted mature height at baseline

[6,25]. While studies have failed to show benefit if treatment is begun after age 8 years [26], this does not take into account subsequent diminution of growth potential without treatment. Some studies suggest that the Bayley-Pinneau method may over-predict adult height among those with advanced skeletal age by several centimeters at baseline [2,7,27]. The 30 patients who had adult heights in this study had a mean HtSDS of -0.1, which indicates that their mean height was within the range of target heights equivalent to that of the normal population. Twenty-four of the 29 patients with target heights reached their target height range.

Similar to previous studies (11, 15, 19, 21, 22, 26-28), we used multiple linear regression to identify factors that may affect height gain from baseline and from the end of treatment and final adult height in females with CPP. Factors having significant correlation by multiple linear regression analyses (Tables 2, 3, and 4) are discussed below.

Factors Influencing Adult Height

The two factors that explained 82% of the variability in adult height were HtSDS score at baseline and average growth rate during treatment. Both were positively correlated and similarly identified as positive factors in a previous study in determining patients who may benefit the most with regard to height gain from leuprolide acetate 1-month depot therapy [20]. The positive correlation between growth rate during treatment and adult height highlights the importance of monitoring the level of growth rate suppression during treatment Adequate growth rates during treatment were associated with positive final growth outcomes in our study population. The growth rates observed in this study (5-6 cm/year during the first 72 weeks of therapy and 4-4.5 cm/year from week 72 to week 192) were similar to growth rates observed in normal prepubertal children of these ages. Unlike prior reports and common expectations, CA at onset of therapy did not predict height outcome. This is likely related to the diversity of age at onset of puberty.

Factors Influencing Height Gain Over PAH at Baseline
In the multiple linear regression for height gain over PAH at baseline, the advancement of BA over CA at baseline was a strong positive predictor, and time to treatment from onset of CPP was a strong negative predictor. This indicates that the greater the advancement of BA over CA at baseline and the shorter the interval between onset of CPP and the initiation of treatment, the greater the height gain (defined as adult height minus predicted mature height at baseline). This observation is similar to results reported by Mul et al. [12]. Overall, the advancement of BA over CA at baseline and the time to treatment from onset of CPP accounted for 41% of the variability in height gain. The finding that advancement in BA at the onset of therapy is a positive predictor of height gain over PAH may seem inconsistent with the previously described inverse relationship of BA at onset of therapy and adult height [20]. Because subjects with a more advanced BA have a lower PAH at the onset of therapy, halting advancement of BA during GnRHa therapy appears to result in a greater gain in height than the initial predicted height. This would explain the positive predictor of height gain, but not actual adult height. Hence, there appears to be a greater "gain back" growth potential among those in this study having more advanced BAs at onset of therapy.

Factors Influencing Height Gain After Stopping Therapy
The duration of therapy had a negative association with the height gain after stopping therapy. Previous studies have shown no association between duration of therapy and height gain after therapy [20,25]. The negative correlation between BA at baseline and height gain after stopping therapy is expected, and was observed by Brito et al [20]. The two factors of treatment duration and BA at baseline explain 72% of the variance in height gain after treatment. The univariate analysis showing a correlation between ΔBA/ΔCA and growth after therapy does not persist with the multiple linear regression analyses; hence, this is not a major factor. The difference in the results between the univariate and multiple linear regression analyses might be explained by the considerable variation in BAs. At the onset of therapy, BA would

be expected to continue to advance until typical pubertal BA is reached. The ratio, therefore, may reflect considerable variation.

In summary, treatment with leuprolide acetate 1-month depot increased adult height over the PAH. In addition, the HtSDS was equivalent to that of the normal population, indicating that these patients had on average nearly achieved the height of their peers without CPP. Overall, treatment with leuprolide acetate 1-month depot preserved adult height potential and resulted in clinically meaningful height gains over PAH. The results of this study confirm that in females, early initiation of treatment from the onset of CPP results in the greatest increase in height. In addition, female patients with the greatest advance in BA experience the most height gain over PAH with GnRHa treatment, and maintaining growth rates within that of normal prepubertal children during GnRHa treatment may result in the highest adult height outcome.

Acknowledgements
Financial support for this study was provided by Abbott Laboratories, formerly TAP Pharmaceutical Products Inc. Medical writing support was provided by Amanda J. Fein, PhD and Theresa J. Peterson, PhD on behalf of Abbott. The authors would like to thank the following authors for their participation in the study: Barry B. Bercu, MD; Clifford Bloch, MD; Stuart A Chalew, MD; Robert Clemons, MD; Felix A. Conte, MD; Raymond Hintz, MD; Michael S. Kappy, MD; Georgeanna J. Klingensmith, MD; and Edward O. Reiter, MD.

Author details
[1]The Milton S. Hershey Medical Center, College of Medicine, Pennsylvania State University, Hershey, PA 17033, USA. [2]Section of Pediatric Endocrinology and Diabetology, James Whitcomb Riley Hospital for Children, School of Medicine, Indiana University, Indianapolis, IN 46202, USA. [3]Division of Pediatric Endocrinology and Diabetes, Room G313, Stanford University Medical Center, Stanford, CA 94305, USA. [4]Abbott Laboratories, 200 Abbott Park Road, Abbott Park, IL 60064, USA.

Authors' contributions
PL was involved in the original protocol, the laboratory assessments, the planning and execution of the phase 4 (follow-up) study as well as the preparation of the manuscript. EKN and JF participated in data collection and interpretation and manuscript preparation. LL and DY performed the statistical analysis and participated in drafting the manuscript. CMG and KC participated in interpreting the data and manuscript preparation. All authors read and approved the final manuscript.

Competing interests
PAL has been a consultant for Abbott and Novo Nordisk with grants from Abbott, Eli Lilly, Novo Nordisk, Pfizer, and Ipsen. EKN has received grant/research support from and has been a consultant and scientific advisory board member for Abbott. JF has been a scientific advisory board member for Abbott. DY, LL, CMG, and KC are all employees of Abbott and LL, CMG, and KC all own Abbott stock.

References
1. Brauner R: **Central precocious puberty in girls: prediction of the aetiology.** *J Pediatr Endocrinol Metab* 2005, **18**(9):845-7.
2. Carel JC, Eugster EA, Rogol A, Ghizzoni L, Palmert MR, Antoniazzi F, *et al*: **Consensus statement on the use of gonadotropin-releasing hormone analogs in children.** *Pediatrics* 2009, **123**(4):e752-62.

3.   Parker KL, Lee PA: **Depot leuprolide acetate for treatment of precocious puberty.** *The Journal of clinical endocrinology and metabolism* 1989, **69(3)**:689-91.
4.   Arrigo T, Cisternino M, Galluzzi F, Bertelloni S, Pasquino AM, Antoniazzi F, et al: **Analysis of the factors affecting auxological response to GnRH agonist treatment and final height outcome in girls with idiopathic central precocious puberty.** *European journal of endocrinology/European Federation of Endocrine Societies* 1999, **141(2)**:140-4.
5.   Brauner R, Adan L, Malandry F, Zantleifer D: **Adult height in girls with idiopathic true precocious puberty.** *The Journal of clinical endocrinology and metabolism* 1994, **79(2)**:415-20.
6.   Carel JC, Roger M, Ispas S, Tondu F, Lahlou N, Blumberg J, et al: **Final height after long-term treatment with triptorelin slow release for central precocious puberty: importance of statural growth after interruption of treatment. French study group of Decapeptyl in Precocious Puberty.** *The Journal of clinical endocrinology and metabolism* 1999, **84(6)**:1973-8.
7.   Kauli R, Galatzer A, Kornreich L, Lazar L, Pertzelan A, Laron Z: **Final height of girls with central precocious puberty, untreated versus treated with cyproterone acetate or GnRH analogue. A comparative study with re-evaluation of predictions by the Bayley-Pinneau method.** *Hormone research* 1997, **47(2)**:54-61.
8.   Kaye D, Frankl W, Arditi LI: **Probable postcardiotomy syndrome following implantation of a transvenous pacemaker: report of the first case.** *American heart journal* 1975, **90(5)**:627-30.
9.   Kreiter M, Burstein S, Rosenfield RL, Moll GW Jr, Cara JF, Yousefzadeh DK, et al: **Preserving adult height potential in girls with idiopathic true precocious puberty.** *The Journal of pediatrics* 1990, **117(3)**:364-70.
10. Lanes R, Soros A, Jakubowicz S: **Accelerated versus slowly progressive forms of puberty in girls with precocious and early puberty. Gonadotropin suppressive effect and final height obtained with two different analogs.** *J Pediatr Endocrinol Metab* 2004, **17(5)**:759-66.
11. Leger J, Reynaud R, Czernichow P: **Do all girls with apparent idiopathic precocious puberty require gonadotropin-releasing hormone agonist treatment?** *The Journal of pediatrics* 2000, **137(6)**:819-25.
12. Mul D, Oostdijk W, Otten BJ, Rouwe C, Jansen M, Delemarre-van de Waal HA, et al: **Final height after gonadotrophin releasing hormone agonist treatment for central precocious puberty: the Dutch experience.** *J Pediatr Endocrinol Metab* 2000, **13(Suppl 1)**:765-72.
13. Pasquino AM, Pucarelli I, Segni M, Matrunola M, Cerroni F: **Adult height in girls with central precocious puberty treated with gonadotropin-releasing hormone analogues and growth hormone.** *The Journal of clinical endocrinology and metabolism* 1999, **84(2)**:449-52.
14. Clemons RD, Kappy MS, Stuart TE, Perelman AH, Hoekstra FT: **Long-term effectiveness of depot gonadotropin-releasing hormone analogue in the treatment of children with central precocious puberty.** *American journal of diseases of children (1960)* 1993, **147(6)**:653-7.
15. Neely EK, Hintz RL, Parker B, Bachrach LK, Cohen P, Olney R, et al: **Two-year results of treatment with depot leuprolide acetate for central precocious puberty.** *The Journal of pediatrics* 1992, **121(4)**:634-40.
16. Tanaka T, Niimi H, Matsuo N, Fujieda K, Tachibana K, Ohyama K, et al: **Results of long-term follow-up after treatment of central precocious puberty with leuprorelin acetate: evaluation of effectiveness of treatment and recovery of gonadal function. The TAP-144-SR Japanese Study Group on Central Precocious Puberty.** *The Journal of clinical endocrinology and metabolism* 2005, **90(3)**:1371-6.
17. Neely EK, Lee PA, Bloch CA, Larsen L, Yang D, Mattia-Goldberg C, et al: **Leuprolide acetate 1-month depot for central precocious puberty: hormonal suppression and recovery.** *Int J Pediatr Endocrinol* 2010, **2010**:398639.
18. Roche AF, Chumlea WC, Thissen D: **Assessing the skeletal maturity of the hand wrist: FELS method.** Springfield, IL: Charles C. Thomas; 1988.
19. Bayley N, Pinneau SR: **Tables for predicting adult height from skeletal age: revised for use with the Greulich-Pyle hand standards.** *The Journal of pediatrics* 1952, **40(4)**:423-41.
20. Brito VN, Latronico AC, Cukier P, Teles MG, Silveira LF, Arnhold IJ, et al: **Factors determining normal adult height in girls with gonadotropin-dependent precocious puberty treated with depot gonadotropin-releasing hormone analogs.** *The Journal of clinical endocrinology and metabolism* 2008, **93(7)**:2662-9.
21. Badaru A, Wilson DM, Bachrach LK, Fechner P, Gandrud LM, Durham E, et al: **Sequential comparisons of one-month and three-month depot**

leuprolide regimens in central precocious puberty. *The Journal of clinical endocrinology and metabolism* 2006, **91(5)**:1862-7.
22. Carel JC, Lahlou N, Jaramillo O, Montauban V, Teinturier C, Colle M, et al: **Treatment of central precocious puberty by subcutaneous injections of leuprorelin 3-month depot (11.25 mg).** *The Journal of clinical endocrinology and metabolism* 2002, **87(9)**:4111-6.
23. Eugster EA, Clarke W, Kletter GB, Lee PA, Neely EK, Reiter EO, et al: **Efficacy and safety of histrelin subdermal implant in children with central precocious puberty: a multicenter trial.** *The Journal of clinical endocrinology and metabolism* 2007, **92(5)**:1697-704.
24. Pasquino AM, Pucarelli I, Accardo F, Demiraj V, Segni M, Di Nardo R: **Long-term observation of 87 girls with idiopathic central precocious puberty treated with gonadotropin-releasing hormone analogs: impact on adult height, body mass index, bone mineral content, and reproductive function.** *The Journal of clinical endocrinology and metabolism* 2008, **93(1)**:190-5.
25. Lazar L, Padoa A, Phillip M: **Growth pattern and final height after cessation of gonadotropin-suppressive therapy in girls with central sexual precocity.** *The Journal of clinical endocrinology and metabolism* 2007, **92(9)**:3483-9.
26. Magiakou MA, Manousaki D, Papadaki M, Hadjidakis D, Levidou G, Vakaki M, et al: **The efficacy and safety of gonadotropin-releasing hormone analog treatment in childhood and adolescence: a single center, long-term follow-up study.** *The Journal of clinical endocrinology and metabolism* 2010, **95(1)**:109-17.
27. Bar A, Linder B, Sobel EH, Saenger P, DiMartino-Nardi J: **Bayley-Pinneau method of height prediction in girls with central precocious puberty: correlation with adult height.** *The Journal of pediatrics* 1995, **126(6)**:955-8.

12

Eating behaviors in obese children with pseudohypoparathyroidism type 1a: a cross-sectional study

Lulu Wang[1] and Ashley H Shoemaker[2]*

Abstract

Background: Children with pseudohypoparathyroidism type 1a (PHP-1a) develop early-onset obesity. These children have decreased resting energy expenditure but it is unknown if hyperphagia contributes to their obesity.

Methods: We conducted a survey assessment of patients 2 to 12 years old with PHP-1a and matched controls using the Hyperphagia Questionnaire (HQ) and Children's Eating Behavior Questionnaire (CEBQ). Results of the PHP-1a group were also compared with an obese control group and normal weight sibling group.

Results: We enrolled 10 patients with PHP-1a and 9 matched controls. There was not a significant difference between the PHP-1a group and matched controls for total HQ score (p = 0.72), Behavior (p = 0.91), Drive (p = 0.48) or Severity (p = 0.73) subset scores. There was also no difference between the PHP-1a group and matched controls on the CEBQ. In a secondary analysis, the PHP-1a group was compared with obese controls (n = 30) and normal weight siblings (n = 6). Caregivers reported an increased interest in food before age 2 years in 6 of 10 PHP-1a patients (60%), 9 of 30 obese controls (30%) and none of the siblings (p = 0.04). The sibling group had a significantly lower Positive Eating Behavior score than the PHP-1a group (2.6 [2.4, 2.9] vs. 3.5 [3.1, 4.0], p < 0.01) and obese controls (2.6 [2.4, 2.9] vs. 3.4 [2.6, 3.8], p = 0.04), but there was not a significant difference between the PHP-1a and obese controls (p = 0.35). The sibling group had a lower Desire to Drink score than both the PHP-1a group (1.8 [1.6, 2.7] vs. 4.3 [3.3, 5.0], p < 0.01) and obese controls (1.8 [1.6, 2.7] vs. 3.3 [3.0, 4.0], p < 0.01) but there was not a significant difference between the PHP-1a and obese control Desire to Drink scores (p = 0.11).

Conclusions: Patients with PHP-1a demonstrate hyperphagic symptoms similar to matched obese controls.

Keywords: Pseudohypoparathyroidism, Obesity, Eating behaviors

Introduction

Pseudohypoparathyroidism type 1a (PHP-1a) is a rare disorder caused by a maternally inherited mutation in the gene *GNAS*. *GNAS* encodes the alpha subunit of the stimulatory G-protein (G$_s$α). In some tissues, the paternal allele is imprinted and only the maternal allele is expressed. Therefore, in imprinted tissues, patients with PHP-1a lack functional G$_s$α and have abnormal G-protein coupled receptor signaling. Examples of known imprinted tissues include kidney, thyroid, hypothalamus and pituitary [1-3]. PHP-1a is usually diagnosed in childhood due to a distinctive phenotype that includes short stature, brachydactyly, cognitive impairment, ectopic ossifications and multi-hormone resistance.

A more recently described feature of PHP-1a is early-onset obesity [4]. This obesity occurs despite adequate treatment of hormone deficiencies, including thyroid hormone and growth hormone replacement. A current hypothesis is that the obesity phenotype is due to abnormal function of the melanocortin-4 receptor (MC4R) in the hypothalamus. The MC4R is a G-protein coupled receptor that plays a critical role in energy homeostasis. Mutations in *MC4R* are the most common cause of monogenic obesity in humans [5].

In a previous study, we showed that children with PHP-1a have decreased resting energy expenditure which

* Correspondence: Ashley.H.Shoemaker@vanderbilt.edu
[2]Monroe Carell Jr. Children's Hospital at Vanderbilt University, Nashville, TN 37232-9170, USA
Full list of author information is available at the end of the article

may contribute to the obesity phenotype [6]. Hyperphagia is seen in humans and mice with abnormal MC4R signaling [5,7] but has not been demonstrated in the PHP-1a mouse model [1]. It is not known if hyperphagia or abnormal eating behaviors are seen in children with PHP-1a. We hypothesized that children with PHP-1a have mild hyperphagia leading to excess caloric intake and abnormal weight gain. To test this hypothesis, we measured eating behaviors and hyperphagia in children with PHP-1a and matched controls.

Methods
Participants
Study participants were recruited from the Vanderbilt adult and pediatric endocrinology clinics as well as online advertisements from August, 2012 through January, 2014. Inclusion criteria were age 2–12 years old, English proficiency and one of the following: clinical diagnosis of PHP-1a or status as a sibling of a PHP-1a patient. Exclusion criteria were: obesity due to another known genetic syndrome (e.g., Prader-Willi syndrome) or current use of appetite-suppressing medications.

Healthy, matched controls were recruited from the Vanderbilt pediatric clinics and the Vanderbilt Childhood Obesity Registry (VCOR). VCOR is a registry for patients with a history of BMI >97th percentile before 6 years old. Controls were matched based on gender, age (±2 years) and BMI Z-score (±0.25). All patients in VCOR age 2–12 years old were included in the general obese control group.

Consent and age appropriate assent were obtained. The study was approved by the Institutional Review Board of Vanderbilt University.

Experimental procedure
All participants completed a medical history form. Children's height and weight were obtained from the most recent endocrinology or primary care clinic visit. BMI height and weight z-scores were calculated as standard deviations from the mean using gender and age specific Centers for Disease Control growth charts. All children had a Hyperphagia Questionnaire (HQ) [8] and Children's Eating Behavior Questionnaire (CEBQ) [9] completed by the primary caregiver.

The HQ was originally developed to assess hyperphagia in Prader-Willi syndrome and contains 11-questions that assess symptoms of hyperphagia in one of three categories (Behavior, Drive and Severity), as rated on a five-point scale (1 = not a problem to 5 = severe and/or frequent problem). The total HQ score has a minimum of 11 points and a maximum of 55. The 35-item CEBQ assesses Positive and Negative Eating Behaviors. The Positive Eating Behavior score is comprised of four

sub-scales: Food Responsiveness, Enjoyment of Food, Emotional Overeating and Desire to Drink.

Data collection
Study data were collected and managed using REDCap electronic data capture tools hosted at Vanderbilt University. REDCap (Research Electronic Data Capture) [10] is a secure, web-based application designed to support data capture for research studies. Questionnaires were completed either online (REDCap survey) or via mail.

Statistical analysis
The primary outcome was the subset scores of the HQ in PHP-1a patients compared with matched controls. Secondary analyses include comparison of CEBQ subset scores and comparison of PHP-1a, sibling and obese control groups. Results are presented as median (interquartile range) unless otherwise specified. Paired analysis was done using Wilcoxon signed rank test. For the secondary analysis of the three groups (PHP-1a, obese controls and sibling controls), continuous variables were compared using the Kruskal-Wallis test. If the p value was <0.05, each group was compared using the Mann–Whitney U test. Categorical variables were compared using Chi-square test. Based on our sample size, we did not use regression or analyses of covariance due to concerns for over-fitting. Internal consistency of the HQ was assessed using Cronbach's alpha. Statistics were performed using SPSS version 22.

Results
Study population
Ten patients with PHP-1a enrolled in the study, including 2 sibling pairs. We identified a matched control for 9 of 10 PHP-1a patients. We enrolled all unaffected siblings (n = 6) to serve as a normal weight control group. The two PHP-1a sibling pairs and one additional PHP-1a subject did not have an unaffected sibling. An additional 21 obese children between 2 and 12 years old had questionnaire data available in VCOR. These children were combined with the matched controls to form an obese control group (n = 30) for secondary analysis.

Baseline characteristics
Patients were matched on age, gender and BMI z-score (Table 1). All PHP-1a patients were white and 6 of 9 matched controls where white, the remaining patients were African American. Table 2 summarizes the baseline characteristics of the subjects. The PHP-1a group age range was 2 to 10 years old, the obese control group was 3 to 12 years old and the sibling control group was 3 to 12 years old. As expected, the PHP-1a and obese control groups were significantly more obese than the sibling controls as measured by BMI z-score (p <0.01) but there

Table 1 Baseline characteristic of the matched pairs

Patient	PHP-1a group		Matched control	
	Age	BMI z-score	Age	BMI z-score
1	2	3.33	---	---
2	3	1.71	3	1.54
3	4	1.16	4	1.08
4	5	2.78	7	2.72
5	5	1.44	5	1.39
6	6	2.98	5	3.01
7	9	3.01	9	2.95
8	9	2.41	10	2.44
9	10	1.85	11	1.74
10	10	2.70	10	2.63

PHP-1a, pseudohypoparathyroidism type 1a; BMI, body mass index. BMI z-scores were calculated as standard deviations from the mean using gender and age specific Centers for Disease Control growth charts.

was no difference between the PHP-1a and obese control groups (p = 0.86). The obese control group was 57% white and 43% African American versus the PHP-1a group that was 100% white (p = 0.02).

Hyperphagia questionnaire

There was not a significant difference between the PHP-1a group and matched controls for total HQ score (p = 0.72), Behavior (p = 0.91), Drive (p = 0.48) or Severity (p = 0.73) (Figure 1). Two PHP-1a patients were outliers with total HQ scores of 39 and 40 (group median 22.5 [17.3, 32.3]) though they were not more obese than the overall group (BMI z-score 2.78 and 2.41, group median 2.55 [1.64, 2.99]). There was also not a significant difference between the PHP-1a, obese control and sibling groups for total HQ score (22.5 [17.3, 32.3] vs. 18.5 [15.8, 27.0] vs. 18.5 [17.3, 20.3], p = 0.40) or subset scores (Figure 2). The HQ includes a question "how old was your child when they first showed an increased interest in food" that is not included in the HQ score. Caregivers reported an increased interest in food before age 2 years in 6 of 10 PHP-1a patients (60%), 9 of 30 obese controls (30%) and none of the siblings (p = 0.04). Internal reliability coefficients (Cronbach's alpha) were 0.86 for the total HQ score, 0.64 for Behavior, 0.84 for Drive and 0.72 for Severity.

Childhood eating behavior questionnaire

There was no significant difference between the PHP-1a group and matched controls for Negative Eating Behaviors (2.9 [2.8, 3.2] vs. 2.9 [2.6, 3.2], p = 0.77) or Positive Eating Behaviors (3.5 [2.9, 4.2] vs. 3.4 [3.1, 3.7], p = 0.86). The subscale scores for Food Responsiveness (p = 1.0), Enjoyment of Food (p = 0.81), Emotional Overeating (p = 0.73) and Desire to Drink (p = 0.31) were not different between matched pairs (Figure 3). One obese control patient did not have CEBQ data available; therefore 29 obese control subjects were included for this subanalysis (Figure 4). The sibling group had a significantly lower Positive Eating Behavior score than the PHP-1a group (2.6 [2.4, 2.9] vs. 3.5 [3.1, 4.0], p < 0.01) and obese controls (2.6 [2.4, 2.9] vs. 3.4 [2.6, 3.8], p = 0.04), but there was not a significant difference between the PHP-1a and obese controls (p = 0.35). There was a difference between the PHP-1a, obese control and sibling groups for the Desire to Drink subscale (p < 0.01, Figure 4). The sibling group had a lower Desire to Drink score than both the PHP-1a group (1.8 [1.6, 2.7] vs. 4.3 [3.3, 5.0], p < 0.01) and obese controls (1.8 [1.6, 2.7] vs. 3.3 [3.0, 4.0], p < 0.01). There was not a significant difference between the PHP-1a and obese control Desire to Drink scores (p = 0.11).

Discussion

To our knowledge, this is the first study to systematically evaluate eating behaviors in children with PHP-1a. While MC4R haploinsufficiency is associated with marked hyperphagia [5,11], our data suggest that children with PHP-1a may not be hyperphagic when compared with other obese children. Similarly, the PHP-1a mouse model shows increased feed efficiency, not increased food intake [1,2]. A recent study in adults found no difference in energy intake between PHP-1a and matched controls using 7-day food records [12]. There is one published case series of parent reported hyperphagia in two young children with PHP-1a [13]. The variability seen in PHP-1a could be due to variable imprinting of MC4R in the hypothalamus, or hyperphagia in MC4R haploinsufficiency may be mediated through non-$G_s\alpha$ signaling pathways. Previously, we have demonstrated that these children have decreased resting

Table 2 Baseline characteristics

	PHP-1a (n = 10)	Obese controls (n = 30)	p value	Siblings (n = 6)	p value
Age (years)	5.5 (3.8, 9.3)	7.0 (5.0-10.0)	0.22	7.5 (4.5, 11.3)	0.43
Gender (% female)	60	70	0.70	100	0.23
Ethnicity (% white)	100	57	0.02	100	1.0
BMI	24.5 (18.2, 30.5)	29.5 (21.6, 35.1)	0.43	*18.4 (14.8, 22.8)	0.05
BMI Z-score	2.55 (1.64, 2.99)	2.50 (1.74, 2.84)	0.86	*0.48 (−0.72, 1.16)	<0.01

PHP-1a, pseudohypoparathyroidism type 1a; BMI, body mass index. Data expressed as median (lower quartile, upper quartile). P-values were determined using Mann-Whitney U test and Fisher's Exact test, comparing the PHP-1a group with each control group. BMI z-scores were calculated as standard deviations from the mean using gender and age specific Centers for Disease Control growth charts. *BMI data was not available for 2 siblings.

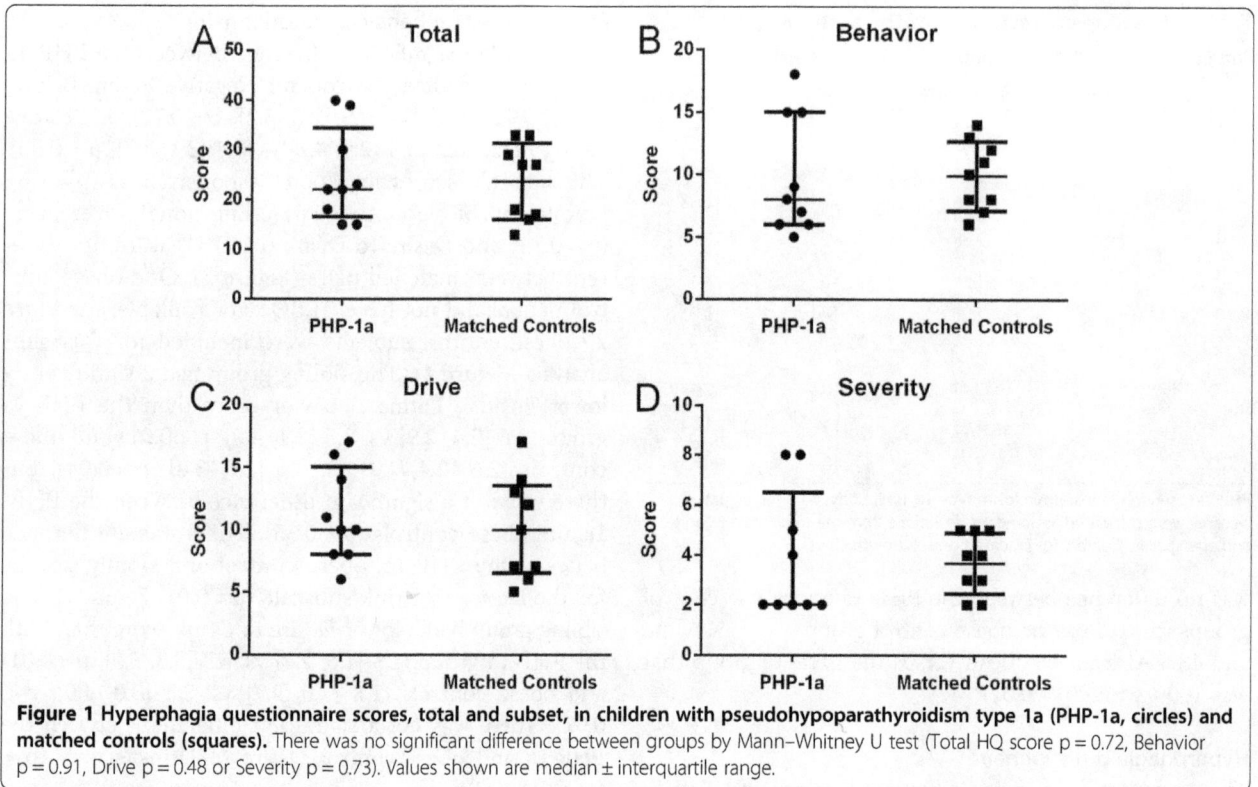

Figure 1 Hyperphagia questionnaire scores, total and subset, in children with pseudohypoparathyroidism type 1a (PHP-1a, circles) and matched controls (squares). There was no significant difference between groups by Mann–Whitney U test (Total HQ score p = 0.72, Behavior p = 0.91, Drive p = 0.48 or Severity p = 0.73). Values shown are median ± interquartile range.

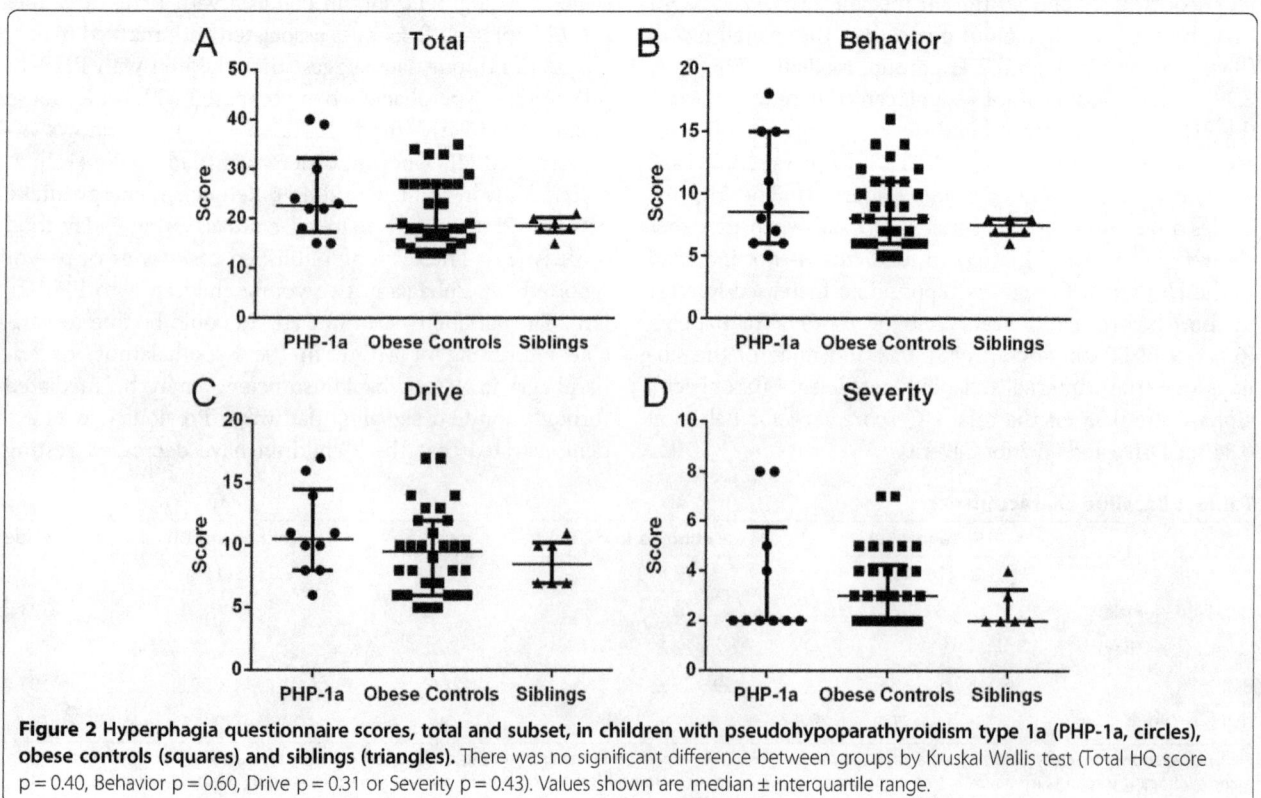

Figure 2 Hyperphagia questionnaire scores, total and subset, in children with pseudohypoparathyroidism type 1a (PHP-1a, circles), obese controls (squares) and siblings (triangles). There was no significant difference between groups by Kruskal Wallis test (Total HQ score p = 0.40, Behavior p = 0.60, Drive p = 0.31 or Severity p = 0.43). Values shown are median ± interquartile range.

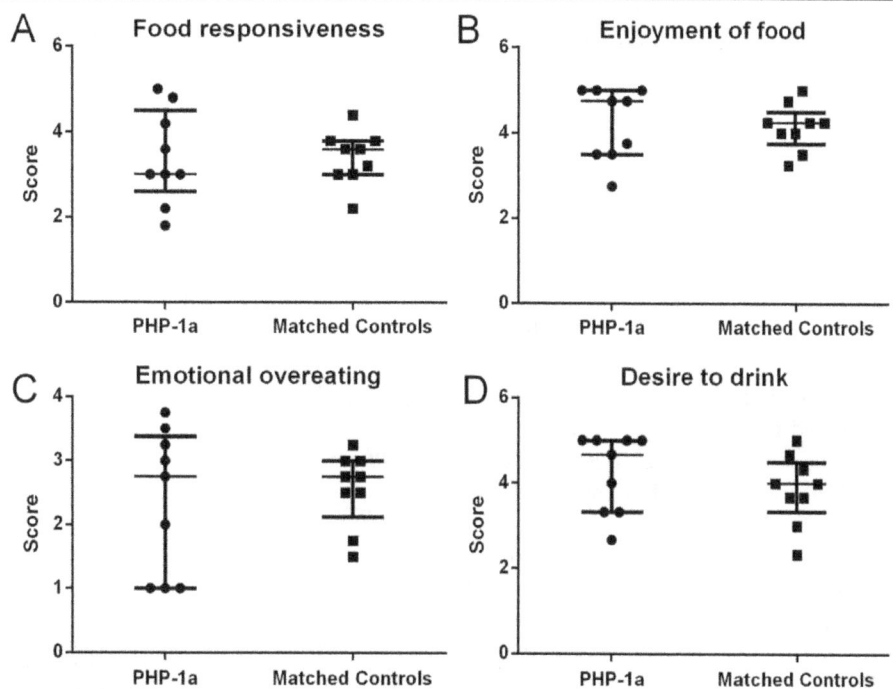

Figure 3 Childhood eating behavior questionnaire positive eating behavior subset scores in children with pseudohypoparathyroidism type 1a (PHP-1a, circles) and matched controls (squares). There was no significant difference between groups by Mann–Whitney U test (Food Responsiveness p = 1.0, Enjoyment of Food p = 0.81, Emotional Overeating p = 0.73 and Desire to Drink p = 0.31). Values shown are median ± interquartile range.

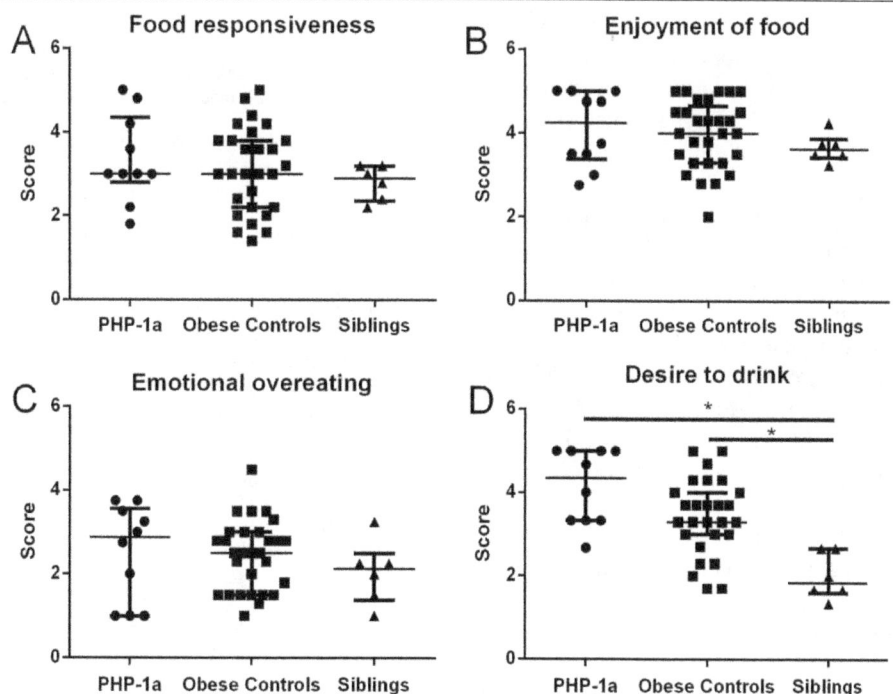

Figure 4 Childhood eating behavior questionnaire positive eating behavior subset scores in children with pseudohypoparathyroidism type 1a (PHP-1a, circles), obese controls (squares) and siblings (triangles). Values shown are median ± interquartile range. *Indicates p value <0.05 by Mann–Whitney U test following a significant Kruskal-Wallis test.

energy expenditure [6]. This energy expenditure imbalance may be the main driver of early-onset obesity in PHP-1a.

The HQ has previously been used to evaluate eating behaviors in other forms of syndromic obesity. The HQ scores for PHP-1a (mean ± SD, total: 24.8 ± 8.9, behavior: 10.0 ± 4.5, drive: 11.1 ± 3.6, severity: 3.7 ± 2.5) were significantly lower than Prader-Willi syndrome (total: 30.5 ± 5.8, behavior: 13.6 ± 4.5, drive: 12.3 ± 3.3, severity: 4.6 ± 1.7) [8], but only slightly lower than brain-derived neurotrophic factor (*BDNF*) haploinsufficiency (total: 26.3 ± 7.3, behavior: 10.6 ± 3.2, drive: 11.5 ± 3.4, severity: 4.2 ± 1.7) [14] and Bardet-Biedl syndrome (total: 27.3 ± 8.2, behavior: 12.3 ± 3.8, drive: 11.1 ± 3.7, severity 3.9 ± 1.6) [8,15]. In contrast with PHP-1a [1,2], mouse models of Bardet-Biedl syndrome [16,17] and *Bdnf* inactivation [18] demonstrate obesity from increased food intake. It is possible that PHP-1a patients are only hyperphagic during specific developmental periods. Rapid weight gain in infancy and parent reported "increased interest in food" at a young age may indicate early, non-progressive hyperphagia in PHP-1a.

PHP-1a and obese controls had increased Positive Eating Behavior and Desire to Drink scores compared with lean siblings, but not compared with obese controls. Heightened preference for and consumption of sugar-sweetened beverages has been linked to increased Desire to Drink scores in children [19] and the motivation for drinking may be desire for the pleasant sensation of sweet taste. Alternatively, these children may demonstrate a drive for high caloric foods, aided by consumption of sugar-sweetened beverages. A reduction in the intake of sugar-sweetened beverages may be an effective strategy to reduce the rate of weight gain in obese children [20,21].

The main limitation of our study was the small sample size. PHP-1a is a rare disorder and it is challenging to identify eligible subjects. We used a matched control group in order to account for possible confounders without over-fitting our statistical model, but a matched control was not available for one child with PHP-1a. In addition, controls were not matched based on race and this may have masked differences between the groups. The HQ was originally designed for children with Prader-Willi syndrome but we believe that it is an appropriate tool for PHP-1a as both disorders cause intellectual disability, multiple medical problems and childhood obesity. An advantage of this questionnaire is that it is completed by the parent which allows the investigation of eating behaviors in young children and those with intellectual disability. The Cronbach's alpha results for our study population (range 0.64-0.86) were all acceptable and similar to those in the original study of Prader-Willi syndrome (range 0.60-0.80) [8].

Conclusion

In summary, our data suggest that children with PHP-1a demonstrate hyperphagic symptoms similar to other obese children. The mild hyperphagia seen in PHP-1a may be common in obese children and not attributable to PHP-1a. Further studies, such as standardized test meals and longitudinal investigations, are needed to confirm our findings. Understanding the pathophysiology of abnormal weight gain in children with PHP-1a may inform our understanding of energy homeostasis in humans and is critical in order to design targeted therapeutic interventions.

Competing interests
The authors have no conflict of interest to disclose.

Authors' contributions
LW generated figures and wrote the manuscript. AHS designed the study, collected and analyzed data and assisted in writing the manuscript. Both authors read and approved the final manuscript.

Acknowledgements
The study was funded by the Vanderbilt Physician Scientist Development Program (AHS) and by CTSA award No. UL1TR000445 from the National Center for Advancing Translational Sciences. Its contents are solely the responsibility of the authors and do not necessarily represent official views of the National Center for Advancing Translational Sciences or the National Institutes of Health.

Author details
[1]School of Medicine, Vanderbilt University, Nashville, TN, USA. [2]Monroe Carell Jr. Children's Hospital at Vanderbilt University, Nashville, TN 37232-9170, USA.

References
1. Chen M, Gavrilova O, Liu J, Xie T, Deng C, Nguyen AT, Nackers LM, Lorenzo J, Shen L, Weinstein LS: **Alternative Gnas gene products have opposite effects on glucose and lipid metabolism.** *Proc Natl Acad Sci U S A* 2005, 102:7386–7391.
2. Chen M, Wang J, Dickerson KE, Kelleher J, Xie T, Gupta D, Lai EW, Pacak K, Gavrilova O, Weinstein LS: **Central nervous system imprinting of the G protein G(s)alpha and its role in metabolic regulation.** *Cell Metab* 2009, 9:548–555.
3. Germain-Lee EL, Schwindinger W, Crane JL, Zewdu R, Zweifel LS, Wand G, Huso DL, Saji M, Ringel MD, Levine MA: **A mouse model of albright hereditary osteodystrophy generated by targeted disruption of exon 1 of the Gnas gene.** *Endocrinology* 2005, 146:4697–4709.
4. Long DN, McGuire S, Levine MA, Weinstein LS, Germain-Lee EL: **Body mass index differences in pseudohypoparathyroidism type 1a versus pseudopseudohypoparathyroidism may implicate paternal imprinting of Galpha(s) in the development of human obesity.** *J Clin Endocrinol Metab* 2007, 92:1073–1079.
5. Farooqi IS, Keogh JM, Yeo GS, Lank EJ, Cheetham T, O'Rahilly S: **Clinical spectrum of obesity and mutations in the melanocortin 4 receptor gene.** *N Engl J Med* 2003, 348:1085–1095.
6. Shoemaker AH, Lomenick JP, Saville BR, Wang W, Buchowski MS, Cone RD: **Energy expenditure in obese children with pseudohypoparathyroidism type 1a.** *Int J Obes (Lond)* 2012, 37:1147–1153.
7. Huszar D, Lynch CA, Fairchild-Huntress V, Dunmore JH, Fang Q, Berkemeier LR, Gu W, Kesterson RA, Boston BA, Cone RD, Smith FJ, Campfield LA, Burn P, Lee F: **Targeted disruption of the melanocortin-4 receptor results in obesity in mice.** *Cell* 1997, 88:131–141.
8. Dykens EM, Maxwell MA, Pantino E, Kossler R, Roof E: **Assessment of hyperphagia in Prader-Willi syndrome.** *Obesity* 2007, 15:1816–1826.
9. Wardle J, Guthrie CA, Sanderson S, Rapoport L: **Development of the children's eating behaviour questionnaire.** *J Child Psychol Psychiatry* 2001, 42:963–970.

10. Harris PA, Taylor R, Thielke R, Payne J, Gonzalez N, Conde JG: **Research electronic data capture (REDCap)–a metadata-driven methodology and workflow process for providing translational research informatics support.** *J Biomed Inform* 2009, **42**:377–381.

11. Valette M, Bellisle F, Carette C, Poitou C, Dubern B, Paradis G, Hercberg S, Muzard L, Clement K, Czernichow S: **Eating behaviour in obese patients with melanocortin-4 receptor mutations: a literature review.** *Int J Obes (Lond)* 2013, **37**:1027–1035.

12. Muniyappa R, Warren MA, Zhao X, Aney SC, Courville AB, Chen KY, Brychta RJ, Germain-Lee EL, Weinstein LS, Skarulis MC: **Reduced insulin sensitivity in adults with pseudohypoparathyroidism type 1a.** *J Clin Endocrinol Metab* 2013, **98**:E1796–E1801.

13. Ong KK, Amin R, Dunger DB: **Pseudohypoparathyroidism–another monogenic obesity syndrome.** *Clin Endocrinol (Oxf)* 2000, **52**:389–391.

14. Han JC, Liu QR, Jones M, Levinn RL, Menzie CM, Jefferson-George KS, Adler-Wailes DC, Sanford EL, Lacbawan FL, Uhl GR, Rennert OM, Yanovski JA: **Brain-derived neurotrophic factor and obesity in the WAGR syndrome.** *N Engl J Med* 2008, **359**:918–927.

15. Sherafat-Kazemzadeh R, Ivey L, Kahn SR, Sapp JC, Hicks MD, Kim RC, Krause AJ: **Hyperphagia in Patients with Bardet Biedl Syndrome.** In *Pediatric Academic Societies Annual Meeting; Washington, D.C.* 2013.

16. Seo S, Guo DF, Bugge K, Morgan DA, Rahmouni K, Sheffield VC: **Requirement of Bardet-Biedl syndrome proteins for leptin receptor signaling.** *Hum Mol Genet* 2009, **18**:1323–1331.

17. Rahmouni K, Fath MA, Seo S, Thedens DR, Berry CJ, Weiss R, Nishimura DY, Sheffield VC: **Leptin resistance contributes to obesity and hypertension in mouse models of Bardet-Biedl syndrome.** *J Clin Invest* 2008, **118**:1458–1467.

18. Fox EA, Byerly MS: **A mechanism underlying mature-onset obesity: evidence from the hyperphagic phenotype of brain-derived neurotrophic factor mutants.** *Am J Physiol Regul Integr Comp Physiol* 2004, **286**:R994–R1004.

19. Sweetman C, Wardle J, Cooke L: **Soft drinks and 'desire to drink' in preschoolers.** *Int J Behav Nutr Phys Act* 2008, **5**:60.

20. de Ruyter JC, Olthof MR, Seidell JC, Katan MB: **A trial of sugar-free or sugar-sweetened beverages and body weight in children.** *N Engl J Med* 2012, **367**:1397–1406.

21. Ebbeling CB, Feldman HA, Chomitz VR, Antonelli TA, Gortmaker SL, Osganian SK, Ludwig DS: **A randomized trial of sugar-sweetened beverages and adolescent body weight.** *N Engl J Med* 2012, **367**:1407–1416.

13

Gender and race influence metabolic benefits of fitness in children: a cross-sectional study

Vanessa A Curtis[1*], Aaron L Carrel[2], Jens C Eickhoff[3] and David B Allen[2]

Abstract

Background: Increasing obesity and poor cardiovascular fitness (CVF) contribute to higher rates of type 2 diabetes mellitus (T2DM) in children. While the relative contributions of fitness and body fat on development of insulin resistance (IR) in children and adolescents remains unresolved, gender- and race-specific differences likely exist in the degree to which CVF influences IR and risk for T2DM. Better understanding of how gender and race affect interactions between body fat, CVF, and metabolic health would be helpful in designing effective and targeted strategies to reduce obesity-associated disease risk. We evaluated whether metabolic benefits of fitness on reducing inflammation and insulin resistance (IR) are affected by gender and race.

Methods: This cross-sectional study included 203 healthy children (mean age 12.2 y, 50% male, 46% non-Hispanic white (NHW), 54% racially diverse (RD)). Fasting insulin, glucose, hsCRP, and adiponectin were measured; race was self-reported; cardiovascular fitness (CVF) was evaluated by the Progressive Aerobic Cardiovascular Endurance Run. Associations between inflammation and gender, race, and CVF were evaluated using analysis of covariance. Multivariate regression analysis identified independent predictors of IR.

Results: Fitness and inflammation were inversely related in both males and females (p < 0.01); this effect was marginally stronger in RD children (p = 0.06) and non-overweight males (p = 0.07). High BMI (p < 0.001), low fitness (p = 0.006), and (female) gender (p = 0.003) were independently associated with higher HOMA-IR. In males, BMI and fitness, but not race independently predicted HOMA-IR. In females, BMI and race, but not fitness independently predicted HOMA-IR.

Conclusions: In middle school children, the beneficial effects of fitness vary based on gender and race. High CVF has an enhanced anti-inflammatory effect in male and RD children. While BMI is the strongest predictor of IR in the study group as a whole, fitness is a significant predictor of IR only in males, and race is a significant predictor of IR only in females.

Keywords: Gender, Race, Cardiovascular Fitness, Insulin Resistance

Background

Increasing obesity and poor cardiovascular fitness (CVF) both contribute to higher rates of type 2 diabetes mellitus (T2DM) in children. While the relative contributions of CVF and % body fat on development of insulin resistance (IR) in children and adolescents remains unresolved, gender- and race-specific differences likely exist in the degree to which CVF influences IR and risk for T2DM [1-4]. Better understanding of how gender and race affect interactions between % body fat, CVF, and metabolic health would be helpful in designing effective and targeted strategies to reduce obesity-associated disease risk.

Adipose tissue, once thought to be an inert energy storage depot, is now known to be an active endocrine organ, secreting bioactive adipokines, both pro- inflammatory (e.g. TNF-α) and anti-inflammatory (e.g. adiponectin), which influence insulin sensitivity and risk for/protection from the metabolic syndrome. Levels of pro-inflammatory cytokines are directly related to fat mass, with visceral adipose tissue mass contributing more robustly than total fat or subcutaneous fat mass [4]. In contrast, anti-inflammatory adiponectin correlates inversely with insulin resistance (IR) and

* Correspondence: vanessa-curtis@uiowa.edu
[1]Department of Pediatrics, University of Iowa Carver College of Medicine, 200 Hawkins Drive, 2859 JPP, Iowa City, IO 52242-1083, USA
Full list of author information is available at the end of the article

progression to T2DM, cardiovascular disease, and hypertension (HTN); [5-11] this inverse relationship persists across gender, race, and age [12-17]. C-reactive protein (CRP) is a general marker of inflammation that reflects the summation of the pro-inflammatory and anti-inflammatory cytokines and has been shown to predict cardiovascular disease in many groups of adult patients [18]. In children, high sensitivity (hs) CRP levels are independently associated with IR [19,20] and, in obese children, are increased before other overt manifestations of the metabolic syndrome are present.[21]. Variations in adipose tissue inflammation response to fitness level may help to explain individual and group differences in metabolic health-promoting responses to fitness interventions.

Increased CVF and physical activity are inversely associated with markers of inflammation [22,23] and attenuate insulin resistance attributable to obesity [24-26]. In obese middle school children, CVF assessed by V0$_2$max consistently and independently predicts IR [1]. This study evaluates whether metabolic benefits of fitness on reducing inflammation and IR are affected by gender and race.

Methods
Study population
Students were recruited from two local middle schools during school registration. All students who attended the official school registration were invited to participate in this cross-sectional study upon arrival at the school. Two hundred and three healthy children, 11-14 years of age were included. Exclusion criteria included insulin or glucocorticoid therapy, acute infection at time of testing, T2DM or chronic illness preventing completion of fitness testing. Consent and racial self-designation for both parents were obtained at that time of recruitment from children's parents. To explore potential influences of race, two groups were identified - non-Hispanic White (NHW) and racially diverse (Hispanic White/Black, Black, Asian, Pacific Islander, American Indian: RD). Subjects in whom both parents identified as non-Hispanic White were allocated to the NHW group. The RD group comprised subjects in whom either parent self-identified as a race other than NHW. The broad racial categorization was based on reported presumed-genetic differences in risk for IR and numbers of subjects needed for sufficiently powerful statistical analysis. Anthropomorphic measurements and venipuncture were completed at the children's' school by the same investigators during early morning visits at the start of the school day after an overnight fast was confirmed. Blood was processed at the school and transported to the University of Wisconsin Hospital laboratory directly for biochemical evaluation of hsCRP, glucose and insulin. A portion of the sample was transported to the University of Wisconsin National Primate Research Center for evaluation of adiponectin. Height was measured using a

stadiometer to the nearest 0.5 cm. Weight was measured without shoes in light clothes on a beam balance platform scale to the nearest 0.1 kg. BMI was calculated and used to divide children into normal weight (BMI <85%ile) and overweight (BMI >85%ile). Homeostasis model of assessment- insulin resistance (HOMA-IR) was calculated from glucose and insulin values (fasting glucose (mg/dL) × fasting insulin (µU/ml)/405). The progressive aerobic cardiovascular endurance run (PACER) fitness testing was conducted by the physical education teacher as part of the students' physical education class within 1 month of the study visit. The procedures were approved by the Human Subjects Committee of the University of Wisconsin.

Measurements
A 10 ml fasting blood sample for insulin, glucose, hsCRP and adiponectin was obtained from an antecubital vein. HsCRP concentrations were determined by the nephelometric method on the Dimension Vista® System, with an analytical measurement range of 0.16-9.50 mg/L. Glucose was determined by hexokinase method and insulin by chemiluminescent immunoassay (University of Wisconsin Hospital and Clinics Laboratory, Madison, WI). Adiponectin concentrations were measured by radioimmunoassay using Linco reagent (National Primate Research Center, University of Wisconsin - Madison).

Fitness testing was done using the 20 m PACER protocol [27,28]. The PACER protocol has been shown to correlate well with laboratory measures of VO2 max [28]. It requires children to run back and forth between two lines set 20 meters apart at progressively faster pace (start at 8.5 km/hr and increase by 0.5 km/hr) with each subsequent level. The test was completed when the participant was not able to complete the distance at the stipulated pace on two consecutive laps. The participant's score was reported as number of laps completed. The test was administered by the same two physical education teachers for all students during their physical education class.

Statistical analysis
Height, weight, BMI z-scores, inflammatory markers, insulin resistance and PACER scores were summarized using standard descriptive statistics. Subject ethnicity was categorized as White if both parents designated race as Non-Hispanic White. Subject race was categorized as non-White if both parents did not self-identify as Non-Hispanic White. The distribution of the hsCRP values was highly skewed to the left due to the truncation (below detection level) at 0.2 mg/L. Sixty-four children had an hsCRP level that was < 0.2 mg/L, but no children had a test designated as invalid. Consequently, hsCRP values were categorized into low/normal category (<0.5 mg/L) and elevated category (≥0.5 mg/L). The 0.5 mg/L threshold value was determined based on the distribution

of hsCRP values for this subject population reported by Cook et al.[29].

The Lambda-Mu-Sigma (LMS) method for constructing normalized curves was used to calculate fitness level z-scores and percentiles [30]. School age children from a large Wisconsin database, with PACER measurements from large cross-sectional study involving approximate 27,000 subjects (our data, unpublished), were used to construct age and gender specific reference values. Subjects were categorized into "low fitness" group (PACER <33th percentile), "moderate fitness" (PACER between 33th and 67th percentile) and "high fitness" group (PACER > 67th percentile). Logistic regression analysis was used to evaluate the associations between gender, race, BMI z-score and hsCRP (low/normal vs. elevated) and adiponectin. Two-way interaction terms were included in the logistic regression analysis models to evaluate interaction effects. The association between gender, BMI z-score, race and insulin resistance was evaluated using univariate and multivariate linear regression analysis. HOMA-IR values were log-transformed before conducting the analyses to satisfy the normality assumption. The lasso (least absolute shrinkage and selection operator) approach will be used to determine whether fitness is an independent predictor for insulin resistance. The lasso regression performs shrinkage of the regression parameters and sets to zero the coefficients for the variables that appear not to contribute to prediction. Shrinkage methods have been shown to be superior for model selection than stepwise or manual selection methods [31].

In order to quantify the strengths of the associations between BMI z-score, PACER z-score and insulin resistance, partial correlation coefficients (r_p) were computed to summarize the results of the multivariate regression analyses and Pearson correlation coefficients (r) for the results of the univariate regression analyses. Least squares adjusted means were computed to compare insulin resistance levels between race and gender groups. All p-values are two-sided, with $p < 0.05$ indicating statistical significance. The data analysis was performed using SAS version 9.2 software (SAS Corp., Cary, NC).

Results

The participants' characteristics are presented in Table 1. Of 203 children who completed the study, 50% (102) were male, and 54% (109; i.e. RD group) had one or both parents who did not identify as non-Hispanic White (races reported included 16.3% Black, 24.6% Hispanic White, 6.4% Asian, 6.4% multiple). The mean age was 12.2 ± 0.9 years (range 11 - 14 years). Mean BMI z-score among participants was 0.64 ± 1.00 with 19.5% (n = 40) classified as overweight (BMI 85-95%ile), and 18.2% (n = 37) classified as obese (BMI > 95%ile). Mean number of PACER laps completed was 32.4 ± 17.2 overall with a

statistically significant ($p < 0.001$) difference between males (37.5 ± 19.5) and females (27.2 ± 12.5). Table 2 shows the distribution of children based on PACER score and hsCRP levels. Forty-three percent of children (n = 88) had elevated hsCRP levels, i.e., hsCRP > 0.5 mg/L. Median HOMA-IR was 3.78 (range 1.41-43.76). Mean adiponectin levels were 13.9 ± 4.6 μ g/ml, with a statistically significant difference (p = 0.04) between males (13.3 ± 4.6) and females (14.5 ± 4.5).

Associations between inflammatory markers and gender, race, and CVF

Results are summarized in Table 3. Fitness and inflammation were strongly ($p < 0.01$) and inversely related in both males and females, and, overall. Specifically, 67% of subjects in the low fitness group had elevated hsCRP (65% in males, 70% in females) versus 18% (11% in males, 25% in females) in the high fitness group. No significant interaction between gender and fitness level was detected (p = 0.282). However, a marginally significant interaction between race and fitness level (p = 0.058) was noted, with RD children demonstrating a trend toward larger effect of fitness on inflammation than NHW children. In the low fitness group, there was no difference in percentage of children with an elevated hsCRP based on race (68% of RD children and 67% of NHW children); in the high fitness group, however, 8% of RD children and 24% of NHW children had elevated hsCRP.

Due to the paucity of overweight children in the high fitness group, specific analysis of the overweight group could not be performed. To assess whether overweight children were disproportionately affecting the analysis, a sub-group analysis of gender effects was performed on non-overweight children (BMI <85%ile, n = 126). In this non-overweight group, only males retained significant effect of fitness on inflammation (p = 0.003). Further, there was a strong trend that gender influenced the response of inflammation to higher CVF, (p = 0.07); specifically, in the high fitness group only 3% of males had an elevated hsCRP compared to 26% of the females. Table 4

Adiponectin levels showed no significant independent associations with fitness or race.

Predictors of HOMA-IR

For the total study group, BMI (r_p = 0.35, $p < 0.001$), PACER z-score (r_p = – 0.19, p = 0.006), and gender (adjusted means for log-transformed HOMA-IR: 1.50 ± 0.5 in females vs. 1.30 ± 0.5 in males, p = 0.003) were identified as independent predictors of HOMA-IR in a multivariate linear regression analysis. When analyzed by gender, BMI in both males (r = 0.41, p = 0.0006) and females (r = 0.42, $p < 0.001$) was independently predictive of HOMA-IR. PACER z-score was independently

Table 1 Participant characteristics

	Total (n = 203)	Male (n = 102)	Female (n = 101)	NHW (n = 94)	Racially diverse (n = 109)
Age (years)	12.2(±0.9)	12.2(±0.8)	12.2(±1.0)	12.2(±0.9)	12.1(±0.9)
BMI z-score	0.64(±1.00)	0.63(±1.07)	0.64(±0.95)	0.37(±0.93)	0.86(±1.01)
Overweight	40(19.7%)	21(20.6%)	19(18.8%)	20(21.3%)	20(18.3%)
Obese	37(18.2%)	20(19.6%)	17(16.8%)	6(6.4%)	31(28.4%)
Fitness (PACER laps)	32.4(±17.2)	37.5(±19.5)	27.2(±12.5)	36.2(±18.5)	29.0(±15.2)

Data are means ± SE. "Overweight" and "Obese" represent the individuals whose BMI is between the 85-95th %ile and >95th %ile, respectively, based on Centers for Disease Control and Prevention statistics for age and sex

predictive of HOMA-IR in males ($r = -0.21$, $p = 0.004$) but not in females. In contrast, race was independently predictive of HOMA-IR in females (adjusted means for log-transformed HOMA-IR: 1.6 ± 0.7 in RD vs. 1.4 ± 0.78 in NHW, $p = 0.02$) but not in males.

Discussion

Many investigators have examined influence of race and gender on insulin resistance and other aspects of cardiovascular health, however, our study is unique in the attempt to examine whether these factors affect the degree to which cardiovascular fitness influences metabolic health. This cross-sectional study of healthy middle school children suggests that the metabolic benefits of fitness are influenced by both gender and race. Differences in the effect of fitness on inflammatory status and insulin sensitivity could provide insight into physiological characteristics that influence risk for metabolic disease in response to caloric excess and poor physical fitness. During times of nutrient scarcity, pro- and anti-inflammatory adipokines circulate in a balance that promotes energy efficiency to varying degrees. However, these same adipokines become detrimental when sedentary lifestyle leads to low fitness and accumulation of adipose tissue. People who evolved to be particularly adapted to expending high levels of energy in the setting of low caloric availability could, therefore, be at higher risk of inflammation and insulin resistance when activity levels are low and calories plentiful.

This study found that inflammation, measured by hsCRP, correlated strongly and inversely with CVF. This relationship was not confined to obese children; among

Table 2 Distribution of subject based on PACER and hsCRp

	N	%
PACER percentile (age/gender specific)		
<33%	46	23%
33-67%	90	44%
>67%	67	33%
hsCRP		
<0.5 mg/L	115	57%
>0.5 mg/L	88	43%

non-overweight boys (BMI < 85th%tile); more than 50% of those with low fitness had an hsCRP level in the elevated range. The effect of higher CVF on reducing inflammation was highly significant in males and females in all racial groups; however this relationship was especially strong in the RD group and in male children. In both of these subgroups the strong effect of fitness on inflammation reflected primarily low inflammation in fit subjects rather than elevated inflammation in children with low fitness.

This study also reports the new finding that gender and race influence the predictors of IR in middle school-aged children. While this study affirms BMI as the strongest identified predictor of IR overall, fitness was found to be a significant predictor of IR only in males, and race to be a significant predictor of IR only in females. This is consistent with previous work suggesting that males may have a stronger relationship between CVF and IR [1]. A conceivable explanation for these findings would be that males were historically selected according to high fitness, rendering them more intolerant to the adverse effects of low fitness. In contrast, if females were in general selected by ability to reproduce in times of nutrient scarcity rather than physical fitness, this could increase susceptibility to adverse effects of over-nutrition.

While there is a strong correlation between an adult's fitness level and physical activity [32], this correlation is much weaker in children [33]. Reasons behind this difference are likely multi-factorial, but may include the fact that a healthy child's fitness is more genetically-determined than that of an adult, and childhood activity is often unstructured, un-sustained and of insufficient intensity to increase VO2 max [34]. VO2 maximal exercise testing (or proxies there-of) measures a fitness level determined by a particular training stimulus that occurs with vigorous physical activity, such as competitive sports, but is much less indicative of habitual activity and leisure time physical activity, which also contribute to metabolic health. Studies repeatedly fail to show a relationship between habitual physical activity and VO2 max [35]. Further complicating this issue is the fact that boys participate in sports at a higher rate than girls, giving them the type of fitness and experience with exercising at or near VO2 max but may not actually result in more daily activity overall. Cardiovascular

Table 3 Percentages of subjects with elevated hsCRP levels by Gender and Race

| | | % Subjects with hsCRP >0.5 mg/L | | | |
		Low fitness (n = 46)	High fitness (n = 67)	p-value[1]	p-value[2]
Gender	Male (n = 58)	65%	11%	<0.001	0.28
	Female (n = 55)	70%	25%	0.0014	
Race	Non-Hispanic White (n = 56)	67%	24%	0.0035	0.06
	Racially Diverse (n = 57)	68%	8%	<0.0001	

[1]p-value for comparison between "low fitness" vs. "high fitness" group
[2]p-value for evaluating interaction between gender and fitness, race and fitness

fitness and habitual activity are both important for health, but the relative contribution of each may depend on an individual's particular genetic make-up and risk factors. Our data suggest that, if habitual activity is effective at preventing excessive weight gain, it may be more important than vigorous activity for overall health, particularly in girls.

Strengths and limitations
Strengths of this study include sample size, subject diversity, and setting. We sampled a large, racially diverse group of children with distribution of overweight/obese status which matched national trends. The school-based (rather than clinic- or lab-based) study design provided data that should be generalizable to other 'healthy' children. The school setting did introduce some limitations due to the "battlefield conditions" of the school setting, as described below, but overall, we feel that this is a major strength. Given the magnitude of the obesity challenge facing pediatrics today, it is important to develop assessments that can be done on a large and easily reproducible scale.

Limitations of this study include the reliability of PACER testing as a measurement of fitness, lack of pubertal stage documentation, and combining of the RD group into a single group. PACER has been shown to correlate very strongly with aerobic fitness measured via VO2 max [27,28,36] when administered by experienced staff, however, the PACER measurement of CVF depends heavily on speed, agility, and effort. Since males participate in competitive sports more than females [37], their ability to have CVF measured accurately by the PACER test could be enhanced compared to females. The effort dependency of the PACER could

be amplified when children perform the test in a peer environment, such as a co-ed physical education class at school.

Puberty hormones have known effects on body composition, markers of inflammation, and insulin sensitivity. Unfortunately, the school-based setting did not allow sufficient privacy to perform pubertal staging. While control for pubertal status would be optimal, the large sample size, distribution of varying stages of puberty amongst fitness levels, and the classification of fitness based on sex- and age-based normative data should all mitigate confounding effects of puberty on study results.

Finally, it is acknowledged that important differences in the relationships between CVF, IR, and inflammation likely exist between the various groups represented in the RD study group. We were prevented by statistical power calculations from performing separate analyses on each of these racial subgroups, and encourage more studies to investigate these potential differences in-depth.

Conclusions
In middle school children, the beneficial effects of fitness vary based on gender and race. With regard to reducing inflammation, high fitness is particularly beneficial for male and RD children. With regard to IR, elevated BMI remains the most important risk factor. However, in females, race appears to be the most influential risk factor after BMI, whereas in males, low fitness appears to be the next most influential risk factor. Screening for and interventions to prevent T2DM could be guided by these additional factors.

Table 4 Percentage of non-overweight subjects with elevated hsCRP in high and low fitness categories

| | % Subjects with hsCRP >0.5 ng/ml | | |
	Low Fitness (n = 17)	High Fitness (n = 60)	p-value
Male (n = 37)	57%	3%	0.003[1]
Female (n = 40)	50%	26%	0.246[1]
p-value	0.026[2]	0.074[3]	

[1]p-value for comparing between fitness levels, stratified by gender
[2]p-value for comparing between gender, stratified by fitness levels
[3]p-value for evaluating interaction between gender and fitness

Abbreviations
CVF: Cardiovascular fitness; IR: Insulin resistance; T2DM: Type 2 diabetes mellitus; RD: Racially diverse; HTN: Hypertension; CRP: C-reactive protein; NHW: Non-Hispanic White; HOMA-IR: Homeostasis model of assessment-insulin resistance; PACER: progressive aerobic cardiovascular endurance run; LMS: lambda-mu-sigma.

Acknowledgements
This study was supported by NIH postdoctoral fellowship training grant T32 DK077586 and The Genentech Center for Clinical Research in Endocrinology. The authors thank the administration and volunteer students of Cherokee Middle School and Sherman Middle School in Madison, Wisconsin for their assistance in performing this project.

Author details
[1]Department of Pediatrics, University of Iowa Carver College of Medicine, 200 Hawkins Drive, 2859 JPP, Iowa City, IO 52242-1083, USA. [2]Department of Pediatrics, University of Wisconsin School of Medicine and Public Health, Madison, WI, USA. [3]Department of Biostatistics and Medical Informatics, University of Wisconsin, Madison, WI, USA.

Authors' contributions
VC, AC, DA conceived the study, participated in its design and coordination and helped to draft the manuscript. JE participated in the design of the study and performed the statistical analysis. All authors read and approved the final manuscript.

Competing interests
The authors declare that they have no competing interests.

References
1. Allen DB, Nemeth BA, Clark RR, Peterson SE, Eickhoff J, Carrel AL: Fitness is a stronger predictor of fasting insulin levels than fatness in overweight male middle-school children. *J Pediatr* 2007, 150:383-387.
2. Gutin B, Barbeau P, Owens S, Lemmon CR, Bauman M, Allison J, Kang HS, Litaker MS: Effects of exercise intensity on cardiovascular fitness, total body composition, and visceral adiposity of obese adolescents. *Am J Clin Nutr* 2002, 75:818-826.
3. Nassis GP, Papantakou K, Skenderi K, Triandafillopoulou M, Kavouras SA, Yannakoulia M, Chrousos GP, Sidossis LS: Aerobic exercise training improves insulin sensitivity without changes in body weight, body fat, adiponectin, and inflammatory markers in overweight and obese girls. *Metabolism* 2005, 54:1472-1479.
4. Hamdy O, Porramatikul S, Al-Ozairi E: Metabolic obesity: the paradox between visceral and subcutaneous fat. *Curr Diabetes Rev* 2006, 2:367-373.
5. Pischon T, Girman CJ, Hotamisligil GS, Rifai N, Hu FB, Rimm EB: Plasma adiponectin levels and risk of myocardial infarction in men. *Jama* 2004, 291:1730-1737.
6. Kumada M, Kihara S, Sumitsuji S, Kawamoto T, Matsumoto S, Ouchi N, Arita Y, Okamoto Y, Shimomura I, Hiraoka H, *et al*: Association of hypoadiponectinemia with coronary artery disease in men. *Arterioscler Thromb Vasc Biol* 2003, 23:85-89.
7. Hotta K, Funahashi T, Arita Y, Takahashi M, Matsuda M, Okamoto Y, Iwahashi H, Kuriyama H, Ouchi N, Maeda K, *et al*: Plasma concentrations of a novel, adipose-specific protein, adiponectin, in type 2 diabetic patients. *Arterioscler Thromb Vasc Biol* 2000, 20:1595-1599.
8. Weyer C, Funahashi T, Tanaka S, Hotta K, Matsuzawa Y, Pratley RE, Tataranni PA: Hypoadiponectinemia in obesity and type 2 diabetes: close association with insulin resistance and hyperinsulinemia. *J Clin Endocrinol Metab* 2001, 86:1930-1935.
9. Stefan N, Vozarova B, Funahashi T, Matsuzawa Y, Weyer C, Lindsay RS, Youngren JF, Havel PJ, Pratley RE, Bogardus C, Tataranni PA: Plasma adiponectin concentration is associated with skeletal muscle insulin receptor tyrosine phosphorylation, and low plasma concentration precedes a decrease in whole-body insulin sensitivity in humans. *Diabetes* 2002, 51:1884-1888.
10. Punthakee Z, Delvin E, O'loughlin J, Paradis G, Levy E, Platt R, Lambert M: Adiponectin, adiposity, and insulin resistance in children and adolescents. *J Clin Endocrinol Metab* 2006, 91:2119-2125.
11. Lu G, Chiem A, Anuurad E, Havel PJ, Pearson TA, Ormsby B, Berglund L: Adiponectin levels are associated with coronary artery disease across Caucasian and African-American ethnicity. *Transl Res* 2007, 149:317-323.
12. Jeffery AN, Murphy MJ, Metcalf BS, Hosking J, Voss LD, English P, Sattar N, Wilkin TJ: Adiponectin in childhood. *Int J Pediatr Obes* 2008, 3:130-140.
13. Hanley AJ, Bowden D, Wagenknecht LE, Balasubramanyam A, Langfeld C, Saad MF, Rotter JI, Guo X, Chen YD, Bryer-Ash M, *et al*: Associations of adiponectin with body fat distribution and insulin sensitivity in nondiabetic Hispanics and African-Americans. *J Clin Endocrinol Metab* 2007, 92:2665-2671.
14. Lindsay RS, Funahashi T, Hanson RL, Matsuzawa Y, Tanaka S, Tataranni PA, Knowler WC, Krakoff J: Adiponectin and development of type 2 diabetes in the Pima Indian population. *Lancet* 2002, 360:57-58.
15. Kantartzis K, Fritsche A, Tschritter O, Thamer C, Haap M, Schafer S, Stumvoll M, Haring HU, Stefan N: The association between plasma adiponectin and insulin sensitivity in humans depends on obesity. *Obes Res* 2005, 13:1683-1691.
16. Martin LJ, Woo JG, Daniels SR, Goodman E, Dolan LM: The relationships of adiponectin with insulin and lipids are strengthened with increasing adiposity. *J Clin Endocrinol Metab* 2005, 90:4255-4259.
17. Arita Y, Kihara S, Ouchi N, Takahashi M, Maeda K, Miyagawa J, Hotta K, Shimomura I, Nakamura T, Miyaoka K, *et al*: Paradoxical decrease of an adipose-specific protein, adiponectin, in obesity. *Biochem Biophys Res Commun* 1999, 257:79-83.
18. Mora S, Musunuru K, Blumenthal RS: The clinical utility of high-sensitivity C-reactive protein in cardiovascular disease and the potential implication of JUPITER on current practice guidelines. *Clin Chem* 2009, 55:219-228.
19. Lambert M, Delvin EE, Paradis G, O'Loughlin J, Hanley JA, Levy E: C-reactive protein and features of the metabolic syndrome in a population-based sample of children and adolescents. *Clin Chem* 2004, 50:1762-1768.
20. Kelly AS, Wetzsteon RJ, Kaiser DR, Steinberger J, Bank AJ, Dengel DR: Inflammation, insulin, and endothelial function in overweight children and adolescents: the role of exercise. *J Pediatr* 2004, 145:731-736.
21. Mauras N, Delgiorno C, Kollman C, Bird K, Morgan M, Sweeten S, Balagopal P, Damaso L: Obesity without established comorbidities of the metabolic syndrome is associated with a proinflammatory and prothrombotic state, even before the onset of puberty in children. *J Clin Endocrinol Metab* 2010, 95:1060-1068.
22. Ischander M, Zaldivar F Jr, Eliakim A, Nussbaum E, Dunton G, Leu SY, Cooper DM, Schneider M: Physical activity, growth, and inflammatory mediators in BMI-matched female adolescents. *Med Sci Sports Exerc* 2007, 39:1131-1138.
23. Fischer CP, Berntsen A, Perstrup LB, Eskildsen P, Pedersen BK: Plasma levels of interleukin-6 and C-reactive protein are associated with physical inactivity independent of obesity. *Scand J Med Sci Sports* 2007, 17:580-587.
24. Kelley DE, Goodpaster BH: Effects of physical activity on insulin action and glucose tolerance in obesity. *Med Sci Sports Exerc* 1999, 31:S619-S623.
25. Kraemer RR, Castracane VD: Exercise and humoral mediators of peripheral energy balance: ghrelin and adiponectin. *Exp Biol Med (Maywood)* 2007, 232:184-194.
26. Solomon TP, Sistrun SN, Krishnan RK, Del Aguila LF, Marchetti CM, O'Carroll SM, O'Leary VB, Kirwan JP: Exercise and diet enhance fat oxidation and reduce insulin resistance in older obese adults. *J Appl Physiol* 2008, 104:1313-1319.
27. Leger LA, Lambert J: A maximal multistage 20-m shuttle run test to predict VO2 max. *Eur J Appl Physiol Occup Physiol* 1982, 49:1-12.
28. Varness T, Carrel AL, Eickhoff JC, Allen DB: Reliable prediction of insulin resistance by a school-based fitness test in middle-school children. *Int J Pediatr Endocrinol* 2009, 2009:487804.
29. Cook DG, Mendall MA, Whincup PH, Carey IM, Ballam L, Morris JE, Miller GJ, Strachan DP: C-reactive protein concentration in children: relationship to adiposity and other cardiovascular risk factors. *Atherosclerosis* 2000, 149:139-150.
30. Cole TJ: The LMS method for constructing normalized growth standards. *Eur J Clin Nutr* 1990, 44:45-60.
31. Tibshirani R: Regression shrinkage and selection via the Lasso. *J Royal Stat Soc Series B-Methodological* 1996, 58:267-288.

32. Pate RR, Pratt M, Blair SN, Haskell WL, Macera CA, Bouchard C, Buchner D, Ettinger W, Heath GW, King AC, *et al*: Physical activity and public health. A recommendation from the Centers for Disease Control and Prevention and the American College of Sports Medicine. *JAMA* 1995, **273**:402-407.

33. Dencker M, Andersen LB: Accelerometer-measured daily physical activity related to aerobic fitness in children and adolescents. *J Sports Sci* 2011, **29**:887-895.

34. Bailey RC, Olson J, Pepper SL, Porszasz J, Barstow TJ, Cooper DM: The level and tempo of children's physical activities: an observational study. *Med Sci Sports Exerc* 1995, **27**:1033-1041.

35. Armstrong N, Tomkinson G, Ekelund U: Aerobic fitness and its relationship to sport, exercise training and habitual physical activity during youth. *Br J Sports Med* 2011, **45**:849-858.

36. Liu NY, Plowman SA, Looney MA: The reliability and validity of the 20-meter shuttle test in American students 12 to 15 years old. *Res Q Exerc Sport* 1992, **63**:360-365.

37. Slater A, Tiggemann M: Gender differences in adolescent sport participation, teasing, self-objectification and body image concerns. *J Adolesc* 2011, **34**:455-463.

14

Metabolic control and bone health in adolescents with type 1 diabetes

Jill H Simmons[1*], Miranda Raines[1], Kathryn D Ness[2], Randon Hall[1], Tebeb Gebretsadik[3], Subburaman Mohan[4] and Anna Spagnoli[5]

Abstract

Background: Adults with type 1 diabetes (T1D) have decreased bone mineral density (BMD) and increased fracture risk, yet the etiologies remain elusive. Early detection of derangements in bone biomarkers during adolescence could lead to timely recognition. In adolescents with T1D, we evaluated the relationships between metabolic control, BMD, and bone anabolic and turnover markers.

Methods: Cross-sectional study of 57 adolescent subjects with T1D who had HbA1c consistently $\geq$ 9% (Poor Control, PC n = 27) or < 9% (Favorable Control, FC n = 30) for two years prior to enrollment. Subjects had T1DM for at least three years and were without diabetes complications, known celiac disease, or other chronic diseases.

Results: There were no differences between HbA1c groups in BMD, components of the IGF system, or 25-hydroxyvitamin D status. The prevalence of 25-hydroxyvitamin D abnormalities was similar to that seen in the general adolescent population. Few patients met the recommended dietary allowance (RDA) for vitamin D or calcium.

Conclusions: These data provide no evidence of association between degree of metabolic control and BMD in adolescents with T1D. Adolescents with T1D have a high prevalence of serum 25-hydroxyvitamin D abnormalities. Longitudinal studies are needed to evaluate the predictive value of vitamin D abnormalities on fracture risk.

Keywords: bone mineral density, intact parathyroid hormone, insulin-like growth factor, type 1 diabetes, adolescent

Introduction

The effects of improved home blood glucose monitoring, pharmacotherapy, and educational interventions have led to a longer lifespan for patients with type 1 diabetes mellitus (T1D). However, bone health remains a problem for many with T1D, as adults with T1D have increased fracture risk and generalized osteoporosis [1,2], and abnormalities in bone mineral density (BMD) have been reported in adolescents with T1D. The underlying mechanisms triggering the changes in BMD in patients with T1D are not well-known. Reports of the relationships between metabolic control, BMD, and bone marker parameters in patients with T1D have been conflicting [3,4]. Evaluations of bone disease in

adults with T1D are generally complicated by the presence of other diabetic complications such as nephropathy, muscle insufficiency, or impaired vision that can affect bone disease. Early detection, prior to other diabetes complications, of derangements in bone markers can provide insight into the pathogenesis of bone disease in patients with T1D.

Bone health is dependent upon appropriate regulation of both anabolic and catabolic processes. Insulin-like growth factor I (IGF-I) is an anabolic regulator of bone metabolism, and BMD has been positively correlated with IGF-I levels in both human and animal studies [5-7]. IGF-I is decreased in patients with T1D, associated with the degree of metabolic control [8-10]. Patients with T1D have dysregulation of the growth hormone-IGF-I axis [9-11] and dysregulation of IGF binding proteins (IGFBP) [9,11], which determine the tissue availability of IGF-I. Parathyroid hormone has both

* Correspondence: jill.h.simmons@vanderbilt.edu
[1]Department of Pediatrics, Division of Endocrinology and Diabetes, Vanderbilt Children's Hospital, Nashville, TN, USA
Full list of author information is available at the end of the article

anabolic and catabolic effects on bone. Low, unaltered or elevated levels of intact parathyroid hormone (iPTH) have previously been reported in patients with T1D [12,13]. However, these studies evaluated few patients and included patients with important confounders such as diabetic nephropathy that may have led to secondary hyperparathyroidism. Aberrations in bone markers may be predictive of osteoporosis and fractures [14]. Bone-specific alkaline phosphatase, which is a bone formation marker reflective of osteoblastic activity, is lower in patients with T1D than controls [15]. In addition, urinary cross linked N-telopeptides of type I collagen (NTX), bone breakdown markers, are decreased in patients with T1D [16]. Bone turnover therefore is decreased in patients with T1D, although the etiologies are unclear.

Peak bone mass is attained by early adulthood [17], and therefore interference with this process in adolescence results in life-long complications. Evaluations of bone disease in adolescents with T1D are limited. This study was designed to evaluate whether in adolescents with T1D: 1) poor metabolic control is associated with reduced BMD; 2) changes in biochemical bone parameters such as IGF-I system components, iPTH, bone turnover markers, and 25-hydroxyvitamin D are associated with metabolic control. We also hypothesized that adolescents with T1D would have a higher prevalence of vitamin D deficiency than the healthy adolescent population.

Materials and methods

Participants

Adolescents (ages 13-18 years) with T1D for ≥ 3 years were recruited from the pediatric clinic in the Eskind Diabetes Center at Vanderbilt Medical Center. All participants were diagnosed with T1D by a pediatric endocrinologist. The study was conducted in accordance with the Declaration of Helsinki and was approved by the Vanderbilt University Medical Center Institutional Review Board. Informed consent was obtained from each participant's parent/legal guardian, and informed assent was obtained from each participant prior to beginning the study. Participants were categorized by the degree of glucose control. Poor control (PC) was defined as all (must have a minimum of 3) HbA1c measurements ≥ 9% and favorable control (FC) was defined as all HbA1c measurements < 9% during the previous 2 years. Exclusion criteria were: presence of microalbuminuria, retinopathy or neuropathy; pre-existing bone disease, cystic fibrosis or celiac disease, eating disorder, estro-progesterone or testosterone treatment including oral contraceptives, smoking, pregnancy, amenorrhea, polycystic ovarian syndrome as diagnosed by a pediatric endocrinologist based upon irregular menses as well as

hirsutism and/or biochemical evidence of androgen excess, obesity [body mass index (BMI) > 95th percentile for age and sex], short stature (< 3rd percentile for age and sex), or delayed/precocious puberty.

Anthropometric Evaluation

Height and weight were obtained, and body mass index was calculated based on the following formula: weight (kg)/height (m)^2.

Response variables

1. Bone measurements

The primary dependent variable was BMD measured by DEXA scan.

Total BMD, lumbar spine (L2-L4) BMD, L2-L4 width, and femoral neck BMD were determined by dual energy radiographic absorptiometry (DEXA, GE Healthcare, Lunar iDEXA, Tube model 40782). Prior to September 2007, DEXA scans were performed using the GE Healthcare Lunar Model 8743. Lumbar (L2-L4) BMD and L2-L4 width were used to determine bone mineral apparent density (BMAD, grams per cubic centimeter), which was calculated based on the following formula: BMD (L2-L4) × (4/[pi x width]) [18]. Results were expressed as z-scores for total body BMD, lumbar BMD, BMAD, and femoral neck BMD. Z-scores were calculated using the means and SD reported for age and gender [19]. Serum pregnancy tests were negative on all females prior to DEXA scan.

2. Laboratory Evaluation

Other dependent variables included components of the IGF system, bone turnover makers, and serum 25-hydroxyvitamin D levels. Venous blood samples were collected after an overnight fast (approximately 10 hours). Participants received their usual evening insulin glargine dose the night prior or were continued on their insulin pump at the usual basal rate. For each participant, serum for IGF-I, IGFBP-3 (insulin-like growth factor binding protein 3), IGFBP-4, IGFBP-5, iPTH, bone-specific alkaline phosphatase (BAP), total 25-hydroxyvitamin D, calcium, phosphorus, and creatinine were obtained. Urine was collected for 24 hours at home prior to arrival for analysis for cross linked N-telopeptides of type I collagen (NTX), creatinine, calcium, and phosphorus.

3. Diet diary

Subjects were asked to keep a diet diary for 72 hours prior to the study visit, in order to ascertain information regarding dietary vitamin D and calcium intake. Each subject was instructed to record type of food/beverage and amount consumed in as much detail as possible. Verbal and written instructions were given to each subject and his/her parents when consented for the study, and logsheets were provided for each subject. The information from these diet diaries was placed into the Nutrition Data System for Research (NDSR, University of Minnesota), and an analysis of calcium and vitamin D intake per day was obtained.

Exposure variable

The primary independent variable was the average of 3or more consistent levels of HbA1c in the 2 years prior to enrollment. Subjects were assigned either to the poor control (PC) group (HbA1c ≥ 9%) or the favorable control group (FC) (HbA1c < 9%). Subjects who had HbA1c values in both categories during the two years prior to potential study enrollment were excluded. The enrollment plan included that an equal number (± 10%) of subjects would be enrolled in the two metabolic groups. This targeted enrollment by HBA1c was to ascertain that subjects in poor control were represented in study.

Assay methods

HbA1c was measured by point-of-care immunoassay using the DCA Vantage Analyzer (Siemens Healthcare Diagnostics, Deerfield, IL, USA). Serum concentration of total IGFI was measured by radioimmunoassay (RIA) (ALPCO Diagnostics, Salem, NH, USA). Inter- and intra-assay coefficients of variation were 3.4-4.2% and 2.6-4.1%, respectively. Serum IGFBP-3 was measured by radioimmunoassay (RIA) using rabbit polyclonal antiserum and human recombinant IGFBP-3 as standard and tracer [20]. Serum IGFBP-4 was measured by a specific RIA using recombinant human IGFBP-4 expressed in Escherichia coli as antigen, tracer and standard [21]. Antibodies against human IGFBP-4 were developed in guinea pigs as described previously [21]. Inter-and intra-assay variations were less than 8%. There was no cross-reactivity with other IGFBPs. Serum IGFBP-5 was measured by a specific RIA using recombinant human IGFBP-5 as antigen, tracer and standard as described [22]. There was no cross-reactivity with other IGFBPs. Inter-and intra-assay variations were less than 8%. Cross-linked N-telopeptides in urine were measured by chemiluminescent immunoassay (ARUP Laboratories, Salt Lake City, UT, USA). Intact PTH was measured using the Roche Cobas electrochemiluminescence assay, BAP was measured by the immunoenzymatic assay Access Ostase, and total 25-hydroxyvitamin D was measured using Liquid Chromatography-Tandem Mass Spectrometry (LC-MS/MS) (Mayo Medical Laboratories, Rochester, MN, USA). The criteria used to define vitamin D sufficiency, insufficiency, and deficiency were 25-hydroxyvitamin D levels ≥ 30 ng/mL, 15-29 ng/mL, and <15 ng/mL, respectively, as was recently reported [23].

Statistical methods

Clinical and demographic variables are presented as number and percent or medians and interquartile ranges [IQR]. Categorical variables were compared by HbA1c degree of control group with χ^2 test and continuous variables with Wilcoxon rank sum test. Spearman correlation coefficients (rho) were used to assess the correlation of continuous BMD measures, components of the IGF system, bone turnover markers, vitamin D and calcium intake, age, and HbA1c. We assessed for the adjusted association between BMD measures, components of the IGF system, bone turnover markers, vitamin D and calcium intake and age with HbA1c as an independent variable with multiple linear regression analyses. Multivariable linear regression assumptions of normality of residuals were checked and were met. Covariates for adjustment were chosen *a priori* and included age, gender and race. All reported *p* values are unadjusted for multiple tests. All analyses used a 5% two-sided significance level and were performed with R version 2.10.10 http://www.r-project.org. To compare the prevalence of vitamin D status with published NHANES study report[23], we calculated the proportion of subjects who were insufficient and deficient in 25-hydroxyvitamin D by gender and calculated the 95% confidence interval (CI) for binomial proportion using the Wilson method. The Wilson method was used as it works better for calculation of 95%CI with small samples and extreme probability (approaching 1 or 0) [24].

Results

Demographic characteristics

The study population included 57 participants, 30 in the FC group and 27 in the PC group (stable HbA1c during the 2 years prior to study participation). There were no significant differences between groups in age, gender, duration of diabetes, or anthropometrics (Table 1). As expected based on selection criteria, the average HbA1c during the two years prior to the study in the PC group was higher than that in the FC group.

BMD, bone markers, and components of the IGF system in FC and PC groups

The FC group had a higher iPTH level [30.5 pg/ml (21.8, 37.8)] compared with the PC group [19 pg/ml (15, 31)], p = 0.04. The FC group also had higher urine n-telopeptides (NTX) than the PC group [238 nM BCE/mM creat (98,366) vs 56 nM BCE/mM creat (41,311), p = 0.03] and a lower urine Ca/Cr than the PC group [0.07 (0.05, 0.15) vs 0.14 (0.09, 0.21), p = 0.02], consistent with higher iPTH levels (Table 2). There were no differences between groups in measurements of BMD, IGFI or IGFBPs, BAP, serum calcium, serum creatinine, eGFR, or 25-hydroxyvitamin D levels.

Table 1 Characteristics of subjects by metabolic control, results shown as median and [IQR] interquartile range.

	Favorable Control (n = 30)	Poor Control (n = 27)	p value*
HbA1C (%)	7.7 [7.3, 7.9]	10.3 [9.9, 11.4]	**
Age (yrs)	15.2 [14.3, 16.1]	16.4 (15.1, 17.8)	0.05
Gender (% female)	37%	59%	0.42
Race (% Caucasian)	87% [26/30]	81%[21/26]	0.55
Duration DM (yrs)	6.5 [4.8,8.0]	6.5[5.5,9.5]	0.40
Height (cm)	169.8 [158.6,178.1]	163.2 [16.03,165.7]	0.22
Weight (kg)	68.5 [55.4,74.0]	67.5 [59.0,77.5]	0.91
BMI (kg/m²)	22.8 [20.4,27.5]	25.0 [21.4,27.9]	0.35

*Wilcoxon rank sum test for continuous variables or χ² test for categorical variables.

** Groups were defined based on HbA1c

Relationship between metabolic control and BMD, bone markers, IGF system components and vitamin D/calcium intake

Univariate analyses (Table 3) demonstrated a positive correlation between HbA1c and % body fat (rho = 0.30, p = 0.02) and urine Ca/Cr (rho = 0.27, p = 0.047) and negative correlations between HbA1c and NTX (rho = -0.36, p = 0.01), intact PTH (rho = -0.28, p = 0.04), and

serum creatinine (rho =-0.27, p = 0.04). There were no other significant correlations between HbA1c and any of the other study variables. After controlling for age, sex, and race, there was a positive association between HbA1c and serum phosphorus and a negative association between HbA1c and serum creatinine that were statistically significant. There were no associations between HbA1c and BMD, bone turnover markers, components of the IGF system, serum 25-hydroxyvitamin D, serum calcium, or dietary intake of calcium and vitamin D.

Dietary Intake of vitamin D and calcium

Subjects with T1D who have favorable metabolic control report consuming a similar amount of vitamin D and calcium as those who have poor metabolic control (Table 2). Only 12% (3/25) of the total subgroup with intake data reported consuming the recommended daily allowance (RDA) of vitamin D (400 IU/day at the time of the study), and 16% (4/25) of the total subgroup reported consuming the RDA for calcium (1300 mg/day), with no differences between groups (18% vs 12%, p = 0.74). When evaluated with the Institute of Medicine's 2011 RDA of 600 IU vitamin D/day [25], only 1 subject reported consuming this amount.

Table 2 Clinical and biochemical features of subjects with T1D

	n	FC (n = 30)	PC (n = 27)	p value†
Lumbar spine BMD*	56	0.01 (-1.14, 1.07)	-0.46 (-0.82, 0.37)	0.58
Volumetric lumbar spine (BMAD)*	56	0.05 (-0.63, 0.69)	-0.14 (-0.48, 0.57)	0.83
Femoral neck BMD*	56	0.12 (-1.23, 0.98)	-0.48 (-1.19, 1.39)	0.66
Total body BMD*	56	0.46 (-1.27, 1.35)	-0.03 (-1.1, 0.72)	0.66
% body fat	56	28.7 (16.7, 35.3)	33.7 (20.2, 40)	0.22
IGF-1 (ng/mL)	56	564 (430, 644)	488 (402, 603)	0.29
IGF BP-3 (μg/L)	54	2883 (2448, 3060)	2901 (2676, 3436)	0.36
IGF BP-4 (μg/L)	54	398.5 (334.8, 439.2)	415.5 ± 57.9	0.17
IGF BP-5 (μg/L)	54	346.0 (300.8, 384.2)	316.5 (273.2, 447.8)	0.55
NTX (nM BCE/mM creat)	**54**	**238 (98, 366)**	**56 (41, 311)**	**0.03**
Bone-Specific Alkaline Phosphatase (ug/L)	53	34 (23, 63)	19 (14.5, 49.5)	0.09
Intact PTH (ρg/mL)	**53**	**30.5 (21.8, 37.8)**	**19 (15, 31)**	**0.04**
Serum 25-hydroxyvitamin D (ng/mL)	52	31 (21, 37)	32 (24, 38.5)	0.76
Serum Calcium (mg/dL)	56	9.4 (9.3, 9.7)	9.4 (9.2, 9.6)	0.99
Serum Phosphorus (mg/dL)	56	4.4 (4.1, 5.0)	4.8 (4.3, 5.2)	0.21
Serum creatinine (mg/dL)	56	0.75 (0.63, 0.8)	0.7 (0.6, 0.8)	0.22
eGFR estimation (ml/min)	56	137.5 (122.7, 149.8)	141.8 (118.2, 166.4)	0.72
uCa/uCr	**54**	**0.07[0.05, 0.15]**	**0.14[0.09,0.21]**	**0.02**
uPhos/uCr	54	0.80[0.64, 0.92]	0.90[0.72, 1.0]	0.22
Average vitamin D intake/day (IU)	25	173 (128, 246)	168 (122, 246)	1
Average calcium intake/day (mg)	25	872 (651, 1136)	686 (574, 927)	0.46

Items in bold p < 0.05.

† Wilcoxon rank sum test for comparison of continuous variables

* z-scores

Abbreviations: FC: Favorable Control, PC: Poor Control, BMD: bone mineral density, BMAD: bone mineral apparent density, eGFR (estimated glomerular filtration rate)

Table 3 Association between HbA1c and bone mineral density measurements, components of the IGF system, bone turnover markers, and dietary intake of calcium and vitamin D

	Spearman correlation coefficient	p value*	Adjusted p value **
Age	0.24	0.08	
Lumbar Spine BMD †	-0.12	0.37	0.63
Volumetric Lumbar Spine † (BMAD)	-0.041	0.76	0.85
Femoral neck BMD †	-0.056	0.68	0.24
Total body BMD †	-0.086	0.53	0.87
% Body fat	**0.30**	**0.02**	0.66
IGF-I (ng/ml)	-0.15	0.27	0.92
IGFBP3 (µg/L)	0.13	0.37	0.33
IGFBP4 (µg/L)	0.23	0.10	0.1
IGFBP5 (µg/L)	-0.09	0.52	0.65
NTX (nM BCE/mM creat)	**-0.36**	**0.01**	0.73
Bone-specific alkaline phosphatase (µg/L)	-0.26	0.06	0.81
Intact PTH (pg/ml)	**-0.28**	**0.04**	0.2
Serum 25-hydroxyvitamin D (ng/ml)	-0.047	0.74	0.89
Serum Calcium (ml/dL)	0.15	0.28	0.19
Serum Phosphorus (mg/dL)	0.2	0.14	**0.01**
Serum creatinine (mg/dL)	**-0.27**	**0.04**	**0.007**
UCa/uCr	**0.27**	**0.047**	**0.05**
uPhos/uCr	0.22	0.1	0.37
Average vitamin D intake/day (IU)	-0.09	0.67	0.55
Average calcium intake/day (mg)	-0.13	0.55	0.42

Items in bold p < 0.05.

*Spearman correlation coefficient p value; ** p value adjusted for age, race, and gender; † z-scores

Hydroxyvitamin D status There were no differences between groups in serum 25-hydroxyvitamin D levels (Table 2), with 14% of the FC group deficient (25-hydroxyvitamin D levels < 15 ng/ml) and 31% insufficient (25-hydroxyvitamin D levels 15-29 ng/ml) and 13% of the PC group deficient and 35% insufficient in serum 25-hydroxyvitamin D, p = 0.96. Together, there were no differences between subjects with T1D and the normal adolescent population [23] in the prevalence of 25-hydroxyvitamin D deficiency, as 11% (95%CI: 2.9%, 31.4%) of girls and 0% (95%CI: 0, 13.3%) of boys with T1D were deficient in 25-hydroxyvitamin D, compared with 5% and 3% of the normal adolescent population, respectively. Thirty-two percent of girls (95%CI: 15.4%, 54.0%) and 40% (95%CI: 23.4%, 59.2%) of boys were insufficient in 25-hydroxyvitamin D, compared with 57% and 63%, respectively, of the general adolescent population. When using the 2011 Institute of Medicine Report's definition of vitamin D inadequacy [25], 21% of the FC group and 17% of the PC group had 25-hydroxyvitamin D levels <20 ng/ml, p = 0.76.

Discussion

This study addresses whether metabolic control has an effect on bone health in patients with T1D who have not yet achieved peak bone mass. Adolescents with T1D in consistently poor metabolic control appear to have lower iPTH levels than a group of adolescents with T1D in favorable metabolic control, although this association was attenuated when adjusted for age, gender and race. After adjustment, urine calcium is associated with metabolic control, consistent with lower iPTH levels. We also explored the prevalence of 25-hydroxyvitamin D abnormalities in adolescents with T1D, as vitamin D abnormalities have been increasingly recognized as a significant health problem both for healthy patients and those with chronic illnesses [26]. Adolescents with T1D have significant 25-hydroxyvitamin D abnormalities, but these abnormalities are not more prevalent than in the general adolescent population.

Poor bone health is a significant problem for many adults with T1D, as is demonstrated by a two-fold increase in fracture risk in the lumbar spine, femoral neck, and distal radius [1]. Women with T1D have more than a 10-fold increase in risk of hip fractures compared with age-matched controls [2]. Almost 20% of patients with T1D ages 20-56 years meet criteria for osteoporosis [27], which is a debilitating illness that impairs functionality and quality of life [28]. However, the etiologies of decreased BMD in adults with T1D have been unclear [29,30]. The mechanisms of osteoporosis associated with T1D differ from the development of osteoporosis associated with aging [31], and several potential mechanisms have been proposed, including effects of advanced glycation end products in bone collagen [32], increased urinary excretion of calcium, phosphate and magnesium [33], inflammatory cytokines [34], low levels of iPTH [12], diabetic microangiopathy with reduced blood flow to bone [35], decreased bone resorption [16], decreased bone formation [36], and vitamin D deficiency [37]. We sought to evaluate whether poor metabolic control during adolescence is associated with abnormal bone health.

Previous studies investigating the role of metabolic control and BMD in patients with T1D have been limited by older BMD measurement methods which may be inaccurate, limited knowledge in the consistency of patients' actual metabolic control (many studies use only a single HbA1c measurement as the index of metabolic control), and confounding factors affecting BMD such as the use of oral contraceptives. In this study, we controlled confounding factors and found no correlations between metabolic control and BMD, similar to others [3,38,39], but differing from some [4]. Although subjects had stable diabetes control for two years prior to the study, two years of poor diabetes control may not be long enough to lead to changes in BMD demonstrated by DEXA scans in adolescents.

The role of IGF-I as a critical anabolic regulator of BMD is clearly demonstrated in animal studies in which genetic manipulation of the IGF system led to osteopenia [7]. In humans, cross-sectional and cohort studies in various populations, including subjects from the Framingham Heart Study, have demonstrated a strong correlation between serum levels of IGF-I and BMD [6,40]. Dysregulation of the IGF-I/IGFBP system has been reported in patients with T1D [9-12,32]. We found no associations between metabolic control and components of the IGFI system, although other studies have reported that IGF-I levels correlate with metabolic control [11]. As we did not have a control group of healthy subjects, IGFI levels may be too low within a population of T1D patients to detect significant differences.

Only 35% of healthy non-Hispanic white adolescents are sufficient in 25-hydroxyvitamin D [23], which plays an important role in the maintenance of bone health. Similar to recent studies, we found a significant prevalence of 25-hydroxyvitamin D abnormalities in adolescents with T1D [37,41], but we did not find a difference in 25-hydroxyvitamin D status between adolescents with T1D and the normal adolescent population [23]. However, the proportions of vitamin D sufficiency status by gender were limited by small numbers which resulted in

proportions with wide confidence intervals. There is not enough evidence to support that metabolic control plays a role in vitamin D status, and other risk factors need to be evaluated.

Only one subject reported consuming the current RDA for vitamin D, with 16% consuming the RDA for calcium. This is not different from the healthy adolescent population, as previous data from NHANES III (1988-1994) demonstrated that only 53-63% of all US children consume at least 200 IU of vitamin D per day from diet and/or supplementation. (200 IU was reported in this paper because it was considered Adequate Intake for vitamin D at that time) [42]. This is of particular concern for adolescent patients with T1D, as vitamin D and calcium intake are modifiable factors that have a significant impact on BMD.

Our study had several limitations. We stratified by design the subjects into poor and favorable metabolic control groups, and we could have missed relationships between HbA1c and study variables due to a lack of a full continuous spectrum of HbA1c values. We did not have a control group of non-diabetic patients. Also, we did not obtain information regarding exercise and specifics regarding pubertal development, which clearly have an effect on BMD and bone turnover. However, we attempted to address this issue by excluding patients with obesity as well as known pubertal delay, amenorrhea, or polycystic ovarian syndrome.

In summary, metabolic control is not associated with BMD as evaluated by DEXA in this adolescent population with T1D, and bone anabolic and turnover markers are not affected by metabolic control, once age, gender, and race are taken into account. Adolescents with T1D are frequently vitamin D insufficient, which is likely also playing an important role in bone metabolism.

Abbreviations
T1D: type 1 diabetes mellitus; HbA1c: hemoglobin A1c; PC: poor control; FC: favorable control; NTX: urinary cross linked N-telopeptides of type I collagen; BAP: bone-specific alkaline phosphatase; IGF-I (insulin-like growth factor I).

Acknowledgements
Supported by Vanderbilt CTSA grant 1 UL1 RR024975 from the National Center for Research Resources (National Institutes of Health), Vanderbilt Clinical Nutrition Research Unit grant, an unrestricted educational grant from Genentech's Center for Clinical Research, and National Institutes of Health AR-048139.

Author details
[1]Department of Pediatrics, Division of Endocrinology and Diabetes, Vanderbilt Children's Hospital, Nashville, TN, USA. [2]Department of Pediatrics, Division of Pediatric Endocrinology, Seattle Children's Hospital, Seattle, WA, USA. [3]Department of Biostatistics, Vanderbilt University Medical Center, Nashville, TN, USA. [4]Musculoskeletal Disease Center, Jerry L Pettis VA Medical Center, and Departments of Medicine and Biochemistry, Loma Linda University, Loma Linda, CA, USA. [5]Department of Pediatrics, Division of Pediatric Endocrinology, University of North Carolina at Chapel Hill, Chapel Hill, NC, USA.

Authors' contributions

JS made substantial contributions to study design, data acquisition, analysis and interpretation of data, and drafted the manuscript. MR, KN, RH, and AS contributed substantially to study design, subject recruitment, data acquisition, and analysis and interpretation of the data. TG contributed through statistical analysis and interpretation of the data. SM contributed through study design and data acquisition. All authors critically revised the manuscript for important intellectual content and approved the final version of the manuscript.

Competing interests

The authors declare that they have no competing interests.

References

1. Hofbauer LC, Brueck CC, Singh SK, Dobnig H: **Osteoporosis in patients with diabetes mellitus**. *J Bone Miner Res* 2007, 22:1317-1328.
2. Nicodemus KK, Folsom AR: **Type 1 and type 2 diabetes and incident hip fractures in postmenopausal women**. *Diabetes Care* 2001, 24:1192-1197.
3. Hamilton EJ, Rakic V, Davis WA, Chubb SA, Kamber N, Prince RL, et al: **Prevalence and predictors of osteopenia and osteoporosis in adults with Type 1 diabetes**. *Diabet Med* 2009, 26:45-52.
4. Heilman K, Zilmer M, Zilmer K, Tillmann V: **Lower bone mineral density in children with type 1 diabetes is associated with poor glycemic control and higher serum ICAM-1 and urinary isoprostane levels**. *J Bone Miner Metab* 2009, 27:598-604.
5. Zhao G, Monier-Faugere MC, Langub MC, Geng Z, Nakayama T, Pike JW, et al: **Targeted overexpression of insulin-like growth factor I to osteoblasts of transgenic mice: increased trabecular bone volume without increased osteoblast proliferation**. *Endocrinology* 2000, 141:2674-2682.
6. Langlois JA, Rosen CJ, Visser M, Hannan MT, Harris T, Wilson PW, et al: **Association between insulin-like growth factor I and bone mineral density in older women and men: the Framingham Heart Study**. *J Clin Endocrinol Metab* 1998, 83:4257-4262.
7. Yakar S, Rosen CJ, Beamer WG, ckert-Bicknell CL, Wu Y, Liu JL, et al: **Circulating levels of IGF-1 directly regulate bone growth and density**. *J Clin Invest* 2002, 110:771-781.
8. Dills DG, Allen C, Palta M, Zaccaro DJ, Klein R, D'Alessio D: **Insulin-like growth factor-I is related to glycemic control in children and adolescents with newly diagnosed insulin-dependent diabetes**. *J Clin Endocrinol Metab* 1995, 80:2139-2143.
9. Spagnoli A, Chiarelli F, Vorwerk P, Boscherini B, Rosenfeld RG: **Evaluation of the components of insulin-like growth factor (IGF)-IGF binding protein (IGFBP) system in adolescents with type 1 diabetes and persistent microalbuminuria: relationship with increased urinary excretion of IGFBP-3 18 kD N-terminal fragment**. *Clin Endocrinol (Oxf)* 1999, 51:587-596.
10. Strasser-Vogel B, Blum WF, Past R, Kessler U, Hoeflich A, Meiler B, et al: **Insulin-like growth factor (IGF)-I and -II and IGF-binding proteins-1, -2, and -3 in children and adolescents with diabetes mellitus: correlation with metabolic control and height attainment**. *J Clin Endocrinol Metab* 1995, 80:1207-1213.
11. Moyer-Mileur LJ, Slater H, Jordan KC, Murray MA: **IGF-1 and IGF-binding proteins and bone mass, geometry, and strength: relation to metabolic control in adolescent girls with type 1 diabetes**. *J Bone Miner Res* 2008, 23:1884-1891.
12. Saggese G, Bertelloni S, Baroncelli GI, Federico G, Calisti L, Fusaro C: **Bone demineralization and impaired mineral metabolism in insulin-dependent diabetes mellitus. A possible role of magnesium deficiency**. *Helv Paediatr Acta* 1989, 43:405-414.
13. Jehle PM, Jehle DR, Mohan S, Bohm BO: **Serum levels of insulin-like growth factor system components and relationship to bone metabolism in Type 1 and Type 2 diabetes mellitus patients**. *J Endocrinol* 1998, 159:297-306.
14. Garnero P, Hausherr E, Chapuy MC, Marcelli C, Grandjean H, Muller C, et al: **Markers of bone resorption predict hip fracture in elderly women: the EPIDOS Prospective Study**. *J Bone Miner Res* 1996, 11:1531-1538.
15. Lumachi F, Camozzi V, Tombolan V, Luisetto G: **Bone mineral density, osteocalcin, and bone-specific alkaline phosphatase in patients with insulin-dependent diabetes mellitus**. *Ann N Y Acad Sci* 2009, 1173(Suppl 1):E64-E67.
16. Gunczler P, Lanes R, Paz-Martinez V, Martins R, Esaa S, Colmenares V, et al: **Decreased lumbar spine bone mass and low bone turnover in children and adolescents with insulin dependent diabetes mellitus followed longitudinally**. *J Pediatr Endocrinol Metab* 1998, 11:413-419.
17. Lehtonen-Veromaa MK, Mottonen TT, Nuotio IO, Irjala KM, Leino AE, Viikari JS: **Vitamin D and attainment of peak bone mass among peripubertal Finnish girls: a 3-y prospective study**. *Am J Clin Nutr* 2002, 76:1446-1453.
18. Boot AM, De MK-S, Pols HA, Krenning EP, Drop SL: **Bone mineral density and body composition before and during treatment with gonadotropin-releasing hormone agonist in children with central precocious and early puberty**. *J Clin Endocrinol Metab* 1998, 83:370-373.
19. van dS, de Ridder MA, Boot AM, Krenning EP, de Muinck Keizer-Schrama SM: **Reference data for bone density and body composition measured with dual energy X ray absorptiometry in white children and young adults**. *Arch Dis Child* 2002, 87:341-347.
20. Nakao Y, Hilliker S, Baylink DJ, Mohan S: **Studies on the regulation of insulin-like growth factor binding protein 3 secretion in human osteosarcoma cells in vitro**. *J Bone Miner Res* 1994, 9:865-872.
21. Honda Y, Landale EC, Strong DD, Baylink DJ, Mohan S: **Recombinant synthesis of insulin-like growth factor-binding protein-4 (IGFBP-4): Development, validation, and application of a radioimmunoassay for IGFBP-4 in human serum and other biological fluids**. *J Clin Endocrinol Metab* 1996, 81:1389-1396.
22. Mohan S, Libanati C, Dony C, Lang K, Srinivasan N, Baylink DJ: **Development, validation, and application of a radioimmunoassay for insulin-like growth factor binding protein-5 in human serum and other biological fluids**. *J Clin Endocrinol Metab* 1995, 80:2638-2645.
23. Kumar J, Muntner P, Kaskel FJ, Hailpern SM, Melamed ML: **Prevalence and Associations of 25-Hydroxyvitamin D Deficiency in US Children: NHANES 2001-2004**. *Pediatrics* 2009.
24. Wilson EB: **Probable Inference, the Law of Succession, and Statistical Inference**. *J Am Statistical Association* 1927, 22:209-212.
25. Institute of Medicine 2011 Dietary reference intakes for calcium and vitamin D. Washington, DC, The National Academies Press. Ref Type: Report; 2011.
26. Ashraf A, Alvarez J, Saenz K, Gower B, McCormick K, Franklin F: **Threshold for effects of vitamin D deficiency on glucose metabolism in obese female African-American adolescents**. *J Clin Endocrinol Metab* 2009, 94:3200-3206.
27. Munoz-Torres M, Jodar E, Escobar-Jimenez F, Lopez-Ibarra PJ, Luna JD: **Bone mineral density measured by dual X-ray absorptiometry in Spanish patients with insulin-dependent diabetes mellitus**. *Calcif Tissue Int* 1996, 58:316-319.
28. Fechtenbaum J, Cropet C, Kolta S, Horlait S, Orcel P, Roux C: **The severity of vertebral fractures and health-related quality of life in osteoporotic postmenopausal women**. *Osteoporos Int* 2005, 16:2175-2179.
29. Valerio G, del PA, Esposito-del PA, Buono P, Mozzillo E, Franzese A: **The lumbar bone mineral density is affected by long-term poor metabolic control in adolescents with type 1 diabetes mellitus**. *Horm Res* 2002, 58:266-272.
30. Heap J, Murray MA, Miller SC, Jalili T, Moyer-Mileur LJ: **Alterations in bone characteristics associated with glycemic control in adolescents with type 1 diabetes mellitus**. *J Pediatr* 2004, 144:56-62.
31. McCabe LR: **Understanding the pathology and mechanisms of type I diabetic bone loss**. *J Cell Biochem* 2007, 102:1343-1357.
32. Paul RG, Bailey AJ: **Glycation of collagen: the basis of its central role in the late complications of ageing and diabetes**. *Int J Biochem Cell Biol* 1996, 28:1297-1310.
33. Ward DT, Yau SK, Mee AP, Mawer EB, Miller CA, Garland HO, et al: **Functional, molecular, and biochemical characterization of streptozotocin-induced diabetes**. *J Am Soc Nephrol* 2001, 12:779-790.
34. Manolagas SC, Jilka RL: **Bone marrow, cytokines, and bone remodeling. Emerging insights into the pathophysiology of osteoporosis**. *N Engl J Med* 1995, 332:305-311.
35. McNair P, Christensen MS, Christiansen C, Madsbad S, Transbol I: **Is diabetic osteoporosis due to microangiopathy?** *Lancet* 1981, 1:1271.

36. Bouillon R, Bex M, Van HE, Laureys J, Dooms L, Lesaffre E, *et al*: **Influence of age, sex, and insulin on osteoblast function: osteoblast dysfunction in diabetes mellitus.** *J Clin Endocrinol Metab* 1995, **80**:1194-1202.

37. Svoren BM, Volkening LK, Wood JR, Laffel LM: **Significant vitamin D deficiency in youth with type 1 diabetes mellitus.** *J Pediatr* 2009, **154**:132-134.

38. Karaguzel G, Akcurin S, Ozdem S, Boz A, Bircan I: **Bone mineral density and alterations of bone metabolism in children and adolescents with type 1 diabetes mellitus.** *J Pediatr Endocrinol Metab* 2006, **19**:805-814.

39. Pascual J, Argente J, Lopez MB, Munoz M, Martinez G, Vazquez MA, *et al*: **Bone mineral density in children and adolescents with diabetes mellitus type 1 of recent onset.** *Calcif Tissue Int* 1998, **62**:31-35.

40. Sugimoto T, Nishiyama K, Kuribayashi F, Chihara K: **Serum levels of insulin-like growth factor (IGF) I, IGF-binding protein (IGFBP)-2, and IGFBP-3 in osteoporotic patients with and without spinal fractures.** *J Bone Miner Res* 1997, **12**:1272-1279.

41. Greer RM, Rogers MA, Bowling FG, Buntain HM, Harris M, Leong GM, *et al*: **Australian children and adolescents with type 1 diabetes have low vitamin D levels.** *Med J Aust* 2007, **187**:59-60.

42. Moore C, Murphy MM, Keast DR, Holick MF: **Vitamin D intake in the United States.** *J Am Diet Assoc* 2004, **104**:980-983.

15

Children's and adolescent's self - assessment of metabolic control versus professional judgment: a cross-sectional retrospective and prospective cohort study

Andreas Bieri, Monika Oser-Meier, Marco Janner, Chantal Cripe-Mamie, Kathrin Pipczynski-Suter, Primus E Mullis and Christa E Flück[*]

Abstract

Background: Morbidity and mortality in T1DM depend on metabolic control, which is assessed by HbA1c measurements every 3–4 months. Patients' self-perception of glycemic control depends on daily blood glucose monitoring. Little is known about the congruence of patients' and professionals' perception of metabolic control in T1DM.

Objective: To assess the actual patients' self-perception and objective assessment (HbA1c) of metabolic control in T1DM children and adolescents and to investigate the possible factors involved in any difference.

Methods: Patients with T1DM aged 8 – 18 years were recruited in a cross-sectional, retrospective and prospective cohort study. Data collection consisted of clinical details, measured HbA1c, self-monitored blood glucose values and questionnaires assessing self and professionals' judgment of metabolic control.

Results: 91 patients participated. Mean HbA1c was 8.03%. HbA1c was higher in patients with a diabetes duration > 2 years ($p = 0.025$) and in patients of lower socioeconomic level ($p = 0.032$). No significant correlation was found for self-perception of metabolic control in well and poorly controlled patients. We found a trend towards false-positive memory of the last HbA1c in patients with a HbA1c > 8.5% ($p = 0.069$) but no difference in patients' knowledge on target HbA1c between well and poorly controlled patients.

Conclusions: T1DM patients are aware of a target HbA1c representing good metabolic control. Ill controlled patients appear to have a poorer recollection of their HbA1c. Self-perception of actual metabolic control is similar in well and poorly controlled T1DM children and adolescents. Therefore, professionals should pay special attention that ill controlled T1DM patients perceive their HbA1c correctly.

Keywords: T1DM, Glycemic control, Self-assessment, HbA1c, Perception

Background

The primary goal of diabetes care for children and adolescents is to achieve an optimal metabolic control to prevent or to minimize the risk of acute (e.g. hypoglycemia) and long-term complications such as retinopathy, nephropathy and neuropathy [1,2]. The recommended everyday treatment regimen for a patient with Type 1 Diabetes Mellitus (T1DM) is complex and demanding. Parents or other adult

care takers initially play a key role in this intensive care system. But as children grow older responsibility for taking care of their chronic condition is placed upon them. During adolescence deteriorations in diabetes management and control are common [3]. These deteriorations raise the risk of acute or long-term complications and are also associated with higher health care costs. It is known that an optimal self-care behavior, independently of age, impacts positively on glycemic control [4]. Therefore, professionals aim to help adolescent patients and their families to become experts in self-management of their disease. A recently

* Correspondence: christa.flueck@dkf.unibe.ch
Pediatric Endocrinology, Diabetology & Metabolism, University Children's Hospital, Inselspital, Freiburgstrasse 15, CH - 3010 Bern, Switzerland

published systematic review investigated demographic and inter- or intrapersonal factors associated with metabolic control and self-care in adolescent patients with T1DM [4]. This revealed that adolescence is associated with both, decreased self-care and deterioration in metabolic control. Factors like a lower socioeconomic status, lower parental responsibility for, and involvement in diabetes-focused daily tasks, higher peer orientation or also intrapersonal characteristics like low conscientiousness and low emotional stability were associated with lower self-care and higher HbA1c values.

Self-care of diabetes in daily routine involves insulin administration, decisions around food – choices and intake, physical activity, timing of glucose measurements and analysis as well as response to the results. This calls for well-organized treatment instructions and continuous coaching by a multidisciplinary team but also for patients cognitive and executive skills. In recent years cognitive and executive functioning in T1DM gained attention in the literature [5,6]. These studies essentially showed only mild differences between the neurocognitive performance of children and adolescents with T1DM when compared to controls. In a meta-analysis of the literature in 2008 only a mildly reduced intellectual quotient was found in children with diabetes [5]. The largest effects, but still within a very small range, were on visuospatial ability, motor speed and writing, and on sustained attention and reading. Most of these investigations focused on cognition.

Overall, there is a body of knowledge about cognitive and executive functioning in T1DM and also of factors associated with self-care, adherence to therapy and metabolic control. By contrast, there is very limited knowledge about the T1DM patients' capacity of self-assessment which obviously is a prerequisite for good self-care. Characteristics of self-assessment for example are self-perception of HbA1c value, patient's memory of the HbA1c value, knowledge on target HbA1c or patients' suggestions on how to improve metabolic control. We found only limited literature concerning the role that recall plays in diabetic management. Only very recently a study investigated the prospective recall and glycemic control in children with T1DM [7]. No clear association between glycemic control and memory was found. Similarly, no literature is available for the difference between patients' and professionals' assessment of metabolic control. Our daily experience suggests that patients' self-assessment of the actual glycemic control depends primarily on the perception of their own diabetes management at home, including daily blood glucose self-monitoring, insulin applications and diet, whereas professionals' assessment depends mainly on measured HbA1c levels and blood glucose measurements from home devices.

Therefore, the aim of our study was to test the hypothesis if there was a difference between patients' self-perception

and an objective assessment (HbA1c) of metabolic control in T1DM children and adolescents; and to investigate factors that may be involved.

Methods
Patients and study design
We performed a cross-sectional, retrospective and prospective cohort study. We recruited patients with T1DM, seen at the outpatient clinic of the University Children's Hospital in Bern between April and September 2011. Inclusion criteria were an age between 8 – 18 years, diagnosis of T1DM for ≥ 12 months, at least 3 regular consultations in our department during the past 12 months and informed consent. Exclusion criteria were a change in the modality of insulin therapy in the past 12 months, less than 3 regular consultations in our department over the past 12 months, other chronic illnesses influencing the metabolic control of T1DM (such as malignancy or neuromuscular disease) and other types of diabetes. The study fulfilled the criteria of the Declaration of Helsinki and was approved by the cantonal ethics committee of Bern, Switzerland. Participating patients and caregivers were informed about the study and gave their written consent.

A total of 91 children (53 boys and 38 girls) were included in the study. 39 T1DM patients between 8 – 18 years did not participate for the following reasons: 3 refused to participate, 33 did not fulfill the inclusion criteria and 3 did not provide full information on the questionnaires. Details on patient characteristics are summarized in Table 1.

Data collection
Clinical and demographic data such as age, duration of disease, modality of insulin therapy and HbA1c of the last consultation were collected from patients' clinical records. Height and weight were measured during the visit at the outpatient clinic. Standard deviation score of the Body Mass Index (BMI) was calculated according to the LMS model taking the Kromeyer-Hauschild percentiles as a reference [8].

Data concerning self-monitored blood glucose levels were taken from memory functions of personal glucometers. Average values per day were calculated over the past 2–4 weeks.

All other information was collected with the help of three specific questionnaires: One for the professional, one for the care taker and one for the patient. Patients were requested to fill in the questionnaires without the help of their care takers.

A classification of the socioeconomic level was performed based on the self-declared educational level and occupational status of both parents as published elsewhere [9]. In brief, the classification "low" consisted of

Table 1 Patient characteristics

Number of patients (n)	All	91	
	Male	53	
	Female	38	
		Mean	**Range**
HbA1c (%)	All	8.03	6.1 - 10.9
	Male	7.99	6.3 - 10.5
	Female	8.09	6.1 - 10.9
Age (years)		13.22	8.23 - 17.81
Duration of T1DM (years)	All	6.13	1.05 - 15.77
Body mass index (SDS)	All	0.06	-2.61 - 1.98
	Male	-0.10	-2.61 - 1.93
	Female	0.28	-1.65 - 1.98
		n	**%**
Modality of therapy	Conventional insulin therapy	9	9.9
	Functional insulin therapy	59	64.8
	Insulin pump	23	25.3
Parental socioeconomic level	Low	8	8.8
	Moderate	64	70.3
	High	17	18.7
	Not determined	2	2.2

public school without professional training; the "intermediate" level included secondary school with completed professional training, and a "high" level was defined as having completed academic studies at a university.

HbA1c was determined by the Latex-Immunagglutination method (DCA 2000 Analyzer, Bayer Corporation, Elkart, IN 46514 USA). For this assay, reference values for healthy, non-diabetic individuals range between 4.0 - 5.6%.

Self assessment score (SAS)

We created a questionnaire and a scoring system to evaluate the quality of the self-assessment of patients' metabolic control. Patients were asked by questionnaire whether they felt that the actual HbA1c might be better, equal or worse than the HbA1c measured 3 months ago. Better or worse were defined as a difference in HbA1c $\geq$ $^{+}/_{-}$ 0.5%. Data were analyzed and categorized as follows. SAS 0 meant, that patient's perception overlapped with the objective result. SAS +1 or +2 meant, that the measured HbA1c value showed an improvement which the patient did not perceive (e.g. the patient meant that the actual HbA1c was worse than the last HbA1c, but in fact it was equal (+1) or better (+2). SAS –1 or –2 meant, that the measured HbA1c value showed a worsening of the metabolic control which the patient did not realize (e.g. the patient meant that the actual HbA1c was equal or better than the last HbA1c, but in fact it was worse (–1 to –2).

Data analysis

Data were analyzed using SPSS 19.0 (IBM® SPSS® Statistics 19). For group comparison the Kruskal-Wallis test was used. A p-value < 0.05 was considered to indicate statistical significance. Most data are shown as boxplots with the top of the box representing the 75th percentile, the bottom of the box representing the 25th percentile, and the line in the middle representing the 50th percentile. The whiskers represent the highest and lowest values, that were not outliers or extreme values.

Results

Patient characteristics and metabolic control in the study cohort

Mean HbA1c of the 91 studied T1DM patients was 8.03% (range 6.1 – 10.9%) (Table 1). In boys the mean HbA1c was 7.99%, in girls 8.09%. Mean duration of T1DM (time since the initial diagnosis) was about 6 years. Two thirds of the patients were treated with a functional insulin therapy using multiple daily injections, 25% of the patients with an insulin pump, and 10% were on a conventional 2–3 insulin injection regimen with fixed meals.

Two thirds of the patients had care givers classified as having a moderate level of socioeconomic status, 17% had a high and 8% a low level.

Figure 1 shows the HbA1c values in the study cohort in relation to age, duration of diabetes, glucose self-

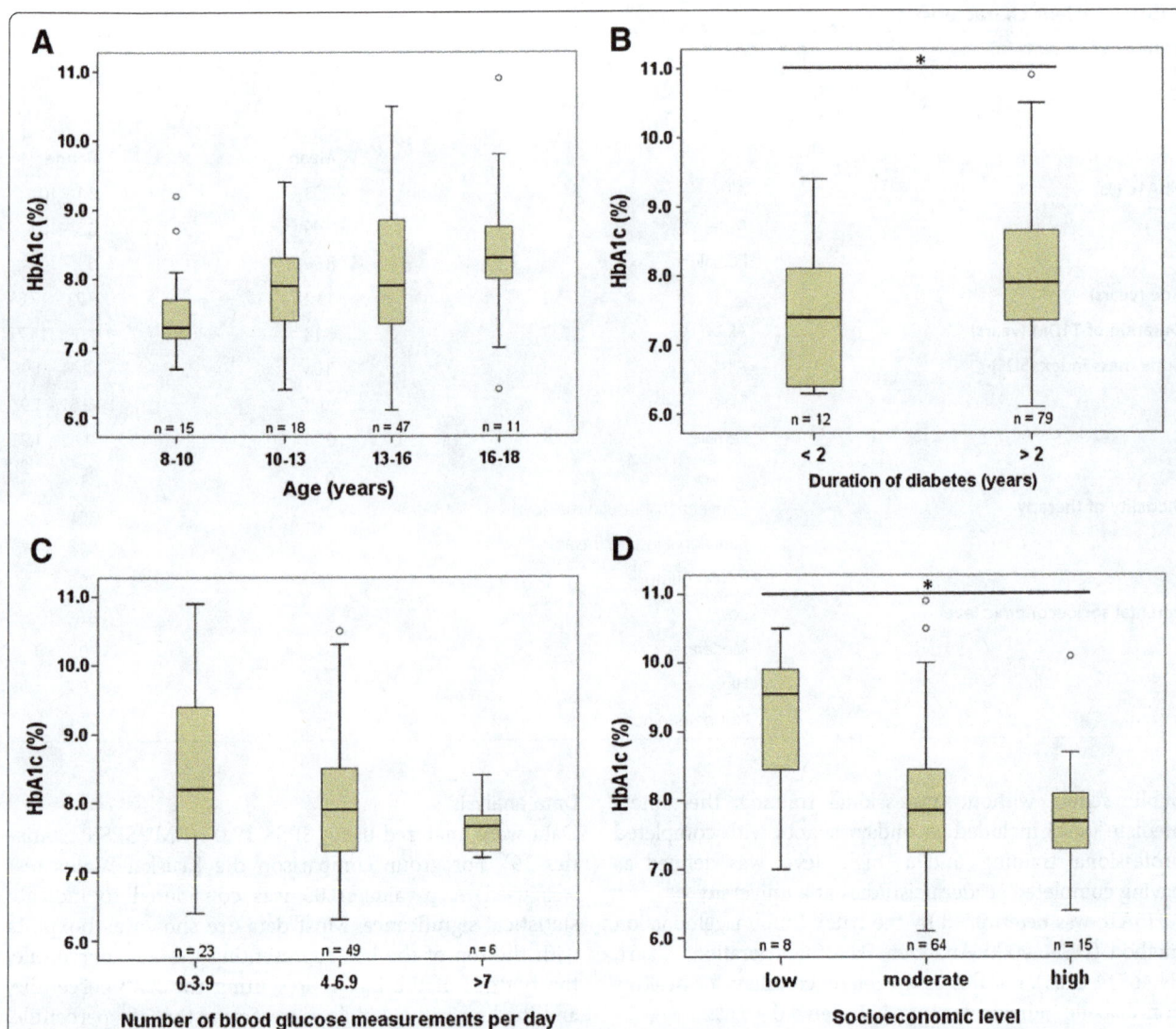

Figure 1 HbA1c in relation to (A) age, (B) duration of diabetes, (C) glucose self-monitoring and (D) socioeconomic level. There is a tendency towards higher HbA1c values with age (p = 0.065). HbA1c values correlate with the duration of diabetes (p = 0.025). HbA1c does not correlate with the number of blood glucose self-measurements (p = 0.173) but correlates with the socioeconomic level (p = 0.032). Data are given as boxplots and were statistically analyzed by Kruskal-Wallis tests with a significance level of p ≤ 0.05.

monitoring and socioeconomic level. We found significant correlations between HbA1c values and the duration of diabetes, with higher HbA1c values in patients with diabetes for > 2 years. Similarly, HbA1c values were significantly higher in the lowest socioeconomic group as compared to the moderate and high socioeconomic group (Figure 1D). Finally, we observed a trend towards higher HbA1c values in older patients (p = 0.065).

Memory of the HbA1c measured at the last consultation

To investigate the impact of regular consultations with diabetes professionals at our center, the memorized HbA1c of the last visit was studied. Recollection of the HbA1c measured during the former visit 3–4 months ago was assessed by questionnaire and compared with

the HbA1c value from the laboratory. The difference between the recalled and the measured HbA1c were then compared to the actual HbA1c, age, frequency of blood glucose self-monitoring, duration of diabetes and socioeconomic level. We found that patients with HbA1c values > 8.5% tended to have a poorer recollection of their last HbA1c than better controlled subjects (p = 0.069) (Figure 2). By contrast no relationship was found between the anamnestic HbA1c and age, frequency of glucose self-monitoring, duration of diabetes and socioeconomic level (data not shown).

Knowledge of target HbA1c

Quality of metabolic control in diabetic patients is followed by regular HbA1c measurements. Internationally a target

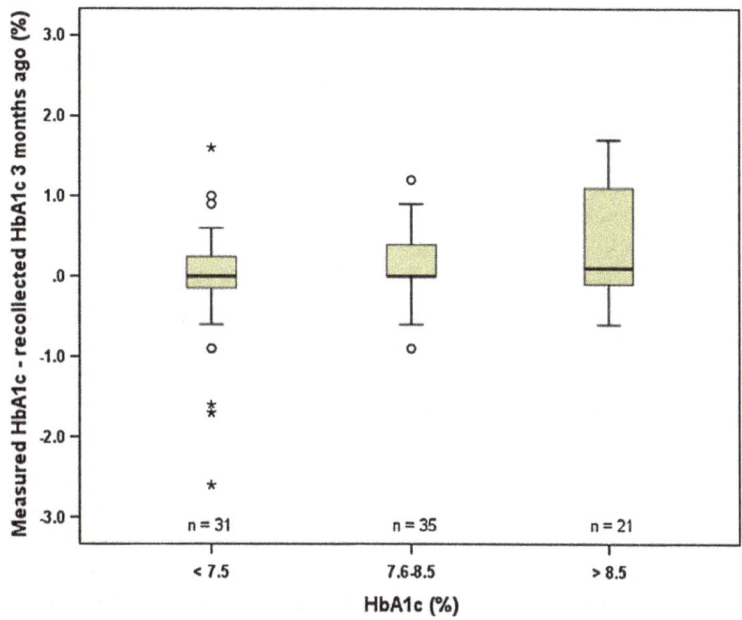

Figure 2 Memory of last HbA1c. The recollection of the last measured HbA1c values was assessed by comparing the objective HbA1c values 3 months ago with the patient's recollection of this HbA1c. The gap between the last measured and remembered HbA1c value was then compared to the actual HbA1c. Data are shown as boxplots with the actual HbA1c in categorized form on the x-axis. Note that there is a tendency towards wrong positive memory of the last HbA1c in patients having an HbA1c > 8.5% (p = 0.069). Data were analyzed by the Kruskal-Wallis test with a significance level of p ≤ 0.05.

HbA1c of < 7.5% is recommended for all age groups [10]. This basic information on diabetes is conveyed to our patients and parents/caregivers by our team during initial instructions and is part of the communication during every follow-up visit. Therefore, we asked our patients for their target HbA1c and then correlated this value with their measured HbA1c value at the time of the visit, age, blood glucose self-monitoring, duration of diabetes and socio-economic level (Figure 3). Overall, we found no relationship between knowledge of target HbA1c and measured HbA1c (Figure 3A). By contrast, older patients indicated higher target values of HbA1c than younger patients (p =

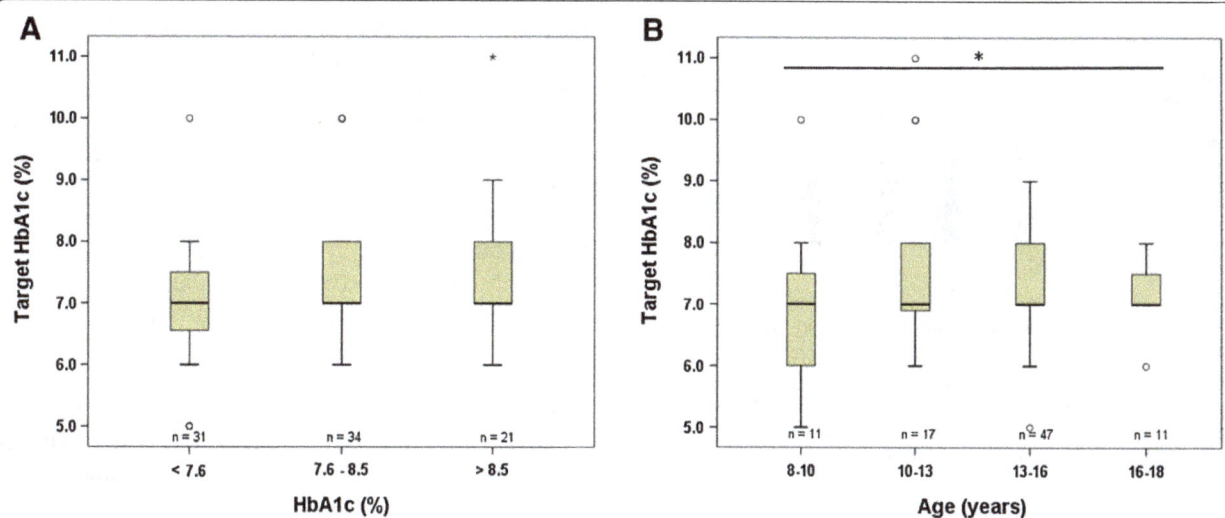

Figure 3 Knowledge of target HbA1c. All patients were asked for the currently recommended HbA1c level for good glycemic control (y-axis). **A)** These data were then compared to the actual HbA1c of each patient (x-axis). No significant difference was found (p = 0.154). **B)** Data were also correlated with the age finding significantly higher target HbA1c levels in older patients (p = 0.017). Data were analyzed by the Kruskal-Wallis test with a significance level of p ≤ 0.05.

0.017) (Figure 3B). No relationship was found between target HbA1c and the frequency of glucose self-monitoring, duration of diabetes and socioeconomic level (data not shown).

Self-perception of metabolic control in T1DM

To assess our patients' self-perception of their metabolic control, we invited them to predict whether the current measured HbA1c would be better, same or worse than the HbA1c assessed during the prior visit. Data were scored (SAS) and related to the actual HbA1c, age, frequency of blood glucose self-monitoring, duration of diabetes and socioeconomic level. For details concerning the SAS see the Methods section. Generally, patients with a SAS of 0 had a perfect fit between their prediction and the actual HbA1c measurement, while patients with a SAS of +/−2 had the biggest difference between their prediction and the objective measurement.

We found that nearly half of the patients with a HbA1c value < 7.6% had a perfect fit showing a SAS of 0, whereas only 36% of the patients with a HbA1c value > 8.5% had a SAS of 0 (Figure 4). However, this effect was not significant (p = 0.99). There was a trend, that patients with a longer duration of diabetes overestimated their actual HbA1c false-positively (p = 0.095) (data not shown).

Interestingly, the largest proportion of patients predicted their metabolic control correctly irrespective of their actual HbA1c (36-45%) while only few made a grossly wrong prediction (Figure 4).

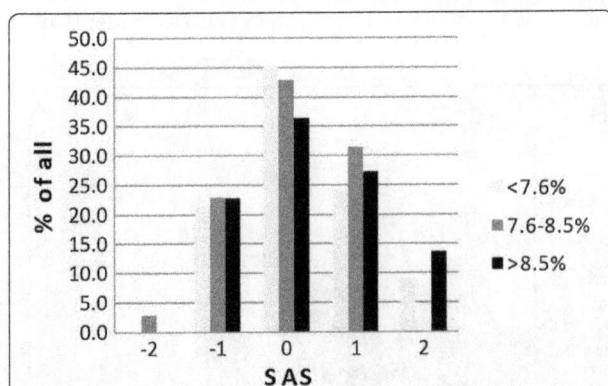

Figure 4 Self-perception of metabolic control in T1DM. HbA1c levels were put in relation to a self assessment score (SAS). Patients were asked to predict their HbA1c qualitatively. Data were collected with questionnaires and categorized from −2 to +2. A SAS 0 meant that patient's perception overlapped with the objective result. A SAS of +1 or +2 meant that the measured HbA1c value was better than the last one but this improvement was not perceived by the patient. A SAS −1 or −2 meant that the actual HbA1c value was worse than the last one but predicted otherwise by the patient. No significant correlation was found between the SAS and the actual HbA1c level (p = 0.99). Data are shown as bar graphs and were analyzed by the Kruskal-Wallis test.

Suggestions for improving metabolic control

Professionals and patients were invited to make suggestions on how to improve or maintain metabolic control. A list of items was given. Data were analyzed descriptively and results are shown as percentage (Figure 5). Professionals often suggested a *Change of the treatment regimen* or *No change*. By contrast, patients more often suggested a change in their daily routine like *Intensified glucose monitoring*, *Modification of nutrition* or *More elaborate self-protocol of therapy*.

Additional analysis revealed a relationship between the number of daily measurements of blood glucose and the age, with a higher number of daily measurements of blood glucose in younger patients (p = 0.012), who also tended to have lower HbA1c levels. On average patients in the age category of 8 – 10 years (n = 12) performed 5.3 glucose self-measurements daily, patients in the age category of 10 – 13 years (n = 16) 5.7, patients in the age category of 13 – 16 years (n = 41) 4.6 and patients in the age category of 16 – 18 years (n = 9) 3.4 only.

Our study questionnaire also included a query concerning the most annoying thing in the patients daily diabetes care: "If you could skip something in your daily diabetes care, what would it be?" We suggested the following items: *Insulin injections*, *Glucose measurements*, *Self-protocol of the therapy in a booklet or electronic device*, *Diet issues* or *Other*. From a total of 87 answers, 39% (n = 34) chose the answer *Insulin injections*, 37.9% (n = 33) chose *Self-protocol of the therapy in a booklet or electronic device*, 10.9% (n = 9) answered with *Glucose measurements*, 6.9% (n = 6) were annoyed with *Diet issues* and 5.7% (n = 5) chose *Other* issues including regular change of catheters of insulin pump or drawing venous blood for recommended laboratory control once a year. When we related these answers to the age of the patients, we observed, that older patients were especially annoyed at having to self-protocol the therapy in a booklet or electronic device and at glucose self-measurements, while younger patients would rather skip insulin injections or diet issues.

Discussion

This study in a small cohort of a single center shows that self-perception of metabolic control is good in children and adolescents with T1DM irrespective if well or poorly controlled.

Little is known about T1DM patients' capacity to self-assess therapy. This includes self-perception of HbA1c value, patient's recall of the HbA1c value, knowledge of target HbA1c level as well as patients' suggestions on how to improve metabolic control. This is in contrast to good knowledge on neurocognitive functioning in T1DM patients and of factors associated with self-care, adherence to therapy and metabolic control.

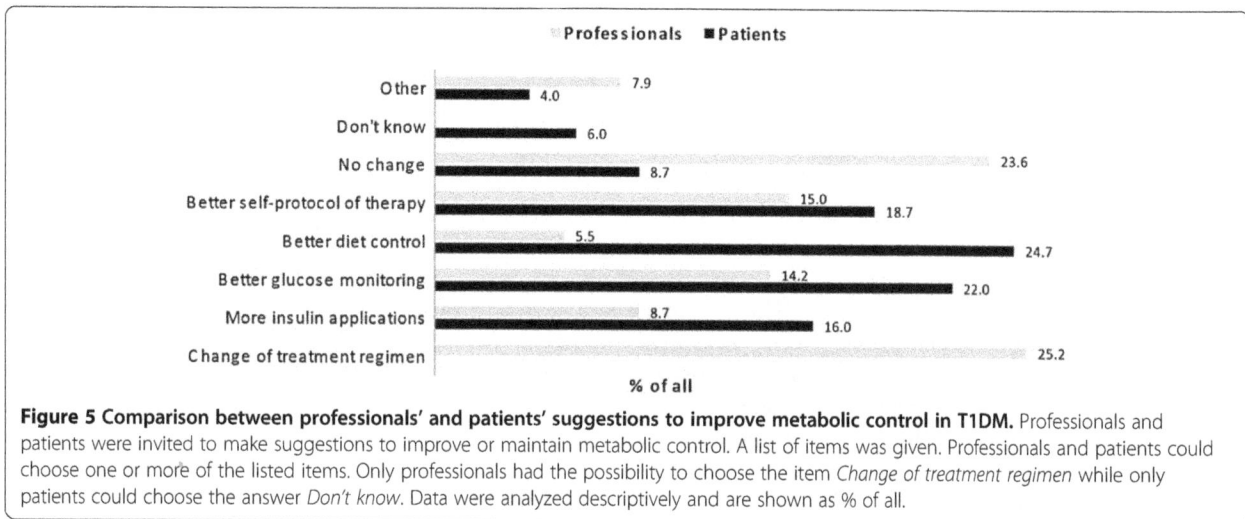

Figure 5 Comparison between professionals' and patients' suggestions to improve metabolic control in T1DM. Professionals and patients were invited to make suggestions to improve or maintain metabolic control. A list of items was given. Professionals and patients could choose one or more of the listed items. Only professionals had the possibility to choose the item *Change of treatment regimen* while only patients could choose the answer *Don't know*. Data were analyzed descriptively and are shown as % of all.

We found that the self-perception of actual metabolic control is similar in well or poorly controlled T1DM patients. This raises the question what factors influence metabolic control, and what factors influence the ability of self-assessment. It is well known, that for example the frequency of blood-glucose self-monitoring, the age of the patients, the duration of disease or the socioeconomic background influence metabolic control [2,11]. Therefore, we wondered whether these same factors were also associated with the ability of self-assessment of metabolic control.

In general, our patients with T1DM have a satisfactory metabolic control with a mean HbA1c of 8.03%. This compares to a cross-sectional study from our center in 2008 with a mean HbA1c of 7.6% [12]. The difference in HbA1c may be explained by the fact that in the study in 2008 all T1DM patients aged 0 – 20 years were enrolled without further limitations. In this study a large proportion (69%) of the patients had a short diabetes duration of 0 – 24 months with presumed residual activity. In line with the actual study the subgroup of diabetic adolescents also had a mean HbA1c of 8.1%. Compared to a large, international multicentre study which reported a mean HbA1c of 8.2% [13], our results are slightly better. Similar to other studies [2,14], we show that metabolic control is better with shorter duration of diabetes and higher socioeconomic level.

We found, that poorly controlled patients (HbA1c > 8.5%) have a worse recollection of their last HbA1c compared to better controlled subjects. Only one recent study investigated the prospective memory in correlation with glycemic control in children with T1DM [7]. Prospective memory was defined as the memory which is required to carry out intended actions. This study employed PROMS, an innovative prospective memory screen and a series of cognitive tests. Overall, this was a largely negative

study which found no association between total PROMS score and glycemic control. Most studies investigating neurocognitive functioning in pediatric T1DM patients conclude that severely low blood glucose levels increase the risk of learning difficulties and a range of cognitive deficits and memory function [5,6]. As we found that poorly controlled patients have a worse recollection of their last HbA1c, we assumed that they overestimated their metabolic control in personal favor. In fact, false-positive recollection of metabolic control can harm the diabetic patient because no actions will be taken to achieve euglycemia (including insulin dose adjustments, intensified glucose monitoring, and diet control). Therefore, regularly measured HbA1c and discussions with professionals are strongly recommended to prevent wrong self-assessment. Factors like age, frequency of glucose self-monitoring, duration of diabetes and socioeconomic level alone don't seem to correlate with the ability of memorizing the personal HbA1c level.

In regards to the knowledge about target HbA1c, no correlation was found with metabolic control. By contrast the personal target HbA1c level correlated with age, with higher personal target levels in older patients. This is inconsistent with the findings of the Hvidoere Childhood Diabetes Study 2005 [13], where reported target HbA1c levels were associated with the actual metabolic control, but not associated with age. The fact that target levels in our study did not correlate with metabolic control, is probably due to the small number of patients in our study. The observation that our older T1DM patients have a higher target HbA1c in mind remains unexplained. It has been reported that, if members of the diabetes care team are consistent in their advice on target HbA1c, adolescents' HbA1c correlates with those targets [13]. So we presume that it is an important teaching point in diabetes care, that patients are aware of the internationally recommended target HbA1c, which is < 7.5% for all age groups [10].

Furthermore, it is discussed in the literature that lower HbA1c levels and longer duration of diabetes might be factors that increase the risk for hypoglycemia in children and adolescents with diabetes [13,15,16]. Therefore, it is conceivable that higher HbA1c levels or a higher personal target HbA1c level might result out of fear of hypoglycemic episodes, especially in patients with hypoglycemia unawareness or recurrent severe hypoglycemia. However, the question whether frequent and/or severe hypoglycemic episodes affect T1DM patients' self-perception of metabolic control is not solved in the literature and remains unsolved as we did not record hypoglycemic episodes for analysis in our study.

We found no correlation between the self-assessment score (SAS) and the actual measured HbA1c or other parameters. Interestingly, the largest proportion of patients in our study predicted their metabolic control correctly irrespective of their actual HbA1c. This may result from the therapeutic approach of our diabetes team to discuss the actual metabolic control with patients and parents and try to support patients in their efforts to improve metabolic control with personal advice. Currently there is no literature to compare these findings. When we assessed professionals' and patients' suggestions to improve actual metabolic control, we found that professionals often suggested a change of treatment regimen or no change, while patients rather suggested changes in their daily routine at home, like improving glucose monitoring or self-protocol or adapting nutrition. This reflects the different perspectives on diabetes management between professionals and patients well. While professionals are primarily preoccupied with values of HbA1c, glucose and insulin doses, patients deal with blood glucose self-monitoring, insulin applications and their diabetes diet regimen and know about their personal compliance. The ideal professional diabetes care has to integrate these two perspectives to reach consensus on what needs to be done to achieve good metabolic control. This goal may only be achieved with a multidisciplinary specialist team consisting of psychologists, social workers, dieticians, diabetes nurse instructors and pediatric diabetologists. Partners of the team may also be pediatricians, teachers or day-care professionals.

Interestingly, when focusing on the answers of the patients concerning our question of the most annoying thing in their daily diabetes care, we found that our patients are just as annoyed by insulin injection as to having self-protocol the therapy in a booklet or electronic device. Especially the older patients were annoyed at the continuous task of keeping a diary. There is hope, that further development of electronic devices will facilitate and simplify patients' self-protocol of therapy in the future.

Conclusion

Self-perception of metabolic control in children and adolescents with T1DM treated according to international standards is good, even if the objective metabolic control does not meet the target. Patients with poor metabolic control are less attentive to their actual HbA1c. In theory, T1DM patients know the target HbA1c levels for excellent metabolic control. Overall, current diabetes care strategies seem to achieve the goal to make T1DM patients experts of their own diabetes.

Abbreviations
T1DM: Type 1 Diabetes Mellitus; IDF: International Diabetes Federation; ISPAD: International Society for Pediatric and Adolescent Diabetes; BMI: Body mass index; LMS: Least mean square; SAS: Self assessment score.

Competing interests
The authors declare that they have no competing interests.

Authors' contribution
The authors' contribution to the paper is as follow: AB and CEF: study concepts and design, data analysis and interpretation, statistical analysis, critical revision of the manuscript for important intellectual content and manuscript preparation; MOM, CCM, KPS, PEM: acquisition of data, critical revision of the manuscript for important intellectual content; MJ: study concepts and statistical analysis. All authors read and approved the final manuscript.

Acknowledgments
We thank all patients and families for participating in this study. We also thank Siemens Healthcare Diagnostics AG, Zürich, Switzerland for their financial support in paying the publication fees.

References
1. Nathan DM, et al: Intensive diabetes treatment and cardiovascular disease in patients with type 1 diabetes. N Engl J Med 2005, 353:25.
2. Global IDF/ISPAD guideline for diabetes in childhood and adolescence: International Diabetes Federation. 2011 (http://www.idf.org/sites/default/files/Diabetes-in-Childhood-and-Adolescence-Guidelines.pdf).
3. Hilliard ME, Wu YP, Rausch J, Dolan LM, Hood KK: Predictors of deteriorations in diabetes management and control in adolescents with type 1 diabetes. J Adolesc Health 2013, 52:28–34.
4. Neylon OM, O'Connell MA, Skinner TC, Cameron FJ: Demographic and personal factors associated with metabolic control and self-care in youth with type 1 diabetes: a systematic review. Diabetes Metab Res Rev 2013, 29(4):257–272.
5. Naguib JM, Kulinskaya E, Lomax CL, Garralda ME: Neuro-cognitive performance in children with type 1 diabetes – a meta-analysis. J Pediatr Psychol 2009, 34(3):271–282.
6. Hannonen R, Tupola S, Ahonen T, Riikonen R: Neurocognitive functioning in children with type-1 diabetes with and without episodes of severe hypoglyaemia. Developmental Medicine & Child Neurology 2003, 24:262–268.
7. Osipoff JN, Dixon D, Wilson TA, Preston T: Prospective memory and glycemic control in children with type 1 diabetes mellitus: a cross-sectional study. Int J Pediatr Endocrinol 2012, 1:29.
8. Kromeyer-Hauschild K, Wabitsch M, Kunze D, et al: Perzentile für den body-mass-Index für das Kindes- und Jugendalter unter Heranziehung verschiedener deutscher Stichproben. Monatsschr Kinderheilkd 2001, 149:807–818.
9. Simonetti GD, Schwertz R, Klett M, Hoffmann GF, Schaefer F, Wühl E: Determinants of blood pressure in preschool children: the role of parental smoking. Circulation 2011, 123:292–298.
10. Rewers M, Pihoker C, Donaghue K, Hanas R, Swift P, Klingensmith GJ: Assessment and monitoring of glycemic control in children and adolescents with diabetes. Pediatr Diabetes 2009, 10(Suppl.12):71–81.

11. Hood KK, Peterson CM, Rohan JM, Drotar D: **Association between adherence and glycemic control in pediatric type 1 diabetes: a meta-analysis.** *Pediatrics* 2009, 124:e1171–1179.

12. Tonella P, Fluck CA, Mullis PE: **Metabolic control of type 1 diabetic patients followed at the University Children's Hospital in Bern: Have we reached the goal?** *Swiss Med Wkly* 2010, 140(July):44.

13. Swift PGF, Skinner TC, De Beaufort CE, *et al*: **Target setting in intensive insulin management is associated with metabolic control: the Hvidoere Childhood Diabetes Study Group Centre Differences Study 2005.** *Pediatr Diabetes* 2010, 11:271–278.

14. Cameron FJ, Skinner TC, De Beaufort CE, *et al*: **Are family factors universally related to metabolic outcomes in adolescents with type 1 diabetes?** *Diabet Med* 2008, 25:463–468.

15. Clarke W, Jones T, Rewers A, Dunger D, Klingensmith GJ: **Assessment and management of hypoglycemia in children and adolescents with diabetes.** *Pediatr Diabetes* 2008, 9:165–174.

16. Blasetti A, Di Giulio C, Tocco AM, *et al*: **Variables associated with severe hypoglycemia in children and adolescents with type 1 diabetes: a population-based study.** *Pediatr Diabetes* 2011, 12:4–10.

16

Insulin detemir in a twice daily insulin regimen versus a three times daily insulin regimen in the treatment of type 1 diabetes in children: A pilot randomized controlled trial

Josephine Ho[1*], Carol Huang[1], Alberto Nettel-Aguirre[1,2] and Danièle Pacaud[1]

Abstract

Background: Children with type 1 diabetes (DM1) often use three daily (TID) injections with intermediate acting insulin at breakfast and bedtime, and rapid acting insulin at breakfast and dinner. Substituting the evening intermediate acting insulin with a long acting insulin analogue (LAIA) at dinner in a twice daily (BID) injection regimen may be as effective as a TID regimen. The objective of this pilot study was to compare HbA1c in children with DM1 using a BID regimen with a LAIA at dinner (intervention) to those using a standard TID regimen (control) over 6 months.

Methods: Randomized controlled trial with main outcome measure being HbA1c at 0, 3 and 6 months. Secondary outcomes were frequency of adverse events (hypoglycemia, diabetic ketoacidosis, weight gain) and scores on the Diabetes Quality of Life Measure for Youth (DQOLY).

Results: 18 subjects (10 control, 8 intervention). Mean years (standard deviations) for control and intervention respectively were: age at diagnosis of DM1 6.31 (2.91) vs 7.76 (3.22), duration of DM1 5.96 (4.95) vs 3.76 (3.37). No significant differences were seen in the mean HbA1c between control and intervention at 0 months [8.48(0.86) vs 8.57(1.13)], 3 months [8.47(0.50) vs 7.99(0.61)], or 6 months [8.42(0.63) vs 8.30(0.76)]. No significant differences were found between groups for frequency of adverse events or DQOLY.

Conclusions: In this pilot study, incorporating LAIA in a BID regimen did not cause deterioration in HbA1c or increases in adverse events; suggesting that this may be a viable option for families where a more simplified insulin regimen would be beneficial and compliance may be improved.

Keywords: type 1 diabetes, glycemic control, pediatric, long acting insulin analogue

Background

Children with type 1 diabetes (DM1) require multiple daily injections of insulin to maintain good glycemic control. The Diabetes Control and Complications Trial (DCCT) has shown that intensive insulin treatment using at least three times daily (TID) injections achieves superior blood glucose control with decreased risk of long term complications than conventional insulin treatment using once daily or twice daily (BID) injections [1,2]. However, this study was done when long acting insulin analogues (LAIA) were not available which limited the types of insulin regimens and there are limited randomized controlled trials assessing analogue insulins in children. Multiple daily injection regimens are not consistently superior in children and other factors including patient support and team cohesion play large roles in glycemic control [3]. Many patients find it difficult to adhere to TID injections since it is an invasive and painful therapy, which results in frequent insulin omission. By replacing bedtime intermediate acting insulin with a LAIA at dinner, this would allow children

* Correspondence: Josephine.ho@albertahealthservices.ca
[1]Department of Pediatrics, University of Calgary, Calgary, T3B 6A8, Canada
Full list of author information is available at the end of the article

Insulin detemir in a twice daily insulin regimen versus a three times daily insulin regimen...

145

with DM1 to maintain their glycemic control with only a BID insulin injection regimen.

The pharmacokinetic properties of the LAIA, detemir, have some potential benefits in the treatment of children with DM1 [4-8]. The longer duration of action would allow this long acting insulin analogue to be incorporated into a BID insulin regimen that could potentially offer equivalent glycemic control to a TID injection regimen. Intermediate and rapid acting insulin could still be given in the morning to avoid a lunchtime injection, while rapid acting and long acting insulin could be given at dinner to cover for the meal plus the background insulin required until the morning. Therefore, children only need to take insulin twice a day, which may result in greater compliance and improved quality of life. Satisfaction with diabetes treatment may also be improved because of more predictable glycemic control and less frequent adverse events. The risk of hypoglycemia may be decreased with detemir [4], because of the flat and protracted pharmacodynamic profile compared to the peak in insulin activity seen with intermediate acting insulins. Less frequent episodes of hypoglycemia may also result in less weight gain that can be seen in intensive insulin therapy.

The primary objective of this pilot, randomized controlled trial is to compare the glycemic control as measured by HbA1c in children with DM1 treated with a BID regimen of insulin using a LAIA overnight versus a TID insulin injection regimen with intermediate acting insulin. Secondary objectives included assessing the satisfaction with treatment of diabetes in each group using the Diabetes Quality of Life Measure for Youths (DQOLY) and determining the frequency of adverse events (severe hypoglycemia, nocturnal hypoglycemia, mild hypoglycemia, diabetic ketoacidosis, and change in body mass index (BMI)).

Methods

Study Design

The study was an open-labelled, randomized controlled trial design with two groups: control group (TID) and intervention group (BID). The trial was registered at *ClinicalTrials.gov Identifier: NCT00522210.*

Subjects

Subjects were recruited from children with DM1 currently being followed at the Alberta Children's Hospital (Calgary, Alberta, Canada). Inclusion criteria were: children aged 6-17 years old, diagnosed with DM1 for at least 1 year and currently being treated with a TID regimen of insulin with rapid acting insulin and intermediate acting insulin. Exclusion criteria were: HbA1c $\geq$ 10% at enrolment, chronic underlying medical conditions that could affect glycemic control (examples: uncontrolled

hypothyroidism, hyperthyroidism, celiac disease, etc.), current participants of other clinical trials, language or psychosocial barrier preventing the family from completing the study.

Protocol

A sample of size of 65 subjects per group was initially calculated based on an estimated baseline HbA1c of 8.4% (SD 1.3%) in each group, a clinically acceptable difference of 10% (absolute difference of 0.84), a power of 90%, and a dropout rate of 20%. Therefore, if one assumed no drop-outs a sample size of 52 patients per arm would have been sufficient.

Subjects were randomized into the control group or intervention group using a computer generated randomization sequence (the sequence was generated in blocks to keep groups as balanced as possible and to help ensure allocation concealment). Subjects were stratified by age groups (6 to 10 years, and greater than 10 years old). Given the nature of the intervention, it was not possible to blind patients, their parents, and caregivers to the treatment allocation.

In the control group (ie. the TID regimen), subjects were asked to continue on their usual insulin regimen (intermediate acting insulin and rapid acting analogue at breakfast, rapid acting analogue at dinner and intermediate acting insulin at bedtime). In the intervention group (ie. the BID regimen), the subjects' usual bedtime dose of intermediate acting insulin was discontinued and replaced with a dose of insulin detemir at dinner time. The intermediate acting insulin used was neutral protamine hagedorn (either Novolin NPH or Humulin N depending on what the patient was currently using). The rapid acting analogues used were lispro insulin (Humalog) or aspart insulin (Novorapid) depending on what the patient was currently using. The detemir was not mixed with the rapid acting insulin and was given as a separate injection. The dose of detemir was approximately 50% of the total daily dose of insulin, with the remaining 50% being comprised of the subject's breakfast dose of intermediate acting insulin and rapid acting analogue and dinner rapid acting analogue. A run-in period of 1 month, with a minimum of a weekly phone contact, was used to facilitate the change in insulin regimen and dose finding for the intervention group and to optimize insulin doses in the control group. No changes were made to the subjects' usual diet and exercise routines.

Throughout the study, monthly phone contact for insulin adjustments was done for both groups. In addition, subjects were assessed in clinic at baseline, 3 months and 6 months (Figure 1). This included height, weight, HbA1c, current insulin doses, episodes of severe hypoglycemia (glucose less than 4 mmol/L associated

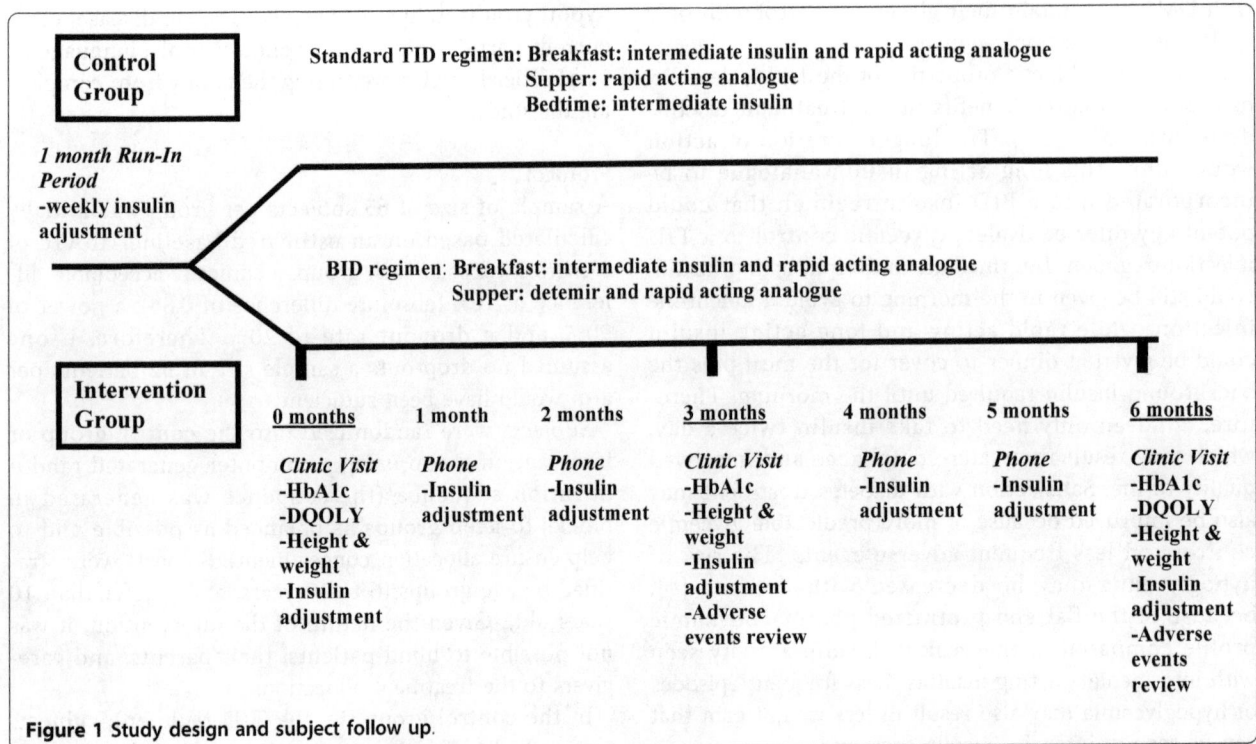

Figure 1 Study design and subject follow up.

with a decreased level of consciousness, seizure, or coma), reported nocturnal hypoglycemia, mild hypoglycemia (glucose less than 4 mmol/L where the patient is able to self treat) and diabetic ketoacidosis (hyperglycemia and ketonuria associated with a pH < 7.3 and/or bicarbonate level < 15 mmol/l).

The Diabetes Quality of Life Measure for Youths (DQOLY) was administered at baseline and again at 6 months. This questionnaire was initially used by the DCCT group and was later revised by Ingersoll et al [9]. It has been validated in youths aged 10-21 years. This instrument has three Likert scales including a 17 item diabetes life satisfaction scale (range of scores 17-85), 23 item disease impact scale (range of scores 23-115), and an 11 item disease related worries scale (range of scores 11-55) [9]. In this study, reverse scores were recorded for the impact and worries scales so that a higher score indicated a better quality of life. For the satisfaction scale, a higher score indicates higher satisfaction.

Data Analysis
Baseline demographic and clinical variables are presented as means with standard deviations (SD) for numerical variables and as proportions for categorical variables. The 95% confidence interval for the difference between groups is presented too. At each time point, HbA1c between the two groups was compared using a two sample t-test and confidence interval for the difference is provided to help assess non-inferiority. The true

expected difference in HbA1c between the control and treatment group was taken to be zero. Based on previous follow up data from the ACH Diabetes Clinic, the mean HbA1C is estimated at 8.4% with a standard deviation of 1.3 for each group. A 10% relative difference was considered a clinically acceptable difference. Therefore, the non-inferiority margin was set at 0.84.

Ethical approval
The protocol, including subject information, informed consent, recruitment procedure, interventions and data collection has been approved by the Conjoint Health Research Ethics Board of the Faculty of Medicine, University of Calgary (Calgary, Alberta, Canada) in accordance with the Declaration of Helsinki and Tri-Council Guidelines.

Results
Table 1 shows the enrolment characteristics of the subjects. There were no significant differences between the groups at baseline. In total, 18 subjects were enrolled (10 control, 8 intervention). The mean age at diagnosis of DM1 was 6.31 years (SD 2.91) for control and 7.76 years (SD 3.22) for intervention. The mean duration of DM1 was 5.96 years (SD 4.95) for control and 3.76 years (SD 3.37) for intervention.

There were no significant differences in the mean HbA1c between control and intervention groups at 0 months [8.48 (SD 0.86) vs 8.57 (SD 1.13)], 3 months

Table 1 Enrolment characteristics of subjects.

Characteristic	Control (TID) N = 10	Intervention (BID) N = 8	Difference between groups (95% confidence interval for the difference)
Gender (Female/Male)	4/6 (40% female)	4/4 (50% female)	10% (-50.02% - 33.36%)
Age groups (children < 10 years old/children ≥ 10 years old)	3/7 (30% children < 10 years old)	3/5 (37.5% children < 10 years old)	7.5% (-47.08% - 33.74%)
Age at study enrolment (years)	12.26 (3.40)	11.52 (2.08)	-0.74 (-3.52 - 2.03)
Age at type 1 diabetes diagnosis (years)	6.31 (2.91)	7.76 (3.22)	1.45 (-1.68 - 4.58)
Duration of diabetes (years)	5.96 (4.95)	3.76 (3.37)	-2.20 (-6.37 - 1.98)
Last HbA1c prior to enrolment (%)	8.54 (0.70)	8.70 (0.58)	0.16 (-0.48 - 0.80)
Insulin dose (units/kg/day)	1.02 (0.40)	0.94 (0.24)	-0.08 (-0.41 - 0.25)
Body Mass Index (kg/m^2)	20.62 (4.07)	20.99 (3.60)	0.38 (-3.46 - 4.22)

No significant differences were found between the groups at baseline. Table shows Number (%) or Mean (Standard deviation). Difference is for intervention minus control.

[8.47 (SD 0.50) vs 7.99 (SD 0.61)], or 6 months [8.42 (SD 0.63) vs 8.30 (SD 0.76)] (Table 2). Adverse events, such as DKA and reported hypoglycemic episodes, were similar in frequency in the control and intervention groups. There were no significant differences in body mass index or quality of life scales between groups (Table 2). The width of the confidence intervals for each of the outcome measures was large, likely due to the

Table 2 Results

	Baseline			3 Months			6 Months		
	Control	Intervention	Difference (95% confidence interval)	Control	Intervention	Difference (95% confidence interval)	Control	Intervention	Difference (95% confidence interval)
HbA1c %	8.48 (0.86)	8.57 (1.13)	0.095 (-0.95 - 1.14)	8.47 (0.50)	7.99 (0.61)	-0.48 (-1.06 - 0.095)	8.42 (0.63)	8.30 (0.76)	-0.12 (-0.84 - 0.60)
Body Mass Index (kg/m2)	20.62 (4.07)	20.99 (3.60)	0.38 (-3.46 - 4.22)	21.81 (6.40)	22.21 (3.48)	0.39 (-4.67 - 5.46)	21.04 (3.87)	21.75 (3.58)	0.71 (-3.03 - 4.45)
DKA (episodes in last 3 months)	0	0	0	0	0	0	0	0	0
Severe Hypoglycemia (episodes in last 3 months)	0.10 (0.32)	0	-0.10 (-0.33 - 0.13)	0.30 (0.67)	0	-0.30 (-0.78 - 0.18)	0.1 (0.32)	0	-0.10 (-0.33 - 0.13)
Mild/Moderate Hypoglycemia #/week	2.11 (1.40)	2.16 (1.65)	0.046 (-1.53 - 1.62)	2.17 (1.76)	1.87 (1.34)	-0.30 (-1.85 - 1.25)	2.12 (1.31)	2.54 (1.36)	0.41 (-0.94 - 1.77)
Nocturnal Hypoglycemia #/week	0.15 (0.34)	0.62 (1.03)	0.47 (-0.39 - 1.34)	0.12 (0.32)	0.72 (0.91)	0.59 (-0.18 - 1.36)	0.26 (0.57)	0.50 (0.72)	0.24 (-0.43 - 0.91)
QOL Impact	83.78 (7.38)	90.37 (8.14)	6.60 (-1.50 - 14.70)	—	—	—	83.70 (17.57)	91.00 (8.45)	7.30 (-6.28 - 20.88)
QOL Worries	41.62 (6.30)	42.00 (5.76)	0.37 (-6.10 - 6.85)	—	—	—	37.90 (8.55)	39.37 (7.29)	1.47 (-6.45 - 9.40)
QOL Satisfaction	67.33 (8.37)	67.00 (10.42)	-0.33 (-10.28 - 9.61)	—	—	—	65.00 (12.62)	72.50 (8.37)	7.50 (-3.06 - 18.06)

Comparison of glycemic control, adverse events and quality of life scores between the control and intervention groups. No significant differences were detected between the groups at baseline, 3 months or 6 months. Dashed line indicates data was not collected at that time point. Control (TID) N = 10. Intervention (BID) N = 8. Difference is for intervention minus control. Table shows Mean (Standard Deviation).

small sample size. However, they do indicate that the intervention was non-inferior when compared to the control group.

Discussion

Currently, a standard TID injection regimen with intermediate acting insulin at breakfast and bedtime, and rapid acting insulin at breakfast and dinner is often used in children. Families that opt for more intensive therapy can choose a continuous subcutaneous insulin infusion or a basal bolus regimen. However, these regimens are costly and require a significant amount of skill and effort from the family. In addition, patient compliance with multiple invasive and painful injections can be an issue when using multiple injections. Another challenge with exogenous insulin administration is hypoglycemia. While the results of the DCCT clearly demonstrated the importance of maintaining a near normal glucose level, the major adverse event reported in the intensive insulin treated subset of patients aged 13-17 years was a nearly three fold increase in severe hypoglycemic events [1,2]. The development of new LAIA offers the opportunity to simplify insulin regimens while achieving similar glycemic control.

Detemir is a LAIA that has prolonged insulin absorption with less intra-patient variability in peak insulin activity as well as very minimal peak activity, in comparison with intermediate acting insulin [10,11]. The pharmacokinetic properties of detemir have been studied in patients with DM1 using a euglycemic glucose clamp technique [5,12]. In comparison to neutral protamine hagedorn (NPH) insulin, detemir resulted in a more stable serum concentration of insulin without the peak seen in NPH [5,12]. In addition, there were less fluctuations in the glucose infusion rates required with detemir in steady state compared to NPH in steady state [5,12]. Detemir has been shown to have a consistent pharmacokinetic profile in children, adolescents, and adults with DM1[7,8].

Recently, a retrospective study by Cengiz et al [13] analyzed the same BID regimen (NPH and rapid acting insulin analogue at breakfast with insulin detemir and rapid acting insulin analogue at dinner) in children with new onset DM1 as an option prior to initiation of insulin pump therapy. They found that by 12 months after diagnosis of DM1, 49 of the patients had changed to pump therapy with a median HbA1c of 6.9% while 59 remained on the BID injection regimen with a median HbA1c of 7.2% [13]. The authors concluded that this BID regimen was effective in children with new onset diabetes and had similar glycemic control [13]. The findings of this retrospective study are consistent with our results, as we also did not find a difference in glycemic control for patients on TID versus the BID regimen.

In contrast to Cengiz et al's study [13], our randomized control trial was aimed at assessing the effectiveness of a BID regimen in children with DM1 greater than 12 months as an option for families where intensive diabetes therapy was not feasible and improved quality of life could be achieved by simplifying the diabetes regimen.

HbA1c changes when using insulin detemir has been studied in children and adolescents with conflicting results [14-17]. Braun et al [16] reported improved HbA1c and fewer severe hypoglycemic episodes in a chart review study of children who were switched from evening NPH insulin to detemir. Interestingly, in this study a subset of children under 12 years of age were treated with a BID regimen and showed an improvement in HbA1c from 8.3% to 7.6% after changing from evening NPH to detemir [16]. Dundar et al [14] reported an improvement in HbA1c in children who changed from a basal bolus regimen with NPH to either glargine or detemir. This study was limited by the fact that it was retrospective and was small with only 15 patients in the detemir treated group [14]. In a large, prospective, 26 week, randomized study of 347 children, Robertson et al [15] reported no difference in HbA1c in children changed to basal bolus therapy with either NPH or detemir compared to pre-basal bolus therapy. Although HbA1c was not better in the detemir group, the risk of nocturnal hypoglycemia was 26% lower [15]. Kurtoglu et al [17] retrospectively assessed children that were initially on basal bolus regimens with NPH or glargine then switched to detemir. After 12 weeks of using detemir, HbA1c was improved and the frequency of hypoglycemic episodes was decreased [17]. Although we did not see a similar improvement in HbA1c in our patients using detemir, these studies examined detemir in basal bolus regimens rather than the BID regimen used in our study. It is also reassuring that our study did not find a worsening of glycemic control despite simplifying the insulin regimen.

Hypoglycemia can be a side effect of intensive insulin therapy. Several studies have demonstrated that detemir is associated with a decreased frequency of hypoglycemia since it does not have a peak activity [4,18]. In a randomized, open, cross-over trial [18], detemir has been compared to NPH insulin in a basal bolus regimen in adults with DM1 and has been found to be as effective as NPH in maintaining glycemic control. Fewer patients experienced hypoglycemia with detemir compared to NPH [18]. Vague et al [4] compared detemir and NPH in 448 adult patients with DM1 in a basal-bolus regimen using twice daily detemir or NPH for basal coverage and rapid acting insulin with each meal. In their detemir group, more predictable glycemic control was seen during night-time plasma glucose monitoring using an intravenous line [4]. A significant reduction in the frequency of hypoglycemia as well as weight gain was also seen in their detemir group [4]. Interestingly, there was no difference in the HbA1c between the two groups after 6 months [4]. In our study, no differences in reported episodes of hypoglycemia were seen between groups.

Weight gain can be a concern when children are on intensified insulin regimens or have frequent hypoglycemia. Home et al [6] conducted a 16 week, randomized control trial of 408 patients with type 1 diabetes. HbA1c improved by 0.18% in the group using insulin detemir as the basal insulin compared to NPH insulin [6]. In addition, there was a decreased frequency of hypoglycemia and no weight gain in the group using insulin detemir compared to the NPH group which did have some weight gain [6]. Although the insulin regimen used in our study was not a basal bolus one, we did not find any significant changes in BMI between the groups.

Diabetic ketoacidosis (DKA) was not seen in either the control or intervention group. This is not necessarily surprising given the short duration of this study and small sample size. Karges et al [19], compared the incidence of DKA in a cohort of 10 682 children and adolescents with DM1 being treated with either NPH insulin or a LAIA. They found that the incidence of DKA was significantly higher in patients using glargine or detemir compared to those using NPH [19]. However, all of the patients studied were on at least three or more insulin injections per day while our patients using detemir were on a BID regimen.

Quality of life measures were not significantly different between the two groups using the DQOLY. A limitation of using the DQOLY was that this questionnaire has only been validated in youths aged 10-21 years [9]. Our study included children aged 6 years and older. However, only 1 subject was 7 years old and 5 subjects were 8 to 9 years old at enrolment and the DQOLY was the most practical and accessible measure to use at the time of this study.

At the time the study was conducted, it was recommended that families could continue mixing the intermediate insulin and rapid insulin analogue in one syringe in the morning. However, at supper time the LAIA and rapid insulin were to be given in two separate injections. Recently, Nguyen et al [20] published a study of 14 children with type 1 diabetes who underwent continuous glucose monitoring and found that mixing insulin detemir with aspart had equivalent effects on blood glucose when compared with giving them as separate injections. The ability to mix insulin detemir with aspart at supper time would again simplify the regimen for families and potentially have a greater impact on satisfaction and compliance.

A significant limitation of this study is the small sample size. Interestingly, recruitment was difficult for this study. Once families received a description of the alternate BID insulin regimen compared to the traditional TID regimen, many did not want to risk being randomized to the control group. The theoretical benefits of decreased nocturnal hypoglycemia and twice daily insulin injection times was very attractive to families; particularly those that struggle with compliance.

Conclusions

The results of this pilot study demonstrate that using a BID insulin regimen incorporating a LAIA allows for maintenance of glycemic control despite a less intensive injection regimen. Ideally, a basal bolus regimen with multiple daily injections or an insulin pump would mimic physiologic insulin secretion most closely, but practically this is often difficult to achieve in young children who are dependent on a responsible adult to be available for injections.

Simplifying to BID insulin regimens incorporating LAIA may be possible with no increase in adverse events and comparable HbA1c compared to standard TID regimens used in children, although larger clinical studies would be required to confirm this finding. Although no significant improvements were seen in DQOLY and nocturnal hypoglycemia, it is important that HbA1c remained stable, and suggests that this regimen is a viable option for families.

Acknowledgements

This study was funded by the Alberta Children's Hospital Foundation. The Alberta Children's Hospital Foundation was not involved in the study design; data collection, analysis or interpretation; writing of the manuscript; or in the decision to publish the manuscript.

Author details

[1]Department of Pediatrics, University of Calgary, Calgary, T3B 6A8, Canada. [2]Department of Community Health Sciences, University of Calgary, Calgary, T3B 6A8 Canada.

Authors' contributions

JH designed the study; collected, analyzed and interpreted the data; and drafted the manuscript. CH, AN and DP significantly contributed in the study design, data analysis, data interpretation and revising of the manuscript. All authors read and approved the final manuscript.

Competing interests

The authors declare that they have no competing interests.

References

1. The Diabetes Control and Complications Trial Research Group: The effect of intensive treatment of diabetes on the development and progression of long-term complications in insulin-dependent diabetes mellitus. *NEJM* 1993, **329**(14):977-986.
2. The Diabetes Control and Complications Trial Research Group: Effect of intensive diabetes treatment on the development and progression of

long-term complications in adolescents with insulin-dependent diabetes mellitus: Diabetes Control and Complications Trial. *J Ped* 1994, 125(2):177-188.

3. Skinner TC, Cameron FJ: Improving glycaemic control in children and adolescents: which aspects of therapy really matter? *Diabet Med* 27(4):369-375.

4. Vague P, Selam JL, Skeie S, De Leeuw I, Elte JW, Haahr H, Kristensen A, Draeger E: Insulin detemir is associated with more predictable glycemic control and reduced risk of hypoglycemia than NPH insulin in patients with type 1 diabetes on a basal-bolus regimen with premeal insulin aspart. *Diabetes Care* 2003, 26(3):590-596.

5. Plank J, Bodenlenz M, Sinner F, Magnes C, Gorzer E, Regittnig W, Endahl LA, Draeger E, Zdravkovic M, Pieber TR: A double-blind, randomized, dose-response study investigating the pharmacodynamic and pharmacokinetic properties of the long-acting insulin analog detemir. *Diabetes Care* 2005, 28(5):1107-1112.

6. Home P, Bartley P, Russell-Jones D, Hanaire-Broutin H, Heeg JE, Abrams P, Landin-Olsson M, Hylleberg B, Lang H, Draeger E: Insulin detemir offers improved glycemic control compared with NPH insulin in people with type 1 diabetes: a randomized clinical trial. *Diabetes Care* 2004, 27(5):1081-1087.

7. Heise T, Nosek L, Ronn BB, Endahl L, Heinemann L, Kapitza C, Draeger E: Lower within-subject variability of insulin detemir in comparison to NPH insulin and insulin glargine in people with type 1 diabetes. *Diabetes* 2004, 53(6):1614-1620.

8. Danne T, Lupke K, Walte K, Von Schuetz W, Gall MA: Insulin detemir is characterized by a consistent pharmacokinetic profile across age-groups in children, adolescents, and adults with type 1 diabetes. *Diabetes Care* 2003, 26(11):3087-3092.

9. Ingersoll GM, Marrero DG: A modified quality-of-life measure for youths: psychometric properties. *The Diabetes Educator* 1991, 17(2):114-118.

10. Hirsch IB: Insulin analogues. *NEJM* 2005, 352(2):174-183.

11. Haffner MC, Kufner MP: Insulin analogues. *NEJM* 2005, 352(17):1822-1824.

12. Bott S, Tusek C, Jacobsen LV, Endahl L, Draeger E, Kapitza C, Heise T: Insulin detemir under steady-state conditions: no accumulation and constant metabolic effect over time with twice daily administration in subjects with Type 1 diabetes. *Diabet Med* 2006, 23(5):522-528.

13. Cengiz E, Sherr JL, Erkin-Cakmak A, Weinzimer SA, Burke EN, Sikes KA, Urban AD, Tamborlane WV: A Bridge to Insulin Pump Therapy: Bid Regimen with NPH and Detemir Insulin During Initial Treatment of Youth with Type 1 Diabetes (T1D). *Endocr Pract* 2011, 1-17.

14. Dundar BN, Dundar N, Eren E: Comparison of the Efficacy and Safety of Insulin Glargine and Insulin Detemir with NPH Insulin in Children and Adolescents with Type 1 Diabetes Mellitus Receiving Intensive Insulin Therapy. *J Clin Res Ped Endo* 2009, 1(4):181-187.

15. Robertson KJ, Schoenle E, Gucev Z, Mordhorst L, Gall MA, Ludvigsson J: Insulin detemir compared with NPH insulin in children and adolescents with Type 1 diabetes. *Diabet Med* 2007, 24(1):27-34.

16. Braun D, Konrad D, Lang-Muritano M, Schoenle E: Improved glycemic control and lower frequency of severe hypoglycemia with insulin detemir; long-term experience in 105 children and adolescents with type 1 diabetes. *Pediatric Diabetes* 2008, 9(4 Pt 2):382-387.

17. Kurtoglu S, Atabek ME, Dizdarer C, Pirgon O, Isguven P, Emek S: Insulin detemir improves glycemic control and reduces hypoglycemia in children with type 1 diabetes: findings from the Turkish cohort of the PREDICTIVE observational study. *Pediatric Diabetes* 2009, 10(6):401-407.

18. Hermansen K, Madsbad S, Perrild H, Kristensen A, Axelsen M: Comparison of the soluble basal insulin analog insulin detemir with NPH insulin: a randomized open crossover trial in type 1 diabetic subjects on basal-bolus therapy. *Diabetes Care* 2001, 24(2):296-301.

19. Karges B, Kapellen T, Neu A, Hofer SE, Rohrer T, Rosenbauer J, Wolf J, Holl RW: Long-acting insulin analogs and the risk of diabetic ketoacidosis in children and adolescents with type 1 diabetes: a prospective study of 10, 682 patients from 271 institutions. *Diabetes Care* 2010, 33(5):1031-1033.

20. Nguyen TM, Renukuntla VS, Heptulla RA: Mixing insulin aspart with detemir does not affect glucose excursion in children with type 1 diabetes. *Diabetes Care* 2010, 33(8):1750-1752.

17

Effects of recombinant human growth hormone (rhGH) administration on body composition and cardiovascular risk factors in obese adolescent girls

Meghan Slattery[1*], Miriam A Bredella[2], Takara Stanley[3], Martin Torriani[2] and Madhusmita Misra[1,3]

Abstract

Background: Obesity is associated with a relative deficiency of growth hormone, which is predictive of greater visceral fat and markers of cardiovascular risk. The study's purpose was to use recombinant human growth hormone (rhGH) as a physiologic probe to assess the effects of reversing obesity-related GH deficiency on body composition, cardiovascular risk markers, and insulin resistance.

Methods: 22 obese girls 13–21 years old were followed for a randomized 6-month trial of rhGH vs. placebo/no treatment. At baseline and 6-months, DXA was performed for body composition, MRI to measure visceral, subcutaneous and total adipose tissue (VAT, SAT and TAT), and fasting blood drawn for IGF-1, inflammatory cardiovascular risk markers [soluble intercellular adhesion molecule (sICAM), high sensitivity CRP], lipids and HbA1C. An oral glucose tolerance test (OGTT) was performed. Twelve girls completed the 6-month visit. Baseline and mean 6-month change were compared between the groups using the Student t-test and the relationship between variables was determined through multiple regression analysis.

Results: After 6-months, the rhGH group maintained IGF-1 levels, and had decreases in total cholesterol (p = 0.03), sICAM-1 (p = 0.04) and HbA1C (p = 0.03) compared to placebo/no treatment. The rhGH group trended towards greater decreases in LDL and 2-hour OGTT glucose. Glucose tolerance did not worsen with rhGH administration.

Conclusions: Administering rhGH in small doses is able to stabilize IGF-1 levels in obesity. We have also shown that rhGH administration leads to an improvement in some markers of cardiovacular risk with without adversely affecting glucose tolerance.

Keywords: Adolescents, Growth hormone, Visceral fat, Body composition, Females, Inflammatory markers

Background

Obesity, a pressing global issue, is characterized by diminished growth hormone (GH) secretion in adults [1,2] and adolescents [3], with decreased frequency and amplitude of GH secretory bursts [4]. Pathological GH deficiency is characterized by a high risk cardiovascular profile [5-8], and similarly, in obese individuals, relatively low GH levels are associated with higher visceral fat [3], which in turn predisposes individuals to components of the metabolic syndrome [9,10], including hyperlipidemia [10,11] and insulin resistance [10,12]. While GH replacement in children with pathologic GH deficiency causes a decrease in visceral adiposity [13], effects of GH administration on body composition have not been examined in an otherwise healthy adolescent obese population that is relatively GH insufficient.

Existing studies examining the effects of rh(GH) on obesity and cardiovascular risk factors have largely been performed either on adults or in children with specific chronic health conditions such as GH deficiency [13] or Prader-Willi Syndrome [14]. Consequently, there is a dearth of data regarding effects of GH replacement on body composition and cardiometabolic risk in otherwise

* Correspondence: mslattery@mgh.harvard.edu
[1]Neuroendocrine Unit, Massachusetts General Hospital and Harvard Medical School, BUL 457B, Neuroendocrine Unit, 55 Fruit Street, MGH, Boston, MA 02114, USA
Full list of author information is available at the end of the article

healthy obese adolescents. This proof-of-concept study used rhGH as a physiologic probe to observe the effects of GH replacement on body composition. We hypothesized that rhGH administration in replacement doses to obese adolescent females would have lipolytic effects without deleterious effects on glucose tolerance.

Methods

The study was approved by the Institutional Review Board of Partners HealthCare system. Written informed consent (for patients ≥18 years) or parental consent with participant assent (for patients <18 years) was obtained from all.

Subject selection

Participants were recruited at Massachusetts General Hospital (MGH) between September 2010 and October 2012 through area pediatric and obesity clinics. Of 32 girls and young women 13–21 years old assessed for study eligibility, 22 obese adolescents met inclusion criteria and were randomized. Inclusion criteria comprised (i) a bone age ≥14 years, (ii) body mass index (BMI) > 95th percentile for age (based on the 2000 Centers for Disease Control and Prevention Growth Charts) [15], or >30 kg/m² if age >18 years, (iii) insulin like growth factor-1 (IGF-1) level below the median for pubertal stage or age, (iv) abdominal obesity with a waist to hip ratio (W/H) >0.85, and (v) stable weight (<5 kg change in weight in the prior 3 months). Exclusion criteria included diabetes mellitus, untreated thyroid dysfunction, chronic renal insufficiency, current or past malignancy, syndromic obesity, pregnancy, breast-feeding, and use of medications known to alter glucose metabolism or body composition (contraceptive pills, daily glucocorticoid use, metformin, sibutramine and Orlistat). Additionally, we excluded girls with new (<6 months) or unstable dosing (dosage change within 3-months) of antipsychotic medications known to cause weight gain. Baseline characteristics for a subset of study participants have been previously published [16].

Eleven subjects were randomized to active rhGH treatment {rhGH (+)} and 11 to rhGH negative {rhGH (–)} treatment. Sixteen subjects {10 rhGH (+) and 6 rhGH (–)} completed the 3-month visit, and 12 subjects {5 rhGH (+) and 7 rhGH (–)} finished the 6-month study period (one rhGH (–) subject missed the 3-month visit but completed other visits). No subject dropped out because of side effects. Of subjects who withdrew (n = 10), one chose to begin an oral contraceptive, 3 withdrew because of personal obligations, and the remaining were considered lost to follow-up (n = 6). Study participants who did or did not complete the study did not differ for baseline characteristics.

Experimental protocol

The study was a 6-month, single-blind, randomized trial, conducted at the Clinical Research Center of MGH. The screening visit included a history and physical examination and blood sampling to ensure participants met inclusion criteria and to rule out exclusion criteria. Diabetes was ruled out via an oral glucose tolerance test (OGTT). Eligible subjects returned for the baseline visit, visits at 1 and 2 weeks (for dose adjustment), and at 1, 3 and 6 months. Subjects were randomized 1:1 to receive once daily subcutaneous rhGH or placebo injections (Somatropin, Genentech, Inc., San Francisco, CA, USA), and taught to self inject medication daily for 6-months. Due to non-availability of placebo (and inability for new placebo to be manufactured) after June 2012, subjects subsequently randomized to placebo (n = 4) were instead randomized to no treatment. Dieticians and the radiologist who performed study related procedures as well as all subjects who enrolled prior to June 2012 (N = 15) remained blinded to randomization status for the entirety of the study. After the placebo expiration necessitated the change in the study design, one subject randomized to rhGH (+) subject and one subject randomized to rhGH (–) treatment dropped out. The subject randomized to rhGH (–) treatment withdrew due to the initiation of an oral contraceptive while the subject randomized to rhGH (+) was lost to follow up after the 3 month visit.

The starting rhGH dose was 0.4 mg and increased at week-1 and week-2 to 0.6 mg and 0.8 mg respectively. The dosing was based on a dose of 12.5 mcg/kg/day for a 16-year-old girl (mean for bone ages 14–18 years) weighing 67 kg (85th percentile for age) [17]. This dosage (0.8 mg at week-2) is at the lower end of the 12.5–25 mcg/kg/day dose used in studies of GH deficient adolescents transitioning from pediatric (40–45 mcg/kg/day) to adult (2–6 mcg/kg/day) replacement rhGH doses [17,18]. We opted for this lower dose as we expected lower GH requirements in this population that is relatively, rather than completely, GH insufficient. The dose was adjusted as needed by 20% at the 1 and 3-month visits to achieve IGF-1 levels in the upper half of the normal range for pubertal stage. When target IGF-1 was achieved, the individualized dose was continued.

Study procedures

Height was measured as the average of three measurements to the nearest 0.1 cm on a single calibrated wall-mounted stadiometer. Participants, wearing a hospital gown, were weighed to the nearest 0.1 kg on a single calibrated electronic scale. BMI was calculated as weight (in kg) divided by height (in meters²) and BMI standard deviation scores (SDS) determined from 2000 CDC charts [15]. Waist measurements were taken with a plastic tape measure to the nearest 0.1 cm at the level of the iliac crest and umbilicus;

the maximum hip circumference was measured. All measurements were taken at the end of expiration with the subject standing. Waist-to-hip ratio (W/H) was calculated as the iliac divided by the hip circumference measurement. An ophthalmoscope was used to rule out papilledema at study onset, and at the 3 and 6-month visits, or if any subject complained of headaches, vision changes, nausea or vomiting. Subjects had a left hand x-ray to assess bone age [19]. Pubertal stage was determined according to the criteria of Tanner [20].

Magnetic resonance imaging (MRI) at the level of L4 was used to determine visceral adipose tissue (VAT) and subcutaneous adipose tissue (SAT) at baseline and 6 months; total abdominal adipose tissue (TAT) was calculated as VAT + SAT [21]. MRI data are available for 11 completers (due to scheduling conflicts one no-treatment subject was unable to perform the MRI component). Body composition was also obtained by dual energy x-ray absorptiometry scans (DXA) at the baseline, 3 and 6-month visits. DXA (Hologic QDR-Discovery A; Hologic Inc., Waltham, MA software version APEX 3.3) was used to assess percent body fat, total, trunk and extremity fat and total and extremity lean mass.

Subjects met with nutritionists of the Clinical Research Center at the baseline, 3 and 6-month visits for (i) basic lifestyle counseling including healthy eating habits and optimizing exercise, and (ii) assessment of prior activity using the Modified Activity Questionnaire (MAQ) [22]. To avoid confounding variables, further dietary or exercise restrictions were not imposed.

Fasting blood samples were drawn for IGF-1 at each visit for rhGH dose adjustment, and a 75-g, 2-hour OGTT performed at screen, 3 and 6-months to determine whether rhGH administration had deleterious effects on glucose tolerance. Fasting blood samples were also assessed for cardiovascular risk markers [lipids, high sensitivity C-reactive protein (hs-CRP), soluble intercellular adhesion molecule-1 (sICAM-1)], HbA1C, glucose and insulin levels at baseline and 6-months.

IGF-1 was analyzed by enzyme-linked immunosorbent assay (ELISA) (Immunodiagnostic systems, Scottsdale, AZ; Limit of Detection (LOD) 3.1 ng/mL, CV < 7%). Fasting insulin was analyzed by immunoassay (Cobas, Roche Diagnostics, Indianapolis, IN; LOD 0.2 µU/mL, CV 0.8 to 4.9%), glucose via an enzymatic *in vitro* test (Cobas, Roche Diagnostics, Indianapolis, IN; LOD 2 mg/dL, intra-assay CV 1.0%), total cholesterol, LDL and HDL via a Roche direct assay (Cobas, Roche Diagnostics, Indianapolis, IN) [total cholesterol (LOD 3 mg/dL, CV 0.8–1.0%), LDL (LOD 3 mg/dL, intra-assay CV 0.71–1.22%) and HDL (LOD 3 mg/dL, intra-assay CV 0.60–0.95%)], triglycerides via the Roche triglyceride assay (Cobas, Roche Diagnostics, Indianapolis, IN; LOD 4 mg/dL, intra-assay CV 0.9–1.5%), and VLDL calculated by subtracting LDL

and HDL from total cholesterol. sICAM-1 was analyzed by ELISA (RnD Systems, Minneapolis, MN; minimum detectable concentration 1 ng/mL, CV < 8%), hsCRP via an immunoradiometric assay (IRMA) (LabCorp, Burlington, NC; LOD 0.3 mg/L, intra-assay CV < 10%). ALT was analyzed by the Architect assay (Abbott, Abbott Park, IL; LOD 2.0 U/L, intra-assay CV < 5.2%). Serum was stored at −80°C for insulin, ALT, and cardiovascular risk factors until analysis. Other samples were analyzed in real time.

Statistical methods

JMP Software (v10: SAS Institute, Inc., Cary, NC) was used for analysis. Results are reported as means ± SD.

Table 1 Baseline characteristics of all obese adolescent girls at study entry

	RhGH + N = 11	RhGH - N = 11	P
Age (years)	16.2 ± 2.6	16.9 ± 2.2	0.50
Bone age (years)	16.9 ± 1.2	17.2 ± 1.3	0.56
Weight (kg)	104.7 ± 24.8	97.4 ± 15.4	0.42
BMI (kg/m²)	40.4 ± 8.4	36.6 ± 6.4	0.25*
BMI SDS	2.3 ± 0.4	2.1 ± 0.4	0.22
Waist circumference (cm)	119.4 ± 17.1	115.0 ± 14.8	0.53
W/H ratio	0.95 ± 0.06	0.93 ± 0.08	0.62
SAT (cm²)	615.6 ± 175.0	580.0 ± 176.9 (N = 9)	0.66
VAT (cm²)	90.6 ± 35.3	87.1 ± 31.8 (N = 9)	0.82
TAT (cm²)	706.2 ± 203.5	667.2 ± 179.8 (N = 9)	0.66
Thigh subcutaneous fat (cm²)	224.2 ± 69.4	221.4 ± 96.3	0.95
Lean mass (grams)	54353 ± 9719	52276 ± 6842	0.57
IGF-1 (ng/mL)	250.6 ± 129.9	271.8 ± 73.1	0.64
2 HR glucose (OGTT) (mg/dL)	107.1 ± 20.5	114.0 ± 18.5	0.42
HbA1c (%)	5.78 ± 0.30	5.49 ± 0.30	**0.03**
Insulin uU/mL	26.4 ± 21.3	40.1 ± 37.2	0.29*
Total cholesterol (mg/dL)	167.6 ± 38.3	156.0 ± 33.5	0.46
LDL (mg/dL)	103.8 ± 28.8	92.6 ± 30.1	0.33*
HDL (mg/dL)	45.1 ± 9.4	43.3 ± 8.5	0.64
VLDL (mg/dL)	18.6 ± 9.4	20.1 ± 8.0	0.70
Triglycerides (mg/dL)	93.0 ± 47.0	100.6 ± 39.8	0.69
hsCRP (mg/L)	4.47 ± 2.76	3.41 ± 3.29	0.25*
sICAM-1 (ng/mL)	268.7 ± 72.5	220.9 ± 56.4	0.10

*P value reported for log transformed values.
RhGH+: Group that received rhGH; RhGH-: Group that received placebo/no treatment.
Abbreviations: BMI body mass index, BMI SDS body mass index standard deviation score, HbA1c hemoglobin A1c, HDL high density lipoprotein, hsCRP high sensitivity C-reactive protein, IGF-1 insulin like growth factor-1, LDL low density lipoprotein, OGTT oral glucose tolerance test, SAT subcutaneous adipose tissue, sICAM-1 soluble intercellular adhesion molecule 1, TAT, VAT total, visceral adipose tissue, VLDL very low density lipoprotein, W/H waist to hip ratio.

Baseline and mean 6-month change were compared using the Student *t*-test or Wilcoxon rank sum test depending on data distribution. A paired *t*-test was also used to compare baseline and 6 month values within groups. Parametric (Pearson) or nonparametric (Spearman) correlations were used as appropriate to determine associations between variables that were or were not normally distributed. Significance was defined as a two-tailed p-value of <0.05. Multivariate regression models were constructed to determine whether significances for changes in endpoints persisted after controlling for weight changes or baseline values of the endpoint (i.e. HbA1c).

Results

Baseline characteristics

Baseline characteristics are summarized in Table 1. Study participants had a mean age of 16.6 ± 2.4 years, mean

weight of 100.1 ± 20.5 kg, and a mean BMI of 38.5 ± 7.5 kg/m². Treatment groups did not differ for baseline characteristics except for a slightly lower HbA1C in the rhGH (–) group. There were no significant baseline differences noted between the blinded (N = 15) and unblinded (N = 7) groups with one exception; the W/H ratio was higher in the group who remained blinded to their treatment allocation (0.96 ± 0.06 vs. 0.90 ± 0.07, p = 0.05). All subjects were Tanner Stage V for breast development at the baseline visit.

Six-month changes in nutritional measures

No differences were noted between rhGH(+) and rhGH(–) groups for changes in calories consumed (142.6 ± 961.0 vs. 193.5 ± 644.0 kcal, p = 0.93), percentage of calories from fat (–8.09 ± 12.04 vs. 0.09 ± 12.95%, p = 0.36), or activity levels (1.64 ± 6.4 vs. 8.83 ± 9.48 hours/week, p = 0.18).

Table 2 Baseline, 6-month and change in body composition and biochemical parameters over 6-months for study completers

	RhGH +			RhGH -			
	Baseline	6-month N = 5	6-month delta	Baseline	6-month N = 7	6-month delta	6 month delta P
Weight (kg)	99.9 ± 29.5	100.6 ± 30.9	0.7 ± 4.3	96.5 ± 18.1	100.4 ± 23.1	3.9 ± 6.6	0.81*
BMI (kg/m²)	39.6 ± 10.2	39.8 ± 10.8	0.2 ± 2.0	36.4 ± 7.3	37.8 ± 9.6	1.4 ± 2.5	0.81*
Waist circumference (cm)	115.4 ± 21.7	113.7 ± 23.1	–1.7 ± 4.0	112.4 ± 17.0	112.5 ± 21.2	0.1 ± 6.5	0.60
W/H ratio	0.94 ± 0.06	0.95 ± 0.06	0.003 ± 0.03	0.91 ± 0.08	0.91 ± 0.08	–0.005 ± 0.04	0.72
SAT (cm²)	578.5 ± 234.8	577.4 ± 232.9	–1.1 ± 60.8	570.0 ± 206.4	606.3 ± 231.1	36.3 ± 51.6 (N = 6)	0.30
VAT (cm²)	92.7 ± 36.6	93.3 ± 47.3	0.6 ± 29.9	90.4 ± 39.6	98.4 ± 43.5	8.0 ± 31.9 (N = 6)	0.70
TAT (cm²)	671.3 ± 264.1	670.7 ± 278.9	–0.5 ± 83.3	660.3 ± 209.1	704.6 ± 234.5	44.3 ± 63.1 (N = 6)	0.34
Thigh subcutaneous fat (cm²)	217.7 ± 72.1	208.7 ± 73.1	–9.0 ± 16.0	228.5 ± 103.4	211.2 ± 72.7	18.6 ± 29.0 (N = 6)	0.08*
Lean mass (grams)	50741.3 ± 7963.2	50758.1 ± 8735.6	17 ± 2160	50659.5 ± 7149.8	51360.7 ± 7309.6	701 ± 2325	0.62
IGF-1 (ng/mL)	235.4 ± 61.9	234.0 ± 48.5	–1.4 ± 79.4	266.0 ± 83.6	185.9 ± 58.0	–80.1 ± 48.8	0.06
2 HR-glucose (OGTT) (mg/dL)	119.8 ± 14.8	113.2 ± 17.6	–6.6 ± 17.0	112.7 ± 14.2	135.1 ± 23.7	22.4 ± 28.8	0.07
HbA1c (%)	5.62 ± 0.30	5.58 ± 0.16	–0.04 ± 0.17	5.47 ± 0.25	5.61 ± 0.30	0.14 ± 0.08	**0.03**
Insulin uU/mL	25.4 ± 25.7	22.6 ± 17.8	–2.8 ± 11.7	41.9 ± 41.0	27.1 ± 22.5	–14.8 ± 38.3	0.94*
Total cholesterol (mg/dL)	189.2 ± 42.6	151.4 ± 27.8	–37.8 ± 23.9	162.1 ± 39.7	153.6 ± 34.8	–8.6 ± 15.5	**0.03**
LDL (mg/dL)	121.2 ± 27.7	95.4 ± 22.4	–25.8 ± 12.8	98.3 ± 35.8	87.6 ± 28.0	–10.7 ± 11.9	0.06
HDL (mg/dL)	48.2 ± 13.4	41.6 ± 8.2	–6.6 ± 6.1	44.0 ± 7.4	45.0 ± 5.2	1.0 ± 5.1	**0.04**
VLDL (mg/dL)	19.8 ± 11.2	14.4 ± 6.0	–5.4 ± 9.6	19.9 ± 7.0	21.0 ± 16.3	1.1 ± 11.7	0.48*
Triglycerides (mg/dL)	99.4 ± 55.7	71.6 ± 29.5	–27.8 ± 46.8	99.1 ± 35.5	105.3 ± 24.9	6.1 ± 58.4	0.57*
hsCRP (mg/L)	3.5 ± 2.1	2.69 ± 1.8	–0.77 ± 2.36	4.4 ± 3.8	4.27 ± 4.6	–0.09 ± 1.79	0.58
sICAM-1 (ng/mL)	226.4 ± 79.3	204.2 ± 74.5	–22.2 ± 30.3	241.1 ± 48.1	262.2 ± 74.8	21.1 ± 33.3	**0.04**

*Wilcoxon rank sum test.
HbA1c, Total Cholesterol, HDL and sICAM were lower after 6 months of rhGH + treatment.
RhGH+: Group that received rhGH; RhGH-: Group that received placebo/no treatment.
Baseline: Mean Baseline values only for study completers.
6-month: Mean 6-month values for study completers.
6-month delta: Change over 6-months from Mean Baseline to Mean 6-month values.
Abbreviations: BMI body mass index, BMI SDS body mass index standard deviation score, HbA1c hemoglobin A1c, HDL high density lipoprotein, hsCRP high sensitivity C-reactive protein, IGF-1 insulin like growth factor-1, LDL low density lipoprotein, OGTT oral glucose tolerance test, SAT subcutaneous adipose tissue, sICAM-1 soluble intercellular adhesion molecule 1, TAT, VAT total, visceral adipose tissue, VLDL very low density lipoprotein, W/H waist to hip ratio.

Six-month changes in IGF-1 levels

Changes in IGF-1 trended higher in the treatment group (Table 2). At the 6-month visit, mean IGF-1 in the rhGH (+) group was non-significantly higher than in the rhGH (−) group (234 ± 24.3 vs. 185.6 ± 20.5 ng/mL, p = 0.16).

Six-month changes in body composition

Body composition changes across treatment groups are presented in Table 2. Although changes in waist circumference and W/H ratio did not differ across groups over the study duration, the increase in IGF-1 between 3–6 months correlated with the decrease in W/H ratio over 6-months (r = −0.74 p = 0.009). A similar finding was also seen in the negative correlation between change in IGF-1 over 3-months and change in body fat percentage over 3-months (r = −0.65 p = 0.009) (Figure 1). SAT and TAT decreased non-significantly in the treatment group compared to an increase in the control group, and VAT showed a negligible increase compared to the control group.

Six-month changes in cardiovascular risk markers
Lipid levels

At 6-months, subjects in the active group had significant reductions in total cholesterol compared with controls (Table 2), and trended to have greater reductions in LDL. The treatment group also had a greater decrease in HDL compared with controls. Six-month changes in IGF-1 correlated negatively with changes in total cholesterol (r = −0.60, p = 0.04) (Figure 2), VLDL (Spearman rho = −0.58, p = 0.05), and triglycerides (Spearman rho = −0.67, p = 0.02) but not HDL (r = −0.37, p = 0.24).

Markers of inflammation

Subjects in the treatment group had a significant decrease in sICAM-1 (a marker of inflammation) compared to an

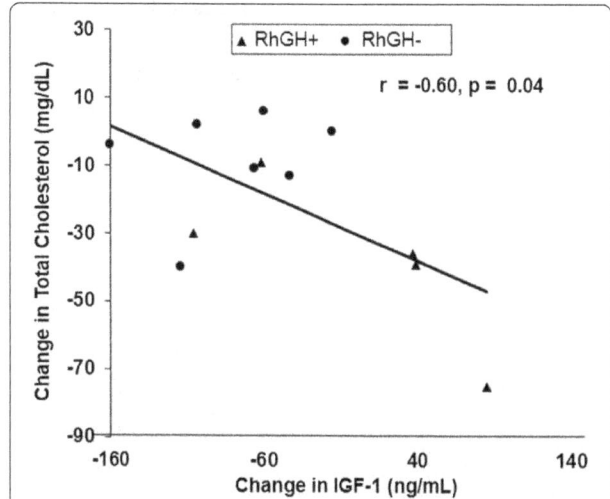

Figure 2 Correlation of 6-month change in IGF-1 with 6-month change in total cholesterol for all subjects. 6-month increase in IGF-1 was associated with the 6-month decrease in total cholesterol.

increase in controls (Table 2 and Figure 3). Mean changes in hsCRP did not differ across groups. Additionally, there was a trend for GH to decrease ALT, a marker of liver inflammation, (−5 ± 5 vs. 3 ± 11 U/L, p = 0.18 for a 2-tailed test and 0.0478 for a one-tailed test).

Six-month changes in glycemic status

At 6-months, subjects in the active group had significant reductions in HbA1c compared to controls (Table 2). This reduction trended to remain significant after controlling for baseline HbA1C (p = 0.06). Subjects in the active group also trended to have greater reductions in 2-hour glucose levels on the OGTT (Table 2). No difference was noted between the groups for 6-month changes in insulin

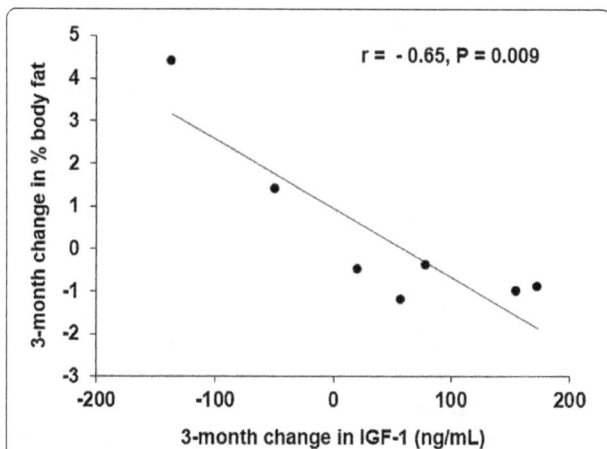

Figure 1 Correlation between 3-month changes in IGF-1 and body fat percentage within the rhGH treated group. 3-month increase in IGF-1 was associated with the 3-month decrease in % body fat.

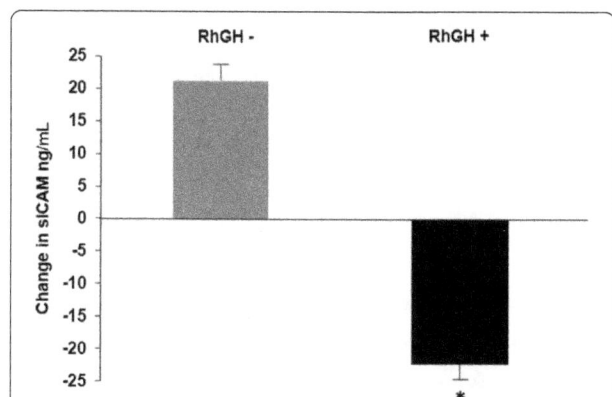

Figure 3 Change in soluble intercellular adhesion molecule-1 (sICAM) levels in obese adolescent females. Change in sICAM levels in obese adolescent females after 6 months of recombinant human growth hormone therapy (rhGH +) (black bar) or placebo/no treatment (rhGH −) (gray bar).

Table 3 Adverse events in treated obese girls (rhGH+) and untreated obese girls (rhGH -)

Event type	Total number of adverse events	Adverse events	
		RhGH + (N)	RhGH - (N)
Serious adverse events	-	-	-
Non-serious adverse events			
Hyperglycemia related events			
IGT at 3 or 6-month (OGTT)	6	2	4
Polyuria/Polydipsia	4	3	1
HbA1c > 6.4%	1	1	-
Symptoms that may relate to raised ICP			
Headache	7	4	3
Nausea with vomiting	1	1	-
Nausea without vomiting	3	3	-
Dizziness without headache	1	-	1
Blurry vision	1	1	-
Arthralgias/Fluid retention related events			
Arthralgia	2	2	-
Back pain	5	4	1
Myalgia	1	1	-
Edema	-	-	-
Menstrual cycle related events			
Change in menstrual Flow	5	3	2
Injection related events			
Bruising/Irritation at injection site	4	2	2
Bruising/Irritation at blood sampling site	1	1	-
Others			
Hypertension	1	-	1
Lightheadedness	-	-	-
ED visit for wheezing with URI	1	-	1
Abdominal pain	2	2	-
Upper respiratory Infection	1	1	-

Table 3 Adverse events in treated obese girls (rhGH+) and untreated obese girls (rhGH -) *(Continued)*

Nasal congestion (with URI)	1	1	-
Fatigue	2	-	2
Eczema	1	-	1

RhGH+: Group that received rhGH; RhGH-: Group that received placebo/no treatment.
Abbreviations: *ED* emergency department, *ICP* intracranial pressure, *IGT* impaired glucose tolerance, *OGTT* oral glucose tolerance test, *URI* upper respiratory infection.
There were no significant differences across the two groups for the various adverse events.

levels. Thus, we did not see the anticipated deleterious effects of rhGH on glucose tolerance.

Adverse events over the 6-month study duration

Adverse events are presented in Table 3. There were no serious adverse events related to study participation. rhGH was well tolerated and no subject required a dose reduction. No subject who complained of headaches, nausea or vomiting had a history or physical exam findings suggestive of pseudotumor cerebri.

Discussion

We have shown that administering rhGH to female adolescents in physiologic doses is able to stabilize IGF-1 in obesity, a state characterized by relative GH insufficiency, without adversely affecting glucose tolerance. We also confirmed the lipolytic effects of endogenous rhGH, administered for the first time to otherwise healthy obese adolescent females, resulting in a decrease in total cholesterol; additionally, we saw a reduction in sICAM-1 as opposed to an increase in sICAM-1 levels in the non-intervention group. Our group has previously reported a relative state of GH insufficiency in obese adolescent girls compared with controls, and that lower GH levels strongly predict higher visceral fat, an important determinant of insulin resistance and hyperlipidemia [3]. Although GH replacement causes a decrease in visceral adiposity in GH deficient children [13], effects of GH administration on body composition and cardiometabolic risk have not been previously examined in a healthy adolescent obese population.

Despite small increases in IGF-1, the dose of rhGH used in our study achieved significant reductions in total cholesterol and sICAM-1. It is thus possible that observed changes represent direct lipolytic effects of GH and direct effects of GH on inflammatory markers, rather than IGF-1 mediated effects. However, we did observe significant inverse associations between 6-month changes in IGF-1 levels and 6-month changes in total cholesterol, triglycerides, and VLDL. Although we observed a decrease in HDL levels in the active arm, no correlation was found between changes in IGF-1 levels and changes in HDL over the 6-month study period.

Of note, by the end of puberty, the increase in insulin resistance that is characteristic of puberty resolves, and returns to prepubertal levels [23]. All subjects in our study were fully pubertal at the start of the study, thus any puberty related variations in insulin resistance parameters were minimized. We speculate that the decrease in sICAM levels in the active arm compared with the increase in the non-treatment arm may represent reduced inflammation in the active arm, compared to a persistent (and potentially worsening) pro-inflammatory state in the non-treatment arm. This may account for the maintenance of HbA1C levels in the intervention group, as opposed to the increase in HbA1C observed over 6 months in the non-intervention group. Given that rhGH studies in adults have found that even at low doses, GH treatment corresponds with elevated glucose and insulin levels [5], adolescence may potentially offer a time period when rhGH replacement (in doses used in this study) will not worsen glucose tolerance.

Given the known inverse associations of GH levels with VAT and hsCRP in obesity, [3,24,25] we expected to see a reduction in VAT content and in hsCRP levels following rhGH administration. However, contrary to our expectations, neither of these parameters decreased, and it is possible that higher doses of rhGH than achieved in this study are necessary to observe such an effect. Following rhGH administration, although the mean IGF-1 level attained in the active arm was higher than in the control arm, this was not statistically significant, and mean levels remained in the lower half of the normal range despite dose titration. Thus, a state of relative GH insufficiency persisted. It is unclear why IGF-1 decreased in the control group. Although variation within the IGF-1 range is an expected finding, it is also possible that the non-significant weight gain in the control group over 6 months contributed to a decrease in GH, and therefore, IGF-1 secretion [3,24,25].

We did observe inverse associations of changes in IGF-1 with changes in the waist/hip ratio, considered to be an excellent surrogate for VAT, which also suggests that a higher dosage of rhGH may have caused improvements in body composition and biochemical parameters overall. The fact that glucose tolerance did not deteriorate in the active arm may also be attributable to the low dosage of rhGH used in the active arm [24,26]. Further studies are necessary based on data from this proof-of-concept study to determine the most appropriate dose of rhGH to improve body composition and cardiometabolic risk markers in obese adolescent girls without significantly worsening insulin resistance.

Limitations of this study include the small sample size and relatively high drop-out rate (common in studies with obese subjects) [27-29]. However, a significant

strength was that we observed changes in lipids and an inflammatory marker despite the small sample size and low GH dose. Many previous studies examining the relationship between IGF-1 and body composition limited their findings to BMI [30,31] and previous prospective rhGH treatment studies focused on obese adults [2,24,25]. The remaining studies that either prospectively or retrospectively analyzed the effects of rhGH on body composition in the pediatric population involved children with Prader-Willi syndrome or GH deficiency [13,14,32]. This current study is the first to examine the effects of rhGH on otherwise healthy obese adolescents.

Conclusions

In conclusion, we have demonstrated that low rhGH doses are easily tolerated with minimal side effects and are able to stabilize IGF-1 levels in obese adolescent girls. Our study confirms the lipolytic effects of growth hormone and suggests that rhGH replacement in viscerally obese adolescent females reduces total cholesterol and sICAM without adversely affecting glycemic status. Further studies are necessary to confirm these findings, and to also better understand the potential clinical role of rhGH as a treatment for obese adolescent girls.

Abbreviations
BMI: Body mass index; CV: Coefficient of variation; DXA: Dual energy x-ray absorptiometry scan; ELISA: Enzyme-linked immunosorbent assay; FAI: Free androgen index; GH: Growth hormone; HbA1c: Hemoglobin A1c; HDL: High density lipoprotein; HOMA-IR: Homeostasis model assessment of insulin resistance; hs-CRP: High-sensitivity C-reactive protein; IGF-1: Insulin-like growth factor 1; IRMA: Immunoradiometric assay; LDL: Low density lipoprotein; LOD: Limit of detection; MAQ: Modified activity questionnaire; MGH: Massachusetts General Hospital; MRI: Magnetic resonance imaging; OGTT: Oral glucose tolerance test; (rh)GH: Recombinant human growth hormone; SAT: Subcutaneous abdominal adipose tissue; SD: Standard deviation; SDS: Standard deviation score; SHBG: Sex hormone binding globulin; sICAM-1: Soluble intercellular adhesion molecule-1; TAT/VAT: Total/visceral abdominal adipose tissue; VLDL: Very low density lipoprotein; W/H: Waist to hip ratio.

Competing interests
The authors state that no competing financial interests exist. This study was funded by an investigator initiated grant (L4716N) from Genentech, San Francisco, CA (with no influence on data collection/analysis). Dr. Misra received support from NIH grants UL1 RR025758 and K24 HD071843-01A1.

Authors' contributions
MM conceived the study; MB, MS and MM carried out study related procedures and performed data collection; MS, MB, MT, TS, and MM analyzed and interpreted data; MS performed the literature search; MS, MB, TS, and MM wrote the manuscript and generated figures; MM had primary responsibility for final content. All authors were involved in manuscript preparation and approved the submitted version.

Acknowledgements
We thank the nursing and bionutrition staff of the MGH Clinical Research Center for their patient care. We also thank the Harvard Clinical and Translational Science Center for the performance of the assays. This study is registered with clinicaltrials.gov, no.: NCT01169103.

Author details
[1]Neuroendocrine Unit, Massachusetts General Hospital and Harvard Medical School, BUL 457B, Neuroendocrine Unit, 55 Fruit Street, MGH, Boston, MA

02114, USA. [2]Department of Radiology, Massachusetts General Hospital and Harvard Medical School, Boston, MA 02114, USA. [3]Pediatric Endocrine Unit, Massachusetts General Hospital for Children and Harvard Medical School, Boston, MA 02114, USA.

References

1. Scacchi M, Pincelli AI, Cavagnini F: Growth hormone in obesity. *Int J Obes Relat Metab Disord* 1999, **23**:260–271.
2. Franco C, Brandberg J, Lonn L, Andersson B, Bengtsson BA, Johannsson G: Growth hormone treatment reduces abdominal visceral fat in postmenopausal women with abdominal obesity: a 12-month placebo-controlled trial. *J Clin Endocrinol Metab* 2005, **90**:1466–1474.
3. Misra M, Bredella MA, Tsai P, Mendes N, Miller KK, Klibanski A: Lower growth hormone and higher cortisol are associated with greater visceral adiposity, intramyocellular lipids, and insulin resistance in overweight girls. *Am J Physiol Endocrinol Metab* 2008, **295**:E385–E392.
4. Kreitschmann-Andermahr I, Suarez P, Jennings R, Evers N, Brabant G: GH/IGF-I regulation in obesity–mechanisms and practical consequences in children and adults. *Horm Res Paediatr* 2010, **73**:153–160.
5. Maison P, Griffin S, Nicoue-Beglah M, Haddad N, Balkau B, Chanson P, Metaanalysis of Blinded RP-CT: Impact of growth hormone (GH) treatment on cardiovascular risk factors in GH-deficient adults: a metaanalysis of blinded, randomized, placebo-controlled trials. *J Clin Endocrinol Metab* 2004, **89**:2192–2199.
6. Rosen T, Bengtsson BA: Premature mortality due to cardiovascular disease in hypopituitarism. *Lancet* 1990, **336**:285–288.
7. Bates AS, Van't Hoff W, Jones PJ, Clayton RN: The effect of hypopituitarism on life expectancy. *J Clin Endocrinol Metab* 1996, **81**:1169–1172.
8. Miller KK, Biller BM, Lipman JG, Bradwin G, Rifai N, Klibanski A: Truncal adiposity, relative growth hormone deficiency, and cardiovascular risk. *J Clin Endocrinol Metab* 2005, **90**:768–774.
9. Demerath EW, Reed D, Rogers N, Sun SS, Lee M, Choh AC, Couch W, Czerwinski SA, Chumlea WC, Siervogel RM, Towne B: Visceral adiposity and its anatomical distribution as predictors of the metabolic syndrome and cardiometabolic risk factor levels. *Am J Clin Nutr* 2008, **88**:1263–1271.
10. Syme C, Abrahamowicz M, Leonard GT, Perron M, Pitiot A, Qiu X, Richer L, Totman J, Veillette S, Xiao Y, Gaudet D, Paus T, Pausova Z: Intra-abdominal adiposity and individual components of the metabolic syndrome in adolescence: sex differences and underlying mechanisms. *Arch Pediatr Adolesc Med* 2008, **162**:453–461.
11. Owens S, Gutin B, Ferguson M, Allison J, Karp W, Le NA: Visceral adipose tissue and cardiovascular risk factors in obese children. *J Pediatr* 1998, **133**:41–45.
12. Weiss R, Dufour S, Taksali SE, Tamborlane WV, Petersen KF, Bonadonna RC, Boselli L, Barbetta G, Allen K, Rife F, Savoye M, Dziura J, Sherwin R, Shulman GI, Caprio S: Prediabetes in obese youth: a syndrome of impaired glucose tolerance, severe insulin resistance, and altered myocellular and abdominal fat partitioning. *Lancet* 2003, **362**:951–957.
13. Roemmich JN, Huerta MG, Sundaresan SM, Rogol AD: Alterations in body composition and fat distribution in growth hormone-deficient prepubertal children during growth hormone therapy. *Metabolism* 2001, **50**:537–547.
14. Carrel AL, Myers SE, Whitman BY, Allen DB: Benefits of long-term GH therapy in Prader-Willi syndrome: a 4-year study. *J Clin Endocrinol Metab* 2002, **87**:1581–1585.
15. Kuczmarski RJ, Ogden CL, Grummer-Strawn LM, Flegal KM, Guo SS, Wei R, Mei Z, Curtin LR, Roche AF, Johnson CL: CDC growth charts: United States. *Adv Data* 2000, **314**:1–27.
16. Slattery MJ, Bredella MA, Thakur H, Torriani M, Misra M: Insulin resistance and impaired mitochondrial function in obese adolescent girls. *Metab Syndr Relat Disord* 2014, **12**:56–61.
17. Attanasio AF, Shavrikova E, Blum WF, Cromer M, Child CJ, Paskova M, Lebl J, Chipman JJ, Shalet SM: Continued growth hormone (GH) treatment after final height is necessary to complete somatic development in childhood-onset GH-deficient patients. *J Clin Endocrinol Metab* 2004, **89**:4857–4862.
18. Mauras N, Pescovitz OH, Allada V, Messig M, Wajnrajch MP, Lippe B: Limited efficacy of growth hormone (GH) during transition of GH-deficient patients

from adolescence to adulthood: a phase III multicenter, double-blind, randomized two-year trial. *J Clin Endocrinol Metab* 2005, **90**:3946–3955.
19. Greulich WW, Pyle SI: *Radiographic Atlas of Skeletal Development of the Hand and Wrist*. 2nd edition. Stanford, Calif: Stanford University Press; 1959.
20. Tanner JM: *Growth at Adolescence*. 2nd edition. Springfield, Ill: Thomas; 1962.
21. Bredella MA, Fazeli PK, Miller KK, Misra M, Torriani M, Thomas BJ, Ghomi RH, Rosen CJ, Klibanski A: Increased bone marrow fat in anorexia nervosa. *J Clin Endocrinol Metab* 2009, **94**:2129–2136.
22. Aaron DJ, Kriska AM, Dearwater SR, Cauley JA, Metz KF, LaPorte RE: Reproducibility and validity of an epidemiologic questionnaire to assess past year physical activity in adolescents. *Am J Epidemiol* 1995, **142**:191–201.
23. Moran A, Jacobs DR Jr, Steinberger J, Hong CP, Prineas R, Luepker R, Sinaiko AR: Insulin resistance during puberty: results from clamp studies in 357 children. *Diabetes* 1999, **48**:2039–2044.
24. Bredella MA, Lin E, Brick DJ, Gerweck AV, Harrington LM, Torriani M, Thomas BJ, Schoenfeld DA, Breggia A, Rosen CJ, Hemphill LC, Wu Z, Rifai N, Utz AL, Miller KK: Effects of GH in women with abdominal adiposity: a 6-month randomized, double-blind, placebo-controlled trial. *Eur J Endocrinol* 2012, **166**:601–611.
25. Bredella MA, Gerweck AV, Lin E, Landa MG, Torriani M, Schoenfeld DA, Hemphill LC, Miller KK: Effects of GH on body composition and cardiovascular risk markers in young men with abdominal obesity. *J Clin Endocrinol Metab* 2013, **98**:3864–3872.
26. Carroll PV, Christ ER, Bengtsson BA, Carlsson L, Christiansen JS, Clemmons D, Hintz R, Ho K, Laron Z, Sizonenko P, Sönksen PH, Tanaka T, Thorne M: Growth hormone deficiency in adulthood and the effects of growth hormone replacement: a review. Growth Hormone Research Society Scientific Committee. *J Clin Endocrinol Metab* 1998, **83**:382–395.
27. Fidler MC, Sanchez M, Raether B, Weissman NJ, Smith SR, Shanahan WR, Anderson CM: A one-year randomized trial of lorcaserin for weight loss in obese and overweight adults: the BLOSSOM trial. *J Clin Endocrinol Metab* 2011, **96**:3067–3077.
28. Chanoine JP, Hampl S, Jensen C, Boldrin M, Hauptman J: Effect of orlistat on weight and body composition in obese adolescents: a randomized controlled trial. *JAMA* 2005, **293**:2873–2883.
29. Foster GD, Wyatt HR, Hill JO, McGuckin BG, Brill C, Mohammed BS, Szapary PO, Rader DJ, Edman JS, Klein S: A randomized trial of a low-carbohydrate diet for obesity. *N Engl J Med* 2003, **348**:2082–2090.
30. Gram IT, Norat T, Rinaldi S, Dossus L, Lukanova A, Téhard B, Clavel-Chapelon F, van Gils CH, van Noord PA, Peeters PH, Bueno-de-Mesquita HB, Nagel G, Linseisen J, Lahmann PH, Boeing H, Palli D, Sacerdote C, Panico S, Tumino R, Sieri S, Dorronsoro M, Quirós JR, Navarro CA, Barricarte A, Tormo MJ, González CA, Overvad K, Paaske Johnsen S, Olsen A, Tiønneland A, *et al*: Body mass index, waist circumference and waist-hip ratio and serum levels of IGF-I and IGFBP-3 in European women. *Int J Obes (Lond)* 2006, **30**:1623–1631.
31. Henderson KD, Goran MI, Kolonel LN, Henderson BE, Le Marchand L: Ethnic disparity in the relationship between obesity and plasma insulin-like growth factors: the multiethnic cohort. *Cancer Epidemiol Biomarkers Prev* 2006, **15**:2298–2302.
32. Fillion M, Deal C, Van Vliet G: Retrospective study of the potential benefits and adverse events during growth hormone treatment in children with Prader-Willi syndrome. *J Pediatr* 2009, **154**:230–233.

18

Congenital hypothyroidism: insights into pathogenesis and treatment

Christine E. Cherella and Ari J. Wassner*

Abstract

Congenital hypothyroidism occurs in approximately 1 in 2000 newborns and can have devastating neurodevelopmental consequences if not detected and treated promptly. While newborn screening has virtually eradicated intellectual disability due to severe congenital hypothyroidism in the developed world, more stringent screening strategies have resulted in increased detection of mild congenital hypothyroidism. Recent studies provide conflicting evidence about the potential neurodevelopmental risks posed by mild congenital hypothyroidism, highlighting the need for additional research to further define what risks these patients face and whether they are likely to benefit from treatment. Moreover, while the apparent incidence of congenital hypothyroidism has increased in recent decades, the underlying cause remains obscure in most cases. However, ongoing research into genetic causes of congenital hypothyroidism continues to shed new light on the development and physiology of the hypothalamic-pituitary-thyroid axis. The identification of *IGSF1* as a cause of central congenital hypothyroidism has uncovered potential new regulatory pathways in both pituitary thyrotropes and gonadotropes, while mounting evidence suggests that a significant proportion of primary congenital hypothyroidism may be caused by combinations of rare genetic variants in multiple genes involved in thyroid development and function. Much remains to be learned about the origins of this common disorder and about the optimal management of less severely-affected infants.

Keywords: Congenital hypothyroidism, Genetics, Central hypothyroidism, Mild hypothyroidism

Background

Thyroid hormone is essential for normal growth and neurologic development, particularly in the first few years of life, and hypothyroidism during this period is a leading cause of preventable intellectual disability worldwide. The implementation of universal newborn screening beginning in the 1970's has been an enormous public health success, virtually eradicating significant intellectual disability due to severe congenital hypothyroidism in the developed world. Following this early success, newborn screening programs have implemented increasingly stringent screening strategies over the past few decades. The resulting detection of milder cases of congenital hypothyroidism is the primary reason for the dramatic increase in the apparent incidence of congenital hypothyroidism from 1:4000 to 1:2000 newborns over the last 20–30 years [1–6]. However, unlike severe congenital hypothyroidism, for which the benefits of early

detection and treatment are indisputable, uncertainty remains about mild disease in terms of the neurodevelopmental risk it poses and whether these risks are mitigated by treatment [7]. Moreover, despite the prevalence of congenital hypothyroidism and our success in treating it, what causes most cases remains a mystery. This review discusses important recent developments in congenital hypothyroidism, focusing on our evolving understanding of its genetics, pathophysiology, and outcomes.

Primary congenital hypothyroidism

Most congenital hypothyroidism is caused by defects in the thyroid gland itself (primary hypothyroidism). Causes of primary congenital hypothyroidism can be broadly classified as failure of the thyroid gland to develop normally (*dysgenesis*) or failure of a structurally normal thyroid gland to produce normal quantities of thyroid hormone (*dyshormonogenesis*). Thyroid dysgenesis—which encompasses the spectrum of thyroid agenesis, hypoplasia, and ectopy—is the most common cause of congenital

* Correspondence: ari.wassner@childrens.harvard.edu
Division of Endocrinology, Boston Children's Hospital, Harvard Medical School, 300 Longwood Avenue, Boston, MA 02115, USA

hypothyroidism, and its incidence (about 1:4000 infants) has not changed significantly over the last several decades [3, 5, 6]. The underlying cause of thyroid dysgenesis, however, remains obscure in the vast majority of cases. Thyroid dysgenesis usually occurs sporadically, with only 2–5% of cases being attributable to identifiable genetic mutations (Fig. 1). Nevertheless, the known genetic causes of thyroid dysgenesis provide an important window into basic thyroid ontogeny. The thyroid-stimulating hormone receptor (TSHR) and the transcription factors PAX8, NKX2–1, and FOXE1 are all expressed in the developing thyroid, and disruption of any of these genes can lead to failure of normal thyroid gland formation [8]. These transcription factors also play important roles in other developing tissues, and mutations in each may be associated with additional syndromic features such as renal abnormalities (PAX8), interstitial lung disease and chorea (NKX2–1), or cleft palate, bifid epiglottis, choanal atresia, and spiky hair (FOXE1) (Table 1).

Several other genes implicated in thyroid dysgenesis offer additional insights into the mechanisms of thyroid development. The transcription factor NKX2–5 is expressed in the developing heart and thyroid, and NKX2–5 mutations are associated with congenital cardiac abnormalities. Deletion of NKX2–5 in mice causes thyroid agenesis, suggesting that this transcription factor plays an important role in thyroid development, but to what degree this finding extends to humans is not clear. Heterozygous variants in NKX2–5 are found in some individuals with thyroid dysgenesis [9, 10]; however, the pathogenicity of these variants is unclear since they do not consistently cosegregate with thyroid disease in families [9] and some may not impair protein function in vitro [11]. Therefore, the precise role of NKX2–5 in thyroid dysgenesis remains to be clarified [8].

Mutations in GLIS3 underlie a complex syndrome of congenital hypothyroidism, neonatal diabetes mellitus, and variable other abnormalities including congenital glaucoma, developmental delay, hepatic fibrosis, and polycystic kidneys [12, 13]. GLIS3 is highly expressed in the thyroid, and congenital hypothyroidism in patients with GLIS3 mutations may be associated with either thyroid dysgenesis or a eutopic but histologically abnormal thyroid gland [13]. GLIS3 may act as a transcriptional activator or repressor, but its precise role in thyroid development and function remains to be determined. Some patients with GLIS3 mutations require unusually high doses of levothyroxine to normalize serum thyroid stimulating hormone (TSH) levels [13, 14], which could imply an additional effect of GLIS3 on central regulation of the hypothalamic-pituitary-thyroid (HPT) axis.

Recently, genetic variants in CDCA8 (also called BOREALIN) were identified in a study of three consanguineous families with thyroid dysgenesis [15]. This gene is expressed in the thyroid and is known to play a key role in the chromosomal passenger complex that stabilizes the mitotic spindle during cell division. Interestingly, however, the CDCA8 variants detected in these patients do not appear to affect mitosis but rather impair cell migration and adhesion in vitro. Thus, the potential mechanistic role of CDCA8 in thyroid dysgenesis is still unclear, and the range of thyroid phenotypes observed in patients carrying CDCA8 variants is broad, ranging from thyroid agenesis or ectopy to euthyroid individuals with asymmetric thyroid lobes or thyroid nodules.

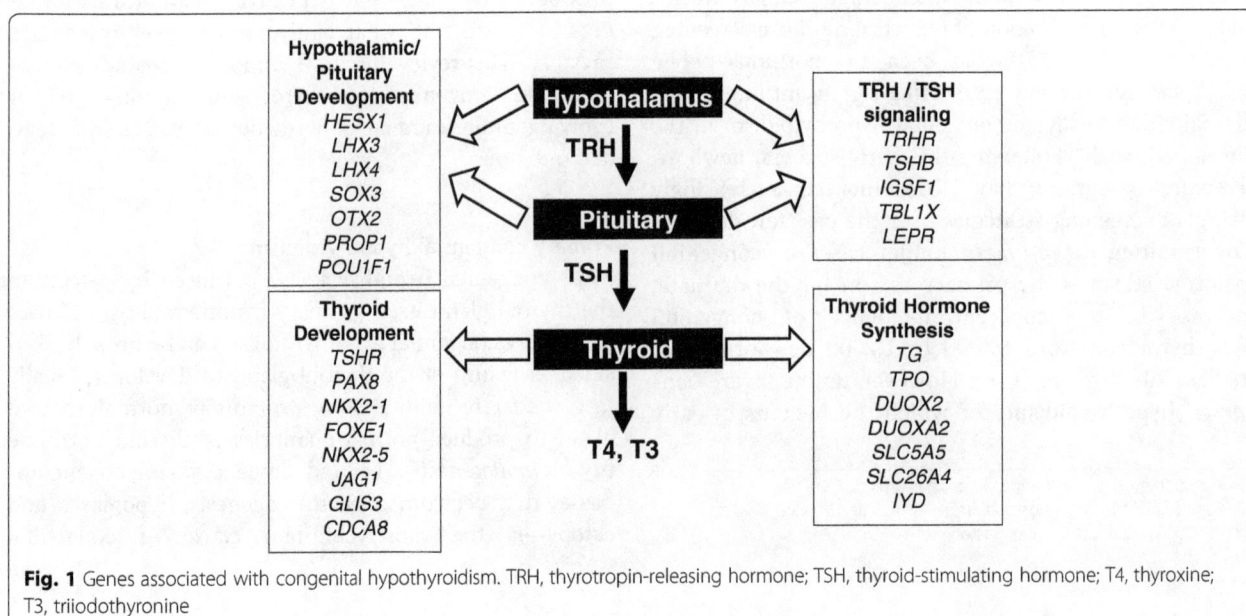

Fig. 1 Genes associated with congenital hypothyroidism. TRH, thyrotropin-releasing hormone; TSH, thyroid-stimulating hormone; T4, thyroxine; T3, triiodothyronine

Table 1 Clinical features of genetic syndromes associated with congenital hypothyroidism

Primary congenital hypothyroidism		Central congenital hypothyroidism	
PAX8	Renal abnormalities	IGSF1	Macro-orchidism, delayed pubertal testosterone rise, PRL deficiency, transient GH deficiency
NKX2–1	Interstitial lung disease, chorea	TBL1X	Hearing deficits
FOXE1	Cleft palate, bifid epiglottis, choanal atresia, spiky hair (Bamforth-Lazarus syndrome)	LEPR	Severe early-onset obesity, delayed puberty
NKX2–5	Congenital heart disease	POU1F1	Combined pituitary hormone deficiency
GLIS3	Neonatal diabetes mellitus, congenital glaucoma, developmental delay, hepatic fibrosis, polycystic kidneys	PROP1	Combined pituitary hormone deficiency
JAG1	Alagille syndrome (variable involvement of liver, heart, eye, skeletal, facial defects), congenital heart disease	HESX1	Combined pituitary hormone deficiency, optic nerve hypoplasia
SLC26A4	Sensorineural hearing loss	LHX3	Combined pituitary hormone deficiency, cervical abnormalities, sensorineural deafness
		LHX4	Combined pituitary hormone deficiency, cerebellar abnormalities
		SOX3	Combined pituitary hormone deficiency, craniofacial abnormalities
		OTX2	Combined pituitary hormone deficiency, micro–/anophthalmia, seizures

While thyroid dysgenesis remains the most common cause of congenital hypothyroidism, the incidence of dyshormonogenesis has been increasing over the last few decades. Whereas dyshormonogenesis accounted for only 15% of congenital hypothyroidism diagnosed in the early days of newborn screening, 30–40% of infants diagnosed by current newborn screening strategies have a eutopic thyroid gland consistent with a form of dyshormonogenesis [3, 5, 6]. [N.B. While the term *dyshormonogenesis* has classically referred to discrete defects in the cellular machinery of thyroid hormone synthesis leading to (often goitrous) congenital hypothyroidism, increasing recognition of the wide spectrum of severity of such defects makes it reasonable to define dyshormonogenesis as inadequate thyroid hormone production from a eutopic thyroid gland].

Unlike thyroid dysgenesis, in which a monogenic cause is present in only a small minority of patients, dyshormonogenesis is frequently due to a genetic defect in some element of thyroid hormone synthesis. Known genetic causes of dyshormonogenesis include mutations in thyroglobulin (*TG*), thyroperoxidase (*TPO*), dual oxidase 2 (*DUOX2*) and its accessory protein (*DUOXA2*), the sodium-iodide symporter (*SLC5A5*), pendrin (*SLC26A4*), and iodotyrosine deiodinase (*IYD*) (Fig. 1). Although dual oxidase 1 (*DUOX1*) is highly homologous to *DUOX2*, isolated defects of *DUOX1* have not been reported to cause congenital hypothyroidism. However, because hypothyroidism due to *DUOX2* mutations tends to be relatively mild, it has been suggested that DUOX1 may partly compensate for DUOX2 deficiency. This hypothesis has been supported by the fact that mice lacking function of both DUOX enzymes have

more severe hypothyroidism than those lacking only DUOX2 [16]. More recently, the first evidence of a physiologic role for DUOX1 in humans was provided by a report of two siblings with homozygous inactivating mutations in both *DUOX1* and *DUOX2* associated with congenital hypothyroidism more severe than is typically observed in DUOX2 deficiency alone [17]. While further data are needed, it appears that DUOX1 may indeed serve a redundant role in the human thyroid, not being required for thyroid function under normal circumstances but able to partly compensate when DUOX2 function is impaired.

Despite the growing number of genes associated with congenital hypothyroidism, precisely what proportion of congenital hypothyroidism is attributable to known genetic causes and the relative prevalence of mutations in specific genes are not known precisely, and estimates vary among studies. These variations are influenced by several factors including cohort selection that differs in terms of patient ethnicity and the type(s) of congenital hypothyroidism studied, and the sequencing approaches used to detect mutations. With regard to ethnicity, for example, *DUOX2* appears to be the most commonly implicated gene in East Asian populations, with *DUOX2* variants reported in 16–32% of congenital hypothyroidism patients in Korea, Japan, and China [18–20]. On the other hand, in a cohort of mostly European and Middle Eastern patients, variants in *TG* were much more common (55%) than *DUOX2* variants, which were found in only 18% [21]. However, the latter study was enriched for familial cases of congenital hypothyroidism and is likely to overestimate the prevalence of genetic mutations; therefore, the reported prevalences are likely not generalizable to sporadic cases, which constitute the majority of congenital hypothyroidism seen in clinical practice.

This demographic difference highlights the important influence of cohort selection on the apparent prevalence of genetic mutations in congenital hypothyroidism. Another illustration comes from studies that include patients with congenital hypothyroidism of varying etiologies. For example, one Korean study of 170 infants with congenital hypothyroidism of any etiology found mutations in 31% (most of whom had dyshormonogenesis) [18], while another study from the same country that included only patients with a eutopic thyroid gland identified mutations in 53.5% [22]. Similarly, the prevalence of *DUOX2* variants in Italy has been reported as 15% in unselected patients with congenital hypothyroidism, 23% in those with a eutopic thyroid gland [23], and to 30–37% in those with a eutopic gland and a documented partial iodine organification disorder [24, 25]. Thus, more refined cohort selection can significantly increase the observed prevalence of variants in relevant genes and must be considered when interpreting these data.

Finally, as might be expected, recent studies examining larger sets of candidate genes (often using next-generation sequencing techniques) are increasingly identifying potentially causative variants in a higher proportion of patients than older studies that analyzed only one or a few genes. For example, a recent analysis of 11 genes associated with congenital hypothyroidism in 177 Italian patients with congenital hypothyroidism of any cause demonstrated an overall variant prevalence of 58%; the prevalence was even higher (about 75%) in patients with a eutopic thyroid gland [23]. Many patients (23%) harbored variants in more than one gene, similar to other reports [18, 20, 22, 26]. This consistent finding suggests that the apparent lack of heritability of congenital hypothyroidism may be explained by a confluence of rare variants in several genes. On the other hand, while this hypothesis is intriguing, it remains at odds with the observed high rate of discordance for thyroid dysgenesis among monozygotic twins (who share nearly all variants in all genes) [27], which implies that it is unlikely for a significant proportion of congenital hypothyroidism to be explained by germline genetic changes alone. Another limitation of this and similar genetic studies is that the functional significance of many reported variants—particularly novel missense variants—has not been rigorously evaluated; accordingly, a causal role for these variants in congenital hypothyroidism must be imputed cautiously.

Another novel aspect of this study was to analyze variants in genes associated with both thyroid dysgenesis and dyshormonogenesis in all patients, regardless of their thyroid anatomy. Somewhat unexpectedly, variants in genes typically associated with dysgenesis (e.g., *NKX2–1*, *FOXE1*) were found in patients with dyshormonogenesis,

and vice versa [23]. This finding highlights the potential overlap in pathogenesis between the classically distinct phenotypes of thyroid dysgenesis and dyshormonogenesis. An example of such cross-over is *JAG1*, which encodes a ligand of the Notch receptor that is critical for normal thyroid gland formation in zebrafish [28]. Recently, anatomic thyroid defects have been found in a series of patients with heterozygous *JAG1* variants, including both patients with classical Alagille syndrome (a multisystem disorder known to be caused by *JAG1* mutations) and patients with congenital hypothyroidism without syndromic features [29]. These variants were confirmed to disrupt JAG1 function in vivo and strongly support a role for JAG1 in thyroid development in humans. Interestingly, however, the etiologies of hypothyroidism in patients with *JAG1* mutations included not only thyroid dysgenesis, as might be expected from the zebrafish model, but also eutopic thyroid glands. Thus, the case of *JAG1* illustrates the complexity of thyroid development and that the genetic abnormalities underlying the phenotypes of thyroid dysgenesis and dyshormonogenesis may overlap to a greater extent than has been previously appreciated.

Central congenital hypothyroidism

In contrast to primary disorders of the thyroid gland, central hypothyroidism is caused by dysfunction of hypothalamic or pituitary control of the thyroid axis that leads to inadequate production and/or bioactivity of TSH. Congenital hypothyroidism of central origin is rare: early estimates of its incidence were between 1:29,000 and 1:110,000 [30–32], although more recent data from the Netherlands suggest that it may occur in as many as 1:16,000 newborns and could represent up to 13% of cases of permanent congenital hypothyroidism [33, 34]. Although this incidence is similar to that of phenylketonuria (1:15,000) [35]—the condition for which newborn screening was originally introduced in the 1960's—central congenital hypothyroidism cannot be detected by the TSH-based screening strategies used by the majority of the newborn screening programs worldwide [1]. Central hypothyroidism may be detected by screening programs that measure T4 concentrations in all infants, along with measurement of TSH either simultaneously or in the subset of infants with low T4. However, this approach may not have optimal sensitivity and may miss some cases of central hypothyroidism [36].

One argument that has been made against routine screening for central hypothyroidism is that it tends to be milder than primary hypothyroidism and is therefore less critical to identify and treat early. Although developmental delays have been reported in small studies of infants who experienced delayed treatment of central congenital hypothyroidism [36, 37], there are no data to demonstrate clearly that early treatment improves outcomes in infants with this condition. However, indirect evidence may be derived from studies of primary congenital hypothyroidism, in which the initial serum concentration of total or free thyroxine (FT4) is one of the most important and consistent predictors of neurodevelopmental outcome [37–40]. In light of this, the premise that central congenital hypothyroidism poses less developmental risk has been challenged by a recent study from the Netherlands demonstrating that 55% of newborns with central hypothyroidism detected on newborn screening had FT4 concentrations sufficiently low (< 10 pmol/L) to warrant treatment according to current consensus guidelines [41, 42]. While few of these patients had the severely low FT4 levels often seen in primary congenital hypothyroidism, their FT4 levels were reduced to a range (5–10 pmol/L) that has been associated with modest deficits at age 10 years [37]. Thus, it appears that a substantial proportion of infants with central congenital hypothyroidism may be at some developmental risk if undetected and untreated, although the precise extent of this risk remains to be determined.

In addition, 75% of infants with central congenital hypothyroidism have additional, potentially life-threatening pituitary hormone deficiencies such as adrenal insufficiency and growth hormone deficiency [34], and detection of these comorbidities represents another argument in favor of screening for central hypothyroidism. Moreover, some have suggested that a carefully designed T4-based screening strategy able to detect these infants may actually be more cost effective than TSH-based screening [33]. In summary, while arguments can be made for routine newborn screening for central hypothyroidism, more compelling evidence is needed to support the need for and feasibility of widespread implementation of such strategies.

Despite its rarity, central congenital hypothyroidism provides an important window into the ontology and physiology of the HPT axis. Normally, thyrotropin-releasing hormone (TRH) from the hypothalamus stimulates thyrotropes in the anterior pituitary to secrete TSH. Congenital defects in this system result from abnormal development of the hypothalamus or pituitary or from genetic alterations that impair the function of TRH or TSH. Developmental or structural anomalies often have broad effects on the hypothalamus and/or pituitary that lead to deficits in multiple pituitary hormones. While some of these cases have no identifiable genetic basis, others can be attributed to mutations in one of several genes critical for the normal early development of these structures, including *HESX1*, *LHX3*, *LHX4*, *SOX3*, and *OTX2* (Fig. 1). These transcription factors have broad effects on fetal development and each is associated with particular syndromic features in addition to combined pituitary hormone deficiency (Table 1). In contrast, the transcription factors *PROP1* and *POU1F1*

are expressed later in anterior pituitary differentiation and their disruption results in combined pituitary hormone deficiency without other syndromic features [43].

While central developmental abnormalities often affect multiple pituitary hormones, specific defects in TRH or TSH signaling lead to isolated central congenital hypothyroidism. Until recently the only known genetic causes of this condition were very rare mutations in the TRH receptor (*TRHR*) [44, 45] or the TSH β-subunit (*TSHB*) [26]. However, in 2012 a study of 11 families with central congenital hypothyroidism identified a novel X-linked cause of central hypothyroidism, *IGSF1* [46]. Numerous cases of IGSF1 deficiency have since been described, making it the most common identifiable genetic cause of isolated central congenital hypothyroidism [47].

In addition to central hypothyroidism, males carrying an inactivating mutation of *IGSF1* manifest a clinical syndrome that includes macro-orchidism (88% of patients) and variable hypoprolactinemia (60% of patients). Testicular enlargement can begin before the onset of puberty and has been observed as early as 3 years of age, and affected adults may have testicular volumes up to 45–50 mL. While the normal pubertal increase in testicular size is accelerated in affected individuals, the pubertal rise in testosterone levels appears to be delayed, and plasma testosterone levels remain in the low-normal range in adults. A few children also appear to have transient growth hormone deficiency that resolves by adulthood. Importantly, although the IGSF1 deficiency syndrome is X-linked, 18% of female mutation carriers have central hypothyroidism, about 20% have biochemical prolactin deficiency (although lactation is apparently normal), and up to one-third have late menarche [48, 49].

At the time of its discovery *IGSF1* was known to encode a plasma membrane glycoprotein expressed in anterior pituitary thyrotropes, but its function was unknown. Recently, two studies have begun to elucidate the role of *IGSF1* in the HPT axis and a potential mechanism by which it may cause central hypothyroidism [50, 51]. Both humans and mice deficient in IGSF1 show impaired secretion of TSH in response to exogenous TRH administration, implying a functional defect in TRH signaling. Further studies indicate that IGSF1 directly stimulates TRHR activity in cell culture [50], while Igsf1-deficient mice have reduced pituitary TRHR expression and increased hypothalamic TRH expression [51]. Thus, both in vitro and in vivo evidence suggest that IGSF1 deficiency may cause central hypothyroidism by impairing expression and downstream signaling of the TRH receptor in pituitary thyrotropes. One mechanism by which IGSF1 may promote TRHR signaling is by blocking the inhibitory effect of TGFβ on TRHR expression [50]. Absence of IGSF1 may permit excessive

TGFβ-mediated suppression of TRHR that leads to central hypothyroidism. Interestingly, IGSF1 appears to have the opposite effect in pituitary gonadotropes of decreasing FSH β-subunit (*FSHB*) expression. Loss of this inhibition and consequent oversecretion of FSH might explain the macro-orchidism observed in males with IGSF1 deficiency. IGSF1 is also expressed in the Leydig cells and germ cells of the testis, where its role remains uncertain [50]. While more research is needed to understand the mechanisms of IGSF1 action, its discovery has opened the door to the study of novel biology in both the thyroid and gonadal axes.

Recently, mutations in *TBL1X* have been found in several families with X-linked central hypothyroidism [52]. This gene is expressed in the human pituitary and the paraventricular nucleus of the hypothalamus (where TRH-secreting neurons are located), and it encodes a protein that is part of the NCoR-SMRT corepressor complex, a key regulator of thyroid hormone-dependent gene expression. A pathogenic role for TBL1X defects is supported by a mouse model in which impaired NCoR function causes central hypothyroidism [53], and further investigation of the potential role of *TBL1X* in central hypothyroidism is now needed.

Mild congenital hypothyroidism

As previously noted, most newborn screening programs around the world use TSH-based strategies that effectively detect the vast majority of congenital hypothyroidism [1]. Over the past 30 years, many programs have lowered their screening TSH cut-offs from 20 - 50 mIU/L to 6–15 mIU/L. These changes have resulted in the diagnosis of many more patients with mild congenital hypothyroidism, most of whom have a eutopic thyroid gland [3, 4]. However, in contrast to the known neurodevelopmental risks of severe congenital hypothyroidism and the obvious benefits conferred by its timely and adequate treatment, much less is known about the risks posed by the milder forms of congenital hypothyroidism that are increasingly being diagnosed [7]. This uncertainty is reflected in current consensus guidelines, which find insufficient evidence to recommend for or against the treatment of infants with persistent modest TSH elevation (6–20 mIU/L in serum) but normal levels of FT4 [42]. Therefore, further defining the risks and appropriate treatment of mild congenital hypothyroidism is important, but a randomized, controlled trial to resolve this issue may be difficult to accomplish given the prevailing bias (and perhaps the ethical duty) not to withhold treatment from these infants [42].

Several recent studies have attempted to address this question. A series of studies in Belgian children that assessed the relationship between newborn screening TSH concentrations and various neurodevelopmental outcomes found no relationship between mild TSH elevation (up to 15 mIU/L) and cognitive or psychomotor development or parent-reported behavior scores at 4–6 years of age [54–56]. However, the power of these studies to detect differences in outcomes was limited by the small number of patients with elevated TSH concentrations, particularly in the 10–15 mIU/L range.

A different conclusion was reached by an Australian study that linked newborn screening results with standardized national assessments of childhood development and school performance [57]. This population-based analysis of over 500,000 children found that the risk of poor educational or developmental outcome rose continuously with increasing newborn screening TSH concentration from the 75th to the 99.9th percentile, even after adjusting for potential confounders. Interestingly, no increased risk was observed among infants with screening TSH levels above the 99.9th percentile (12–14 mIU/L), perhaps due to these patients being diagnosed with and treated for congenital hypothyroidism. This study has limitations, including the lack of many patient-level details (including the possibility of diagnosis and treatment of congenital hypothyroidism), inability to account for the potential confounding effect of iodine deficiency, and the inability to establish causality from the observational study design. Nevertheless, the results suggest that mild congenital hypothyroidism may be associated with identifiable neurodevelopmental risks.

Despite the unresolved question of whether infants with mild congenital hypothyroidism benefit from treatment, detecting mild TSH elevations on newborn screening may have other advantages. In particular, a proportion of infants with mild TSH elevation at screening may actually have congenital hypothyroidism that requires treatment. For example, about 12% of infants confirmed to have permanent congenital hypothyroidism—including both dysgenesis and dyshormonogenesis—have only mild TSH elevation at screening [3–5]. Conversely, among infants with mild initial TSH elevation, between 3% and 30% (depending on the specific cut-off used) prove to have permanent congenital hypothyroidism [58, 59]. In a substantial number of these patients, TSH concentrations are much higher when measured in the confirmatory serum sample than was suggested by an initial mild abnormality that would be missed by a higher TSH cut-off [4, 59]. This issue may be particularly significant in preterm and low birth-weight infants with congenital hypothyroidism, in whom the TSH rise may be delayed [60]. Still, these potential advantages of lower TSH cut-offs come at the expense of increased costs of screening, increased parental anxiety over abnormal results of uncertain significance, and the potential for overtreatment with levothyroxine, which itself may be associated with adverse neurodevelopmental outcomes [61]. Thus, in light of currently available data, the true balance of benefits and costs derived from more stringent screening thresholds continues to be debated [62].

Conclusions

The past 50 years have witnessed extraordinary advancements in the diagnosis, treatment, and outcomes of patients with congenital hypothyroidism. While we still do not understand what causes the majority of congenital hypothyroidism, increasing evidence suggests that a complex interplay of genetic variants in multiple thyroid-related genes may be involved, and the ongoing search for novel genetic causes continues to shed new light on the development and physiology of the hypothalamic-pituitary-thyroid axis. Meanwhile, strong evidence is lacking to guide the management of patients with mild congenital hypothyroidism who have increasingly been diagnosed in recent years. Further high-quality studies are needed to assess the neurodevelopmental risks to these infants and to what extent they may benefit from treatment.

Abbreviations
FT4: Free thyroxine; HPT: Hypothalamic-pituitary-thyroid; TRH: Thyrotropin-releasing hormone; TRHR: Thyrotropin-releasing hormone receptor; TSH: Thyroid-stimulating hormone; TSHR: Thyroid-stimulating hormone receptor

Acknowledgements
We are grateful to Dr. Joseph Wolfsdorf for his critical reading of this manuscript.

Funding
Not applicable.

Authors' contributions
CEC and AJW composed, read, and approved the final manuscript.

Authors' information
AJW is Director of the Thyroid Program at Boston Children's Hospital, Boston, MA.

Competing interests
The authors declare that they have no competing interests.

References
1. Ford G, LaFranchi SH. Screening for congenital hypothyroidism: A worldwide view of strategies. Best Pract Res Clin Endocrinol Metab. 2014;28:175–87.
2. Corbetta C, Weber G, Cortinovis F, Calebiro D, Passoni A, Vigone MC, et al. A 7-year experience with low blood TSH cutoff levels for neonatal screening reveals an unsuspected frequency of congenital hypothyroidism (CH). Clin Endocrinol. 2009;71:739–45.
3. Deladoey J, Ruel J, Giguere Y, Van Vliet G. Is the incidence of congenital hypothyroidism really increasing? A 20-year retrospective population-based study in quebec. J Clin Endocrinol Metab. 2011;96:2422–9.
4. Olivieri A, Corbetta C, Weber G, Vigone MC, Fazzini C, Medda E. Congenital hypothyroidism due to defects of thyroid development and mild increase of TSH at screening: Data from the Italian national registry of infants with congenital hypothyroidism. J Clin Endocrinol Metab. 2013;98:1403–8.
5. Olivieri A, Fazzini C, Medda E, Collaborators. Multiple factors influencing the incidence of congenital hypothyroidism detected by neonatal screening. Horm Res Paediatr. 2015;83:86–93.
6. Wassner AJ, Brown RS. Congenital hypothyroidism: Recent advances. Curr Opin Endocrinol Diabetes Obes. 2015;22:407–12.
7. Grosse SD, Van Vliet G. Prevention of intellectual disability through screening for congenital hypothyroidism: How much and at what level? Arch Dis Child. 2011;96:374–9.
8. Szinnai G. Clinical genetics of congenital hypothyroidism. Endocr Dev. 2014; 26:60–78.
9. Dentice M, Cordeddu V, Rosica A, Ferrara AM, Santarpia L, Salvatore D, et al. Missense mutation in the transcription factor NKX2-5: A novel molecular event in the pathogenesis of thyroid dysgenesis. J Clin Endocrinol Metab. 2006;91:1428–33.
10. Wang F, Liu C, Jia X, Liu X, Xu Y, Yan S, et al. Next-generation sequencing of NKX2.1, FOXE1, PAX8, NKX2.5, and TSHR in 100 Chinese patients with congenital hypothyroidism and athyreosis. Clin Chim Acta. 2017;470:36–41.
11. van Engelen K, Mommersteeg MT, Baars MJ, Lam J, Ilgun A, van Trotsenburg AS, et al. The ambiguous role of NKX2-5 mutations in thyroid dysgenesis. PLoS One. 2012;7:e52685.
12. Senee V, Chelala C, Duchatelet S, Feng D, Blanc H, Cossec JC, et al. Mutations in GLIS3 are responsible for a rare syndrome with neonatal diabetes mellitus and congenital hypothyroidism. Nat Genet. 2006;38:682–7.
13. Dimitri P, Habeb AM, Gurbuz F, Millward A, Wallis S, Moussa K, et al. Expanding the clinical spectrum associated with GLIS3 mutations. J Clin Endocrinol Metab. 2015;100:E1362–9.
14. Alghamdi KA, Alsaedi AB, Aljasser A, Altawil A, Kamal NM. Extended clinical features associated with novel GLIS3 mutation: A case report. BMC Endocr Disord. 2017;17:14.
15. Carre A, Stoupa A, Kariyawasam D, Gueriouz M, Ramond C, Monus T, et al. Mutations in BOREALIN cause thyroid dysgenesis. Hum Mol Genet. 2017;26: 599–610.
16. Grasberger H, De Deken X, Mayo OB, Raad H, Weiss M, Liao XH, et al. Mice deficient in dual oxidase maturation factors are severely hypothyroid. Mol Endocrinol. 2012;26:481–92.
17. Aycan Z, Cangul H, Muzza M, Bas VN, Fugazzola L, Chatterjee VK, et al. Digenic DUOX1 and DUOX2 mutations in cases with congenital hypothyroidism. J Clin Endocrinol Metab. 2017;102(9):3085–90.
18. Park KJ, Park HK, Kim YJ, Lee KR, Park JH, Park JH, et al. DUOX2 mutations are frequently associated with congenital hypothyroidism in the Korean population. Ann Lab Med. 2016;36:145–53.
19. Matsuo K, Tanahashi Y, Mukai T, Suzuki S, Tajima T, Azuma H, et al. High prevalence of DUOX2 mutations in Japanese patients with permanent congenital hypothyroidism or transient hypothyroidism. J Pediatr Endocrinol Metab. 2016;29:807–12.
20. Fan X, Fu C, Shen Y, Li C, Luo S, Li Q, et al. Next-generation sequencing analysis of twelve known causative genes in congenital hypothyroidism. Clin Chim Acta. 2017;468:76–80.
21. Nicholas AK, Serra EG, Cangul H, Alyaarubi S, Ullah I, Schoenmakers E, et al. Comprehensive screening of eight known causative genes in congenital hypothyroidism with gland-in-situ. J Clin Endocrinol Metab. 2016;101:4521–31.
22. Jin HY, Heo SH, Kim YM, Kim GH, Choi JH, Lee BH, et al. High frequency of DUOX2 mutations in transient or permanent congenital hypothyroidism with eutopic thyroid glands. Horm Res Paediatr. 2014;82:252–60.

23. de Filippis T, Gelmini G, Paraboschi E, Vigone MC, Di Frenna M, Marelli F, et al. A frequent oligogenic involvement in congenital hypothyroidism. Hum Mol Genet. 2017;26(13):2507–14.

24. Rabbiosi S, Vigone MC, Cortinovis F, Zamproni I, Fugazzola L, Persani L, et al. Congenital hypothyroidism with eutopic thyroid gland: Analysis of clinical and biochemical features at diagnosis and after re-evaluation. J Clin Endocrinol Metab. 2013;98:1395–402.

25. Muzza M, Rabbiosi S, Vigone MC, Zamproni I, Cirello V, Maffini MA, et al. The clinical and molecular characterization of patients with dyshormonogenic congenital hypothyroidism reveals specific diagnostic clues for DUOX2 defects. J Clin Endocrinol Metab. 2014;99:E544–53.

26. Nicholas AK, Jaleel S, Lyons G, Schoenmakers E, Dattani MT, Crowne E, et al. Molecular spectrum of TSH-beta subunit gene defects in central hypothyroidism in the UK and Ireland. Clin Endocrinol. 2017;86(3):410-418.

27. Perry R, Heinrichs C, Bourdoux P, Khoury K, Szots F, Dussault JH, et al. Discordance of monozygotic twins for thyroid dysgenesis: Implications for screening and for molecular pathophysiology. J Clin Endocrinol Metab. 2002;87:4072–7.

28. Porazzi P, Marelli F, Benato F, de Filippis T, Calebiro D, Argenton F, et al. Disruptions of global and jagged1-mediated notch signaling affect thyroid morphogenesis in the zebrafish. Endocrinology. 2012;153:5645–58.

29. de Filippis T, Marelli F, Nebbia G, Porazzi P, Corbetta S, Fugazzola L, et al. JAG1 loss-of-function variations as a novel predisposing event in the pathogenesis of congenital thyroid defects. J Clin Endocrinol Metab. 2016; 101:861–70.

30. Fisher DA, Dussault JH, Foley TP Jr, Klein AH, LaFranchi S, Larsen PR, et al. Screening for congenital hypothyroidism: Results of screening one million north american infants. J Pediatr. 1979;94:700–5.

31. Hanna CE, Krainz PL, Skeels MR, Miyahira RS, Sesser DE, LaFranchi SH. Detection of congenital hypopituitary hypothyroidism: Ten-year experience in the northwest regional screening program. J Pediatr. 1986;109:959–64.

32. Persani L. Central hypothyroidism: Pathogenic, diagnostic, and therapeutic challenges. J Clin Endocrinol Metab. 2012;97:3068–78.

33. Lanting CI, van Tijn DA, Loeber JG, Vulsma T, de Vijlder JJ, Verkerk PH. Clinical effectiveness and cost-effectiveness of the use of the thyroxine/thyroxine-binding globulin ratio to detect congenital hypothyroidism of thyroidal and central origin in a neonatal screening program. Pediatrics. 2005;116:168–73.

34. van Tijn DA, de Vijlder JJ, Verbeeten B Jr, Verkerk PH, Vulsma T. Neonatal detection of congenital hypothyroidism of central origin. J Clin Endocrinol Metab. 2005;90:3350–9.

35. National Institutes of Health Consensus Development P. National institutes of health consensus development conference statement: Phenylketonuria: Screening and management, october 16-18, 2000. Pediatrics. 2001;108:972–82.

36. Nebesio TD, McKenna MP, Nabhan ZM, Eugster EA. Newborn screening results in children with central hypothyroidism. J Pediatr. 2010;156:990–3.

37. Kempers MJ, van der Sluijs Veer L, Nijhuis-van der Sanden RW, Lanting CI, Kooistra L, Wiedijk BM, et al. Neonatal screening for congenital hypothyroidism in the Netherlands: Cognitive and motor outcome at 10 years of age. J Clin Endocrinol Metab. 2007;92:919–24.

38. Oerbeck B, Sundet K, Kase BF, Heyerdahl S. Congenital hypothyroidism: Influence of disease severity and l-thyroxine treatment on intellectual, motor, and school-associated outcomes in young adults. Pediatrics. 2003; 112:923–30.

39. Bongers-Schokking JJ, de Muinck Keizer-Schrama SM. Influence of timing and dose of thyroid hormone replacement on mental, psychomotor, and behavioral development in children with congenital hypothyroidism. J Pediatr. 2005;147:768–74.

40. Kempers MJ, van der Sluijs VL, Nijhuis-van der Sanden MW, Kooistra L, Wiedijk BM, Faber I, et al. Intellectual and motor development of young adults with congenital hypothyroidism diagnosed by neonatal screening. J Clin Endocrinol Metab. 2006;91:418–24.

41. Zwaveling-Soonawala N, van Trotsenburg AS, Verkerk PH. The severity of congenital hypothyroidism of central origin should not be underestimated. J Clin Endocrinol Metab. 2015;100:E297–300.

42. Leger J, Olivieri A, Donaldson M, Torresani T, Krude H, van Vliet G, et al. European Society for Paediatric Endocrinology consensus guidelines on screening, diagnosis, and management of congenital hypothyroidism. Horm Res Paediatr. 2014;81:80–103.

43. Schoenmakers N, Alatzoglou KS, Chatterjee VK, Dattani MT. Recent advances in central congenital hypothyroidism. J Endocrinol. 2015;227:R51–71.

44. Collu R, Tang J, Castagne J, Lagace G, Masson N, Huot C, et al. A novel mechanism for isolated central hypothyroidism: Inactivating mutations in the thyrotropin-releasing hormone receptor gene. J Clin Endocrinol Metab. 1997;82:1561–5.

45. Bonomi M, Busnelli M, Beck-Peccoz P, Costanzo D, Antonica F, Dolci C, et al. A family with complete resistance to thyrotropin-releasing hormone. N Engl J Med. 2009;360:731–4.

46. Sun Y, Bak B, Schoenmakers N, van Trotsenburg AS, Oostdijk W, Voshol P, et al. Loss-of-function mutations in IGSF1 cause an X-linked syndrome of central hypothyroidism and testicular enlargement. Nat Genet. 2012;44: 1375–81.

47. Persani L, Bonomi M. The multiple genetic causes of central hypothyroidism. Best Pract Res Clin Endocrinol Metab. 2017;31:255–63.

48. Joustra SD, Schoenmakers N, Persani L, Campi I, Bonomi M, Radetti G, et al. The IGSF1 deficiency syndrome: Characteristics of male and female patients. J Clin Endocrinol Metab. 2013;98:4942–52.

49. Joustra SD, Heinen CA, Schoenmakers N, Bonomi M, Ballieux BE, Turgeon MO, et al. IGSF1 deficiency: Lessons from an extensive case series and recommendations for clinical management. J Clin Endocrinol Metab. 2016; 101:1627–36.

50. Garcia M, Barrio R, Garcia-Lavandeira M, Garcia-Rendueles AR, Escudero A, Diaz-Rodriguez E, et al. The syndrome of central hypothyroidism and macroorchidism: IGSF1 controls TRHR and FSHB expression by differential modulation of pituitary TGF-beta and activin pathways. Sci Rep. 2017;7: 42937.

51. Turgeon MO, Silander TL, Doycheva D, Liao XH, Rigden M, Ongaro L, et al. TRH action is impaired in pituitaries of male Igsf1-deficient mice. Endocrinol. 2017;158:815–30.

52. Heinen CA, Losekoot M, Sun Y, Watson PJ, Fairall L, Joustra SD, et al. Mutations in TBL1X are associated with central hypothyroidism. J Clin Endocrinol Metab. 2016;101:4564–73.

53. Costa-e-Sousa RH, Astapova I, Ye F, Wondisford FE, Hollenberg AN. The thyroid axis is regulated by Ncor1 via its actions in the pituitary. Endocrinol. 2012;153:5049–57.

54. Trumpff C, De Schepper J, Vanderfaeillie J, Vercruysse N, Van Oyen H, Moreno-Reyes R, et al. Thyroid-stimulating hormone (TSH) concentration at birth in belgian neonates and cognitive development at preschool age. Nutrients. 2015;7:9018–32.

55. Trumpff C, De Schepper J, Vanderfaeillie J, Vercruysse N, Van Oyen H, Moreno-Reyes R, et al. Neonatal thyroid-stimulating hormone concentration and psychomotor development at preschool age. Arch Dis Child. 2016;101:1100–6.

56. Trumpff C, De Schepper J, Vanderfaeillie J, Vercruysse N, Tafforeau J, Van Oyen H, et al. No association between elevated thyroid-stimulating hormone at birth and parent-reported problem behavior at preschool age. Front Endocrinol (Lausanne). 2016;7:161.

57. Lain SJ, Bentley JP, Wiley V, Roberts CL, Jack M, Wilcken B, et al. Association between borderline neonatal thyroid-stimulating hormone concentrations and educational and developmental outcomes: A population-based record-linkage study. Lancet Diabetes Endocrinol. 2016;4:756–65.

58. Langham S, Hindmarsh P, Krywawych S, Peters C. Screening for congenital hypothyroidism: Comparison of borderline screening cut-off points and the effect on the number of children treated with levothyroxine. Eur Thyroid J. 2013;2:180–6.

59. Jones JH, Smith S, Dorrian C, Mason A, Shaikh MG. Permanent congenital hypothyroidism with blood spot thyroid stimulating hormone <10 mu/l. Arch Dis Child. 2016. [Epub ahead of print].

60. Woo HC, Lizarda A, Tucker R, Mitchell ML, Vohr B, Oh W, et al. Congenital hypothyroidism with a delayed thyroid-stimulating hormone elevation in very premature infants: Incidence and growth and developmental outcomes. J Pediatr. 2011;158:538–42.

61. Bongers-Schokking JJ, Resing WC, de Rijke YB, de Ridder MA, de Muinck Keizer-Schrama SM. Cognitive development in congenital hypothyroidism: Is overtreatment a greater threat than undertreatment? J Clin Endocrinol Metab. 2013;98:4499–506.

62. Lain S, Trumpff C, Grosse SD, Olivieri A, Van Vliet G. Are lower TSH cutoffs in neonatal screening for congenital hypothyroidism warranted? A debate. Eur J Endocrinol. 2017.

19

Increasing incidence of premature thelarche in the Central Region of Denmark - Challenges in differentiating girls less than 7 years of age with premature thelarche from girls with precocious puberty in real-life practice

Mia Elbek Sømod[1*†], Esben Thyssen Vestergaard[2,3†], Kurt Kristensen[1] and Niels Holtum Birkebæk[1]

Abstract

Background: Premature thelarche (PT) seems to be increasing and it is difficult to differentiate its early stages from precocious puberty (PP). Clinical and biochemical parameters are warranted to differentiate the two diagnoses.

Methods: One hundred ninety-one girls aged 0.5–7 years were included. Diagnoses were validated and the girls were categorized to the groups PP ($n = 27$) and PT ($n = 164$). Anthropometry, Tanner stages, ethnicity, bone age, and biochemistry, were recorded. Conventional variables for diagnosing PP were compared between the groups at time of referral to identify parameters predictive for the diagnosis.

Results: The referral rate of PT increased from 1998–2013. Girls with PT and PP differed with regards to age at referral, body mass index standard deviation scores (BMISDS), ethnicity, bone age advancement, basal luteinizing hormone (LH), gonadotropin releasing hormone (GnRH) stimulated LH and follicle stimulating hormone (FSH), basal and stimulated LH/FSH ratio, and sex-hormone binding globulin (SHBG). Apart from SHBG there was considerable overlap of the variables between the PT and the PP groups.

Conclusions: First, the incidence of PT appears to increase. Second, SHBG was the variable which best discriminated PT from PP. Third, stimulated LH in 1–3 years old girls with PT is similar to stimulated LH in 5–7 years old girls with PP. Age, BMISDS, ethnicity, bone age, stimulated gonadotropins and LH/FSH and SHBG are all useful variables for differentiating PP from PT. However normative data for stimulated LH and FSH in the age group 0.5–7 years are warranted.

Keywords: Sex hormone binding globulin, Premature thelarche, Incidence, Gonadotropins, Precocious puberty

Background

Onset of puberty before eight years of age for girls, so-called precocious puberty (PP), is increasing [1–3]. PP is associated with reduced adult height [4], psychosocial problems [5, 6], and may be associated with breast cancer [7] and the metabolic syndrome [8]. The first clinical

sign of puberty in girls is usually breast development (thelarche). Thelarche is accompanied with accelerated growth velocity and bone age advancement. Early stages of PP in girls are, therefore, difficult to differentiate from premature thelarche (PT), which is defined as isolated breast development before eight years of age [9].

The frequency of PT seems dependent on ethnicity and may be increasing [10]. In an U.S. study the incidence rate of PT in the period 1940–1984 was 2.1 per 10,000 person years [11]. PT is a self-limiting condition in the majority of girls, but it may progress into PP in a

* Correspondence: mies@clin.au.dk
†Equal contributors
[1]Department of Pediatrics, Aarhus University Hospital, Skejby, Palle Juul Jensens Boulevard 99, DK-8200 Aarhus N, Denmark
Full list of author information is available at the end of the article

subset of girls [12–14]. De Vries et al. and Pasquino et al. reported that 13 % and 14 %, respectively, of girls with PT progressed into PP [13, 14]. It is of great importance to identify the girls with PT, who progress into PP [9], and to initiate medical treatment to circumvent the negative implications of PP [15].

Unfortunately, robust clinical, biochemical and imaging indicators to help clinicians differentiate PT from PP are lacking, and no single test can predict the progression from PT to PP [12–14]. Diagnostic tests that may help to differentiate PT from PP include pelvic ultrasound measurements [16], bone age evaluation, basal luteinizing hormone (LH), and gonadotropin releasing hormone (GnRH) test, although normative data for the GnRH test in the first years of life have not yet been established.

The aim of this study was to test the hypothesis that the incidence of PT in girls in the Central Region of Denmark is increasing. A further aim was to describe challenges in differentiating girls with PT from girls with early PP using conventional variables for diagnosing PP in real-life practice.

Methods

We identified girls aged 0.5–7 years referred for breast development between January 1998 and September 2013 to the pediatric departments in the Central Region of Denmark (population 1,277,538).

For screening purposes, all patient files of girls who were registered in the Danish National Patient Registry with the ICD10 codes as listed in Table 1, were carefully reviewed.

The girls were included in the study, if they presented with uni- or bilateral breast development corresponding to Tanner stage 2 or more. Ninety-four girls did not meet the inclusion criteria and were subsequently excluded from further analysis. Girls were excluded because 1) they did not have breast development at the first visit (either because of regression or misdiagnosis or they had isolated adrenarche) and 2) data on breast development were missing in the patient file. Girls were assigned to the PP group if they, at the time of referral or before their seventh year, were diagnosed with PP by a pediatric endocrinologist. For validating girls into the PP group they were required to meet the following criteria: breast Tanner stage 2 or more combined with one or more of the following: pubic hair, accelerated growth velocity and bone age greater than 2 SD above the chronological age. Further, they should have a pubertal response (primarily assessed by the peak LH/FSH ratio and the LH response > 5 IU/L) if they underwent a GnRH test at time of referral and data were available. For validating girls into the PT group they were required to have breast development corresponding to Tanner stage 2 or more, without any other signs of puberty.

Table 1 ICD10-diagnosis codes used for the registry extraction

ICD10-code	Description
N60.X	Disorders of breast
N62.X	Hypertrophy of breast
N63.X	Unspecified lump in breast
N64.9	Disorder of breast, unspecified
E30.X	Disorders of puberty, not elsewhere classified
Q78.1	McCune Albright
E22.8	Central precocious puberty
E25.0	Congenital adrenal hyperplasia
E270B	Premature adrenarche
E25.X	Pseudopuberty

Codes where a diagnosis of premature thelarche or precocious puberty could potentially have been misclassified were included

The following parameters were extracted from the patient charts: Ethnicity, anthropometry, Tanner stages of breast and pubic hair, bone age [17], magnetic resonance imaging of the brain (MRI) and biochemistry: Estradiol, inhibin B, sex hormone-binding globulin (SHBG), thyroid stimulating hormone (TSH) luteinizing hormone (LH), follicle stimulating hormone (FSH), and the FSH and LH concentrations 30 min after an intravenous injection of 0.1 mg/m^2 Relefact® (a GnRH agonist), hereafter designated stimulated LH and FSH concentrations.

Some turned 7 years before a GnRH test was performed. The presented biochemical data represent the results from the first blood samples after referral.

The number of newborn girls per year and girls in the age group 0–7 years in the Central Region of Denmark from 1998 to 2013, were obtained from 'Statistics Denmark.'

The study was approved by the National Research Ethics Committee (reference number 1-10-72-186-13) and the Danish Data Protection Agency (reference number 1-16-02-118-13).

Assays

Up to March 2008 LH, FSH, estradiol and TSH levels were measured by chemilu-minescence immunoassay (Siemens Bayer Advia Centaur CP Immunoassay). Since March 2008 LH, FSH, estradiol and TSH were measured by electro-chemiluminescence immunoassay (Roche Cobas E 601, module immunology analyzer). SHBG levels were measured by chemiluminescence immunoassay (Siemens Bayer Advia Centaur CP Immunoassay) up to November 2010 and since then by electrochemiluminescence immunoassay (Roche Cobas E 601, module immunology analyzer). Serum levels of Inhibin B were measured by the Beckman Coulter GenII assay.

Statistics

Statistical analysis was performed by SPSS software version 21. Linear distributed data are presented as mean and SD, while nonlinear distributed data are presented as median and range. Body mass index standard deviation score (BMI SDS) was calculated according to Nysom et al. [18]. An independent samples T test was used to compare the means of the parametric variables in the two groups (PP vs. PT). Some parameters were ln-transformed to obtain normal distribution. Non-parametric variables were compared using Mann-Whitney U test. Binary variables were analyzed using chi-square test. A difference was considered statistically significant at $p < 0.05$.

Results

In total 285 patients were identified. Ninety-four patients did not meet the inclusion criteria and the remaining 191 girls (0.5 to 6.9 years) were included in the study and allocated to the PP group ($n = 27$) or the PT group ($n = 164$). One girl with PP was diagnosed with central PP (hamartoma of tuber cinereum), and the rest were diagnosed with idiopathic central PP. None of the girls was diagnosed with peripheral PP.

Incidence

The annual incidence ranged from 0 to 1 and from 1 to 4 per 10,000 girls for PP and PT, respectively, (Fig. 1).

Non-biochemical characteristics

Girls with PP were older at referral ($p < 0.001$) (Table 2): 14.8 % ($n = 4$) were in the age group 0.5–2 years, whereas 77.7 % ($n = 21$) were 5–7 years old. For girls with PT the majority (70.7 %, $n = 116$) was referred at age 0.5–2 years, Fig. 2.

A greater percentage of girls with PP were of non-European origin ($p = 0.012$) and presented with a higher BMI SDS ($p < 0.001$) compared to the girls with PT.

85.2 % of the girls with PP and 38.4 % of the girls with PT had a bone age examination. Bone age was advanced in all of the PP girls with a median advance of 23 months and in the PT girls bone age deviated from chronological age with a median of plus 4 months ($p < 0.001$).

Biochemical characteristics

SHBG levels were decreased in the PP group ($p = 0.007$), and there was no overlap between the PT and the PP group (Table 2). No between-group differences were observed for estradiol, inhibin B, and TSH (Table 2).

Nineteen girls (70.4 %) with PP, median age 6.0 years, and 47 girls (28.7 %) with PT, median age 2.3 years, underwent a GnRH test. Basal LH and stimulated values were significantly increased in the PP group compared with the PT group ($p = 0.016$ and $p < 0.001$, respectively), whereas the stimulated FSH value was decreased in the PP group compared with the PT group ($p = 0.001$) (Table 2). A stimulated LH-response ≥5 IU/l was recorded in 57.9 % of the girls with PP and in 38.3 % of the girls with PT.

Stimulated LH/FSH ratio was 0.7 (0.3; 2.7) for the PP-group and 0.2 (0.05; 1.3) for the PT-group ($p < 0.001$), Table 2. The LH/FSH ratio was ≥1 for 8 (42.1 %) of the PP girls and 1 (2.1 %) of PT girls (due to a low stimulated FSH value). The basal LH/FSH ratio also indicated a significant difference between the groups ($p = 0.03$), Table 2. The stimulated LH and FSH concentrations are presented

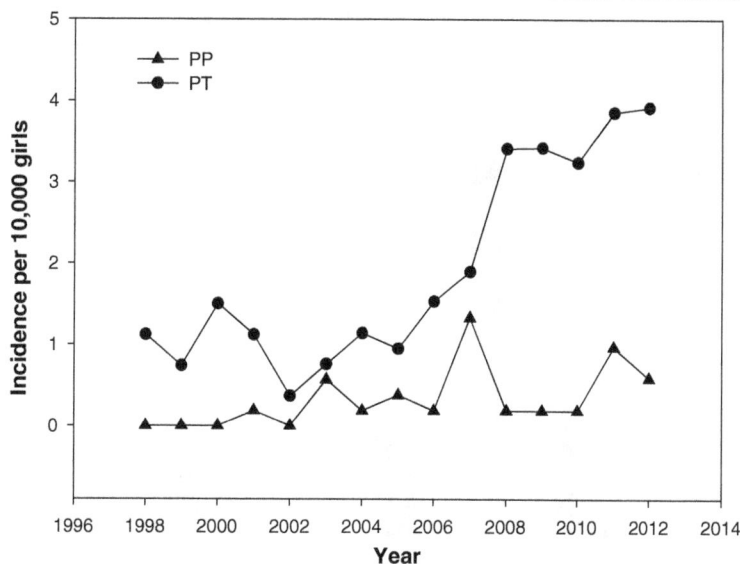

Fig. 1 Incidence of precocious puberty and premature thelarche expressed as an incidence rate and defined as:

$$\frac{\textit{No. of girls who got a diagnosis of PP or PT in a certain year}}{\textit{Total no. of girls } 1/2\text{–}7 \textit{ years living in the region}}$$

Table 2 Clinical and biochemical data of girls with precocious puberty (PP) and premature thelarche (PT)

Variable	PP	n=	PT	n=	P-value
Age at referral (years)[a]	5.9 (1.0-6.9)	27	1.3 (0.5-6.9)	164	0.000
European origin (%)	70.4	27	89.6	164	0.012
BMI SDS	+0.8 (0.3-1.3)	27	-0.3 (-0.5-(-) 0.1)	132	0.000
Bone age advancement (months)[b]	23.0 (3.0-48.0)	23	4.0 (1.0-19.0)	64	0.000
Estradiol (pg/mL)[a]	30.0 (18.0-137.0)	13	18.4 (13.0-85.0)	77	0.288
Inhibin B (pg/mL)	44.2 (23.9-64.4)	12	30.2 (25.6-34.7)	50	0.165
TSH (IU/L)	2.6 (2.1-3.1)	17	2.5 (2.2-2.8)	73	0.827
SHBG (nmol/L)	81.1 (60.2-101.9)	12	114.5 (102.3-126.8)	37	0.007
LH0 (IU/L)[b]	0.4 (0.1-3.0)	19	0.3 (0.05-1.0)	46	0.016
LH30 (IU/L)[b]	7.2 (3.0-45.0)	19	3.8 (0.6-24.0)	47	0.000
FSH0 (IU/L)[b]	2.9 (0.9-8.4)	19	2.85 (0.6-17.3)	46	0.891
FSH30 (IU/L)[b]	9.3 (2.3-27.7)	19	18.9 (0.8-77.9)	47	0.001
Basal LH/FSH ratio[b]	0.2 (0.02-0.71)	19	0.1 (0.02-1.25)	46	0.031
Peak LH/FSH ratio[b]	0.7 (0.26-2.67)	19	0.2 (0.05-1.25)	47	0.000

Results are presented as mean values with 95 % confidence intervals
[a]Indicates non-parametric tests where results are presented as median values and ranges. [b]Indicates parametric test with ln-tranformed data where results are presented as the untransformed median values and ranges

in Figs. 3 and 4, respectively. The youngest girls exhibited the largest stimulated FSH responses. Some girls with PT in the age group ½-3 years had a stimulated LH response comparable to the stimulated LH response in girls presenting PP 5–7 years old. The stimulated LH/FSH ratios was less than 0.6 in 46 of 47 girls with PT and higher than 0.6 in 11 of 19 girls with PP, Fig. 5.

Discussion

Breast development before the age of 7 years of age is often an isolated and self-limiting condition. It can, however, also be the first sign of precocious puberty, which needs further examinations and medical treatment to prevent psychosocial, metabolic, and cardiovascular adverse events. While it is well known that the incidence of premature thelarche was increasing in the period from 1940 to 1984 [11] and that the timing of pubarche is still declining [3, 19, 20] it remains to be investigated, if the incidence of premature thelarche has continued to increase. We addressed this question and the novel finding of our study is that the incidence of girls referred because of premature thelarche before the

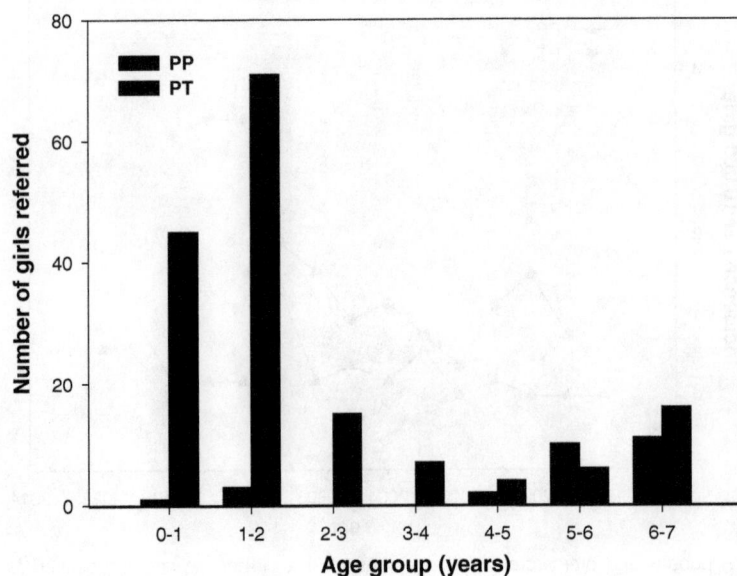

Fig. 2 Number of girls with precocious puberty (PP) and premature thelarche (PT) in the age groups ½-7 years

PP+PT LH30

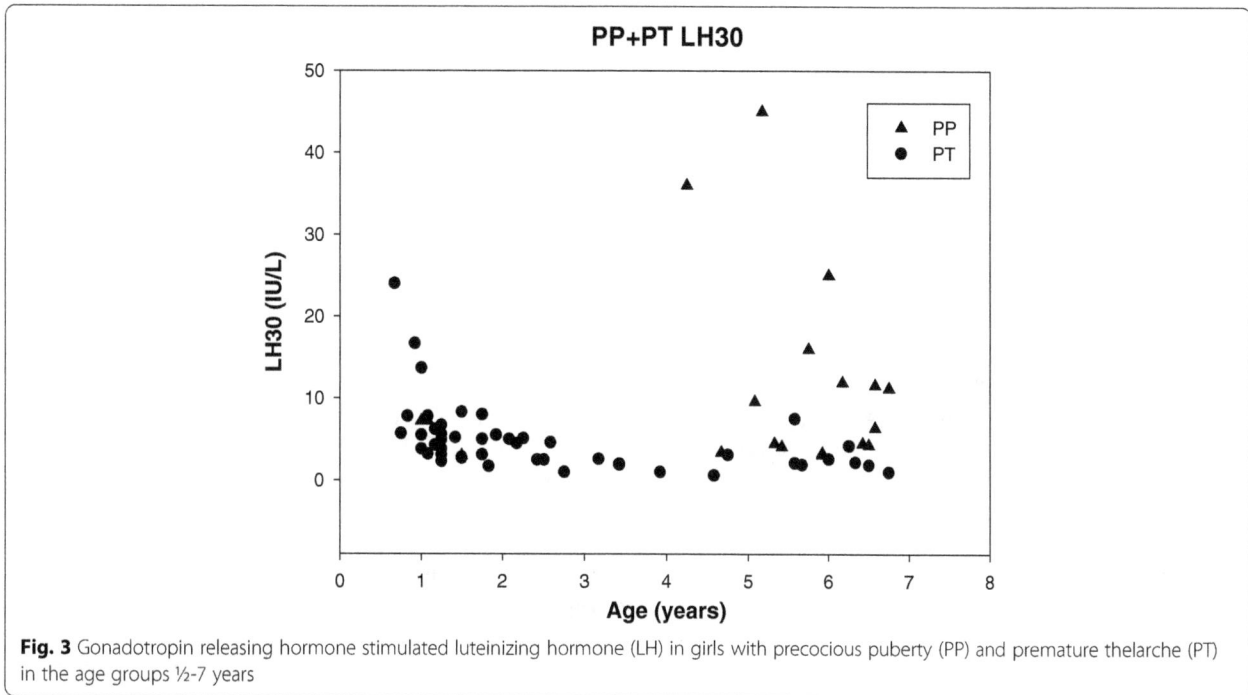

Fig. 3 Gonadotropin releasing hormone stimulated luteinizing hormone (LH) in girls with precocious puberty (PP) and premature thelarche (PT) in the age groups ½-7 years

age of 7 years is increasing. We excluded girls below 6 months of age because precocious puberty in this age group is extremely rare i.e. in a study of 302 girls with thelarche at birth or during the first 6 months of life, none of them developed precocious puberty [12]. Girls older than 7 years were also excluded because of the trend towards onset of pubertal development in this age group ("nonprogressive precocious puberty") as a part of the normal puberty [21]. The continuous increase in girls referred for premature thelarche has also been observed in France as published at a major international congress on pediatric endocrinology [22]. The increasing number of referrals in our study indicates a higher incidence of PT and may have several explanations such as changes in the ethnic composition, increasing BMI and increased number of referrals for premature thelarche

PP+PT FSH30

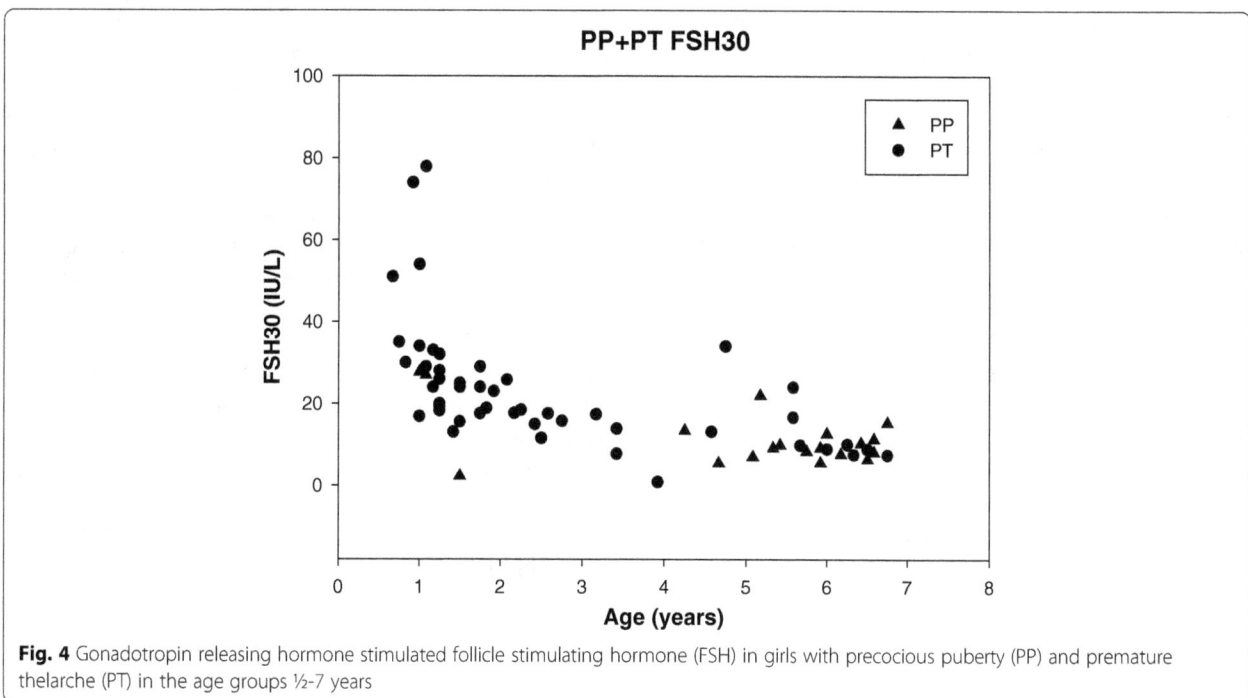

Fig. 4 Gonadotropin releasing hormone stimulated follicle stimulating hormone (FSH) in girls with precocious puberty (PP) and premature thelarche (PT) in the age groups ½-7 years

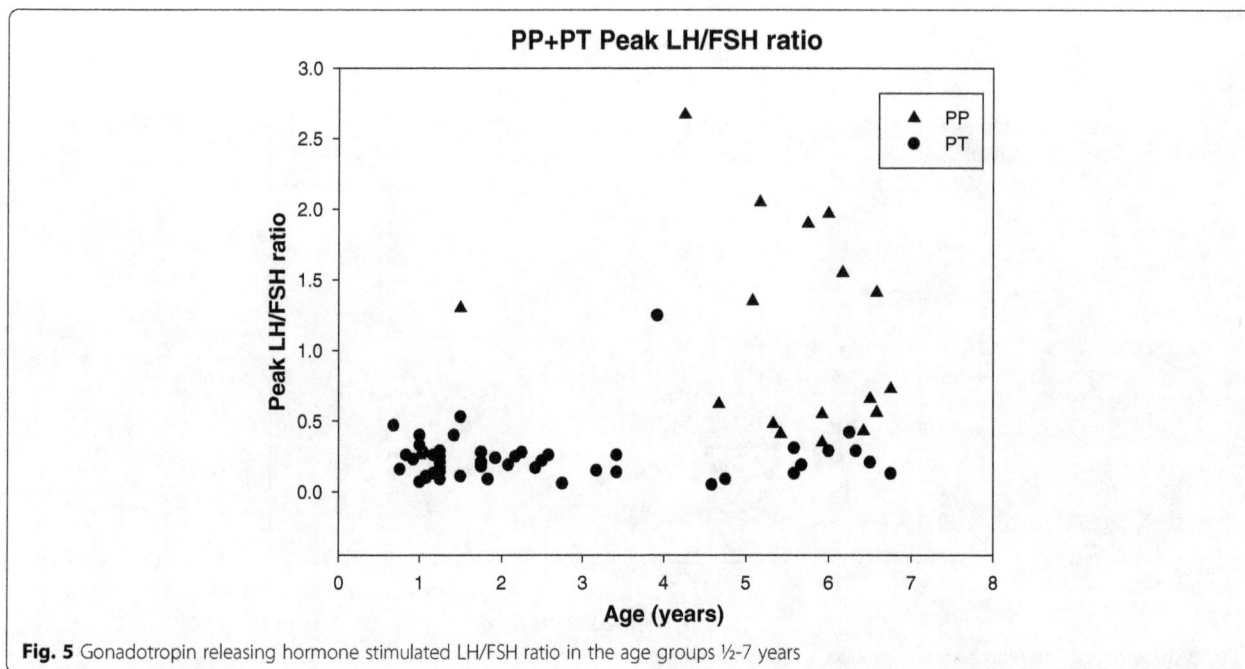

Fig. 5 Gonadotropin releasing hormone stimulated LH/FSH ratio in the age groups ½-7 years

because of greater awareness of the condition in the general population and by the general practitioners.

Differentiating premature thelarche from early stages of precocious puberty in girls is difficult. Therefore, for improving future clinical care of girls with premature thelarche and precocious puberty, we constructed a database on clinical and biochemical data of the girls in our study cohort. Our aim was to identify signs, which can help differentiate girls with premature thelarche from girls with early stages of precocious puberty, but also to draw attention to the challenges in using conventional variables for PP diagnostics in distinguishing PT and PP in the age group ½-7 years.

The most interesting and clinical useful discovery in our study was, that we observed decreased SHBG levels in girls with precocious puberty and observed no overlap of SHBG concentrations in the two groups. Circulating levels of SHBG and androgens correlate inversely and SHBG usually plateau until puberty where after a decline is recorded [23]. We did not routinely measure androgens in our cohort but speculate that a puberty-associated increase of androgen levels caused a decrease of systemic SHBG in girls with precocious puberty. 25 % of the PP girls who underwent a SHBG analysis had pubic hair Tanner stage 2.

Several other parameters also differed between the groups: Chronological age, BMI SDS, ethnic origin, bone age advancement, basal and stimulated LH, stimulated FSH, basal and stimulated LH/FSH ratio.

Fourteen percent of the girls, who were referred because of breast development, progressed to precocious

puberty, but the risk was strongly dependent on the age as only 3 % of girls between 6 months and 3 years, and 41 % girls older than 3 years of age developed precocious puberty. This supports the notion that breast development in the first few years of life is most often a physiological condition that stabilizes or regresses spontaneously [11, 14, 24–26] and why clinical follow-up without hormonal examinations may be the primary option in most cases in the youngest age group. Our data are in line with two earlier reports, where 13 and 14 % of girls with premature thelarche, respectively, developed precocious puberty [13, 14], but contrasts another study, that reported a larger proportion of girls e.g. 6.1 % out of 148 aged 6 months to 3 years progressed from premature thelarche to precocious puberty [12].

Non-European origin was associated with increased risk for precocious puberty in our study, which supports previous reports on the positive association between precocious puberty and ethnic origin [27, 28].

Advanced bone age is a hallmark of precocious puberty [9] and was quite increased in our group of girls with precocious puberty as compared with the girls with premature thelarche.

According to Bizzarri et al. [12] the combined measurement of basal LH and longitudinal diameter of the uterus represents a reliable screening approach to identify subjects who should undergo GnRH testing. Our data set revealed that only a small proportion of our study cohort had an ultrasonography examination and the data quality was low, and ultrasound data were therefore not included in our study.

The gold standard confirmatory laboratory test for central idiopathic precocious puberty for girls older than 6 years of age is a GnRH stimulated LH response in the pubertal range [29], but, so far, no reference interval exists for girls below 6 years of age. When comparing the group of girls progressing to precocious puberty with the group of girls with premature thelarche, we observed an increased basal and stimulated LH response and an increased basal and stimulated LH/FSH ratio. Neely et al. reported that basal LH concentrations were above 0.3 IU/L in all girls in late puberty [30]. This was indeed in line with 89.5 % of the girls in our cohort with precocious puberty, but 69.6 % of the girls with premature thelarche also exhibited increased LH concentrations leaving basal LH measurements inadequate to identify girls with premature thelarche. Bizzarri et al. reported that a basal LH concentration above 0.2 IU/L was the best positive and negative predictor of premature thelarche progressing into precocious puberty in 0 to 3 year old girls [12], but contrasts the basal LH concentrations in our study, where girls in that age group with premature thelarche presented with a median basal LH concentration of 0.3 IU/L. Only 57.9 % of our girls with precocious puberty had a stimulated LH above 5.0 IU/L, and girls with premature thelarche in age group ½-3 years exhibited a stimulated LH comparable to the stimulated LH in the precocious puberty group in 5–7 year old girls. A GnRH-stimulated LH/FSH ratio ≥1 has been considered to have high sensitivity and specificity for differentiating between precocious puberty and premature thelarche [31]. However, applying a stimulated LH/FSH ratio ≥1 as a cut-off value could not discriminate all our girls with precocious puberty from girls with premature thelarche, which was also observed in a recent study [12].

Surprisingly, we did not observe changes in estradiol, inhibin B, and TSH levels in girls with precocious puberty, and speculate that the lack of significance is attributed to a limited data set and a large inter-individual variability. E.g. the girl with the highest estradiol and increased LH response to the GnRH test, who was assigned to the premature thelarche group, underwent an extensive diagnostic program and an appropriate observation period and proved not to have precocious puberty, but rather premature thelarche, unsustained precocious puberty [32] or prolonged minipuberty. Usually minipuberty is considered to affect girls up 6 months of age but may last for a prolonged period [33].

The retrospective study design is a limitation and implies that data are not homogenous for the enrolled girls causing some missing information. The missing data on some of the girls, especially in the group with premature thelarche, also made comparison of the studied parameters difficult and indicates a selection bias for performing for example GnRH testing, bone age examination,

and pelvic ultrasonography. Furthermore, only girls born before 2006 had a 7-year follow up, resulting in an underestimated incidence in the years 2006 to 2012. The assay for LH, FSH, SHBG and TSH changed from chemiluminescence immunoassay to electrochemiluminescence immunoassay during the study period, however reference values did not change for our age-group.

Conclusion

We observed that the incidence of referral for premature thelarche is increasing in the Central Region of Denmark. It remains to be investigated if this earlier breast development over time will advance the entire sexual maturation. The incidence for premature thelarche in our study may serve as reference for future studies investigating secular trends of clinical signs of early pubertal development.

SHBG concentrations appeared to be useful to differentiate girl with premature thelarche from girls with precocious puberty. The sensitivity and specificity of SHBG in differentiating PT from PP needs to be further tested in future prospective studies. No other isolated clinical characteristic or hormonal parameter predicted the progression of premature thelarche to precocious puberty in girls below 7 years of age. Age, BMISDS, ethnicity, bone age, stimulated and basal LH/FSH ratio are all useful variables for differentiating PP from PT, but with considerable overlap between the PT and the PP group. It is notable that the stimulated LH value in 1–3 years old girls with PT may be as high as in 5–7 years old girls with PP. Therefore, in clinical practice, hormonal and x-ray testing in the younger girls should be limited to those with atypical or clearly progressive findings during follow-up. The GnRH test may, in future studies, also be useful to differentiate between premature thelarche and precocious puberty in girls below 6 years of age, but requires establishing of a reference interval in this age group.

Competing interests
The authors have no competing interests to declare.

Authors' contributions
MES: literature research, wrote protocol, data collection, chart reviews, constructed database, data analysis and interpretation, wrote manuscript, created tables and figures. ETV: conceptualized study, study design, wrote protocol, designed and constructed database, collected data, interpreted results, edited and revised manuscript, literature research, approved the final manuscript. KK: conceptualized study, collected data, interpreted results, revised manuscript. NBV: conceptualized study, wrote protocol, collected data, interpreted results, edited and revised manuscript. All authors read and approved the final manuscript.

Acknowledgements
The study was funded by Aarhus University. A special thank to the pediatric departments in the Central Region of Denmark: Randers, Herning, Viborg and Skejby.

Author details
[1]Department of Pediatrics, Aarhus University Hospital, Skejby, Palle Juul Jensens Boulevard 99, DK-8200 Aarhus N, Denmark. [2]Medical Research Laboratory, Aarhus University, Nørrebrogade 44 building 3B, DK-8000 Aarhus

C, Denmark. ³Department of Pediatrics, Randers Regional Hospital, DK-8930 Randers, Denmark.

References

1. Teilmann G, Pedersen CB, Jensen TK, Skakkebæk NE, Juul A. Prevalence and incidence of precocious pubertal development in Denmark: an epidemiologic study based on national registries. Pediatrics. 2005;116(6):1323–8.
2. Sørensen K, Mouritsen A, Aksglade L, Hagen CP, Mogensen SS, Juul A. Recent secular trends in pubertal timing: implications for evaluation and diagnosis of precocious puberty. Horm Res Paediatr. 2012;77:137–45.
3. Aksglaede L, Sorensen K, Petersen JH, Skakkebaek NE, Juul A. Recent decline in age at breast development: the Copenhagen Puberty Study. Pediatrics. 2009;123:e932–9.
4. Carel JC, Lahlou N, Roger M, Chaussain JL. Precocious puberty and statural growth. Hum Reprod Update. 2004;10(2):135–47.
5. Michaud PA, Suris JC, Deppen A. Gender-related psychological and behavioural correlates of pubertal timing in a national sample of Swiss adolescents. Mol Cell Endocrinol. 2006;254-255:172–8.
6. Mrug S, Elliott MN, Davies S, Tortolero SR, Cuccaro P, Schuster MA. Early puberty, negative peer influence, and problem behaviors in adolescent girls. Pediatrics. 2014;133(1):7–14.
7. Ahlgren M, Melbye M, Wohlfahrt J, Sørensen TIA. Growth patterns and the risk of breast cancer in women. N Engl J Med. 2004;351:1619–26.
8. Frontini MG, Srinivasan SR, Berenson GS. Longitudinal changes in risk variables underlying metabolic syndrome X from childhood to young adulthood in female subjects with a history of early menarche: the Bogalusa Heart study. Int J Obes Relat Metab Disord. 2003;27:1398–404.
9. Carel JC, Léger J. Precocious puberty. N Engl J Med. 2008;358:2366–77.
10. Atay Z, Turan S, Guran T, Furman A, Bereket A. The prevalence and risk factors of premature thelarche and pubarche in 4- to 8-year-old girls. Acta Paediatr. 2012;101:71–5.
11. Van Winter JT, Noller KL, Zimmerman D, Melton LJ. Natural history of premature thelarche in Olmsted County, Minnesota, 1940 to 1984. J Pediatr. 1990;116:278–90.
12. Bizzarri C, Spadoni GL, Botarro G, Montanari G, Giannone G, Cappa M, et al. The response to gonadotropin releasing hormone (GnRH) stimulation test does not predict the progression to true precocious puberty in girls with onset of premature thelarche in the first three years of life. J Clin Endocrinol Metab. 2014;99(2):433–9.
13. Pasquino AM, Pucarelli I, Passeri F, Segni M, Mancini MA, Municchi G. Progression of premature thelarche to central precocious puberty. J Pediatr. 1995;126:11–4.
14. De Vries L, Guz-Mark A, Lazar L, Reches A, Phillip M. Premature thelarche: age at presentation affects clinical course but not clinical characteristics or risk to progress to precocious puberty. J Pediatr. 2010;156(3):466–71.
15. Carel JC, Eugster EA, Rogol A, Ghizzoni L, Palmert MR, Antoniazzi F, et al. Consensus statement on the use of gonadotropin-releasing hormone analogs in children. Pediatrics. 2009;123:752–62.
16. De Vries L, Horev G, Schwartz M, Phillip M. Ultrasonographic and clinical parameters for early differentiation between precocious puberty and premature thelarche. Eur J Endocrinol. 2006;154:891–8.
17. Marshall WA, Tanner JM. Variations in pattern of pubertal changes in girls. Arch Dis Child. 1969;44:291–303.
18. Nysom K, Mølgaard C, Hutchings B, Michaelsen KF. Body mass index of 0 to 45-y-old Danes: reference values and comparison with published European reference values. Int J Obes. 2001;25:177–84.
19. Sun SS, Schubert CM, Chumlea WC, Roche AF, Kulin HE, Lee PA, et al. National estimates of the timing of sexual maturation and racial differences among US children. Pediatrics. 2002;110(5):911–9.
20. Wu T, Mendola P, Buck GM. Ethnic differences in the presence of secondary sex characteristics and menarche among US girls: the Third National Health and Nutrition Examination Survey, 1988-1994. Pediatrics. 2002;110(4):752–7.
21. Chauhan A, Grissom M. Disorders of childhood growth and development: precocious puberty. FP Essent. 2013;410:25–31.
22. Gaspari L, Morcrette E, Jeandel C, Valé FD, Paris F, Sultan C. Dramatic rise in the prevalence of precocious puberty in girls over the past 20 years in the south of France. Horm Res Ped. 2014;82 suppl 1:291–92.
23. Elmlinger MW, Kühnel W, Ranke MB. Reference ranges for serum concentrations of Lutropin (LH), follitropin (FSH), estradiol (E"), prolactin, progesterone, sex hormone-binding globuline (SHBG), dehydroepiandrosterone sulfate (DHEAS), cortisol and ferritin in neonates, children and young adults. Clin Chem Lab Med. 2002;40(11):1151–60.
24. Curfman AL, Reljanovic SM, McNeils KM, Dong TT, Lewis SA, Jackson LW, et al. Premature thelarche in infants and toddlers: prevalence, natural history and environmental determinants. J Pediatr Adolesc Gynecol. 2011;24(6):338–41.
25. Pasquino AM, Tebaldi L, Cioschi L, Cives C, Finocchi G, Maciocci M, et al. Premature thelarche: a follow up study of 40 girls. Natural history and endocrine findings. Arch Dis Child. 1985;60(12):1180–2.
26. Batubara JRL, Suranto A, Sastroasmoro S, Tridjaja B, Pulungan AB. Natural history of premature thelarche: review of 60 girls. Paediatr Indones. 2001;41:279–83.
27. Teilmann G, Petersen JH, Gormsen M, Damgaard K, Skakkebæk NE, Jensen TK. Early puberty in internationally adopted girls: hormonal and clinical markers of puberty in 276 girls examined bianually over two years. Horm Res. 2009;72:236–46.
28. Kaplowitz PB, Slora EJ, Wasserman RC, Pedlow SE, Herman-Giddens ME. Earlier onset of puberty in girls: relation to increased body mass index and race. Pediatrics. 2001;108(2):347–53.
29. Neely EK, Hintz RL, Wilson DM, Lee PA, Gautier T, Argente J, et al. Normal ranges for immunochemiluminometric gonadotropin assays. J Pediatr. 1995;127:40–6.
30. Neely EK, Wilson DM, Lee PA, Stene M, Hintz RL. Spontaneus serum gonadotropin concentrations in the evaluation of precocious puberty. J Pediatr. 1995;127:47–52.
31. Pescovitz OH, Hench KD, Barnes KM, Loriaux DL, Cutler Jr GB. Premature thelarche and central precocious puberty: the relationship between clinical presentation and the gonadotropin response to luteinizing hormone-releasing hormone. J Clin Endocrinol Metab. 1988;67(3):474–9.
32. Palmert MR, Malin HV, Boepple PA. Unsustained or slowly progressive puberty in young girls: initial presentation and long-term follow-up of 20 untreated patients. J Clin Endocrinol Metab. 1999;84(2):415–23.
33. Kuiri-Hänninen T, Sankilampi U, Dunkel L. Activation of the hypothalamic-pituitary-gonadal axis in infancy: minipuberty. Horm Res Paediatr. 2014;82:73–80.

20

Influences of gender on cardiovascular disease risk factors in adolescents with and without type 1 diabetes

Talia L. Brown[1,2], David M. Maahs[2], Franziska K. Bishop[2], Janet K. Snell-Bergeon[2] and R. Paul Wadwa[2*]

Abstract

Background: Women with type 1 diabetes (T1D) have a four-fold increased risk for cardiovascular disease (CVD) compared to non-diabetic (non-DM) women, as opposed to double the risk in T1D men compared to non-DM men. It is unclear how early in life CVD risk differences begin in T1D females. Therefore, our objective was to compare CVD risk factors in adolescents with and without T1D to determine the effects of gender on CVD risk factors.

Methods: The study included 300 subjects with T1D (age 15.4±2.1 years, 50 % male, 80 % non-Hispanic White (NHW), glycated hemoglobin (A1c) 8.9±1.6 %, diabetes duration 8.8±3.0 years, BMI Z-score 0.62±0.77) and 100 non-DM controls (age 15.4±2.1 years, 47 % male, 69 % NHW, BMI Z-score 0.29±1.04). CVD risk factors were compared by diabetes status and gender. Multivariate linear regression analyses were used to determine if relationships between diabetes status and CVD risk factors differed by gender independent of differences in A1c and BMI.

Results: Differences in CVD risk factors between T1D subjects and non-DM controls were more pronounced in girls. Compared to boys with T1D and non-DM girls, T1D girls had higher A1c (9.0 % vs. 8.6 % and 5.1 %, respectively), BMI Z-score (0.70 vs. 0.47 and 0.27), LDL-c (95 vs. 82 and 81 mg/dL), total cholesterol (171 vs. 153 and 150 mg/dL), DBP (68 vs. 67 and 63 mmHg), and hs-CRP (1.15 vs. 0.57 and 0.54 mg/dL) after adjusting for Tanner stage, smoking status, and race/ethnicity (p <0.05 for all). In T1D girls, differences in lipids, DBP, and hs-CRP persisted even after adjusting for centered A1c and BMI Z-score.

Testing interactions between gender and T1D with CVD risk factors indicated that differences were greater between girls with T1D and non-DM compared to differences between boys with T1D and non-DM. Overall, observed increases in CVD risk factors in T1D girls remained after further adjustment for centered A1c or BMI Z-score.

Conclusions: Interventions targeting CVD risk factors in addition to lowering HbA1c and maintaining healthy BMI are needed for youth with T1D. The increased CVD risk factors seen in adolescent girls with T1D in particular argues for earlier intervention to prevent later increased risk of CVD in women with T1D.

Keywords: Type 1 diabetes, Cardiovascular, Adolescent, Gender differences

Background

Although microvascular outcomes for people with type 1 diabetes (T1D) have improved, cardiovascular disease (CVD) remains the leading cause of death for people with T1D [1] and mortality is still higher than in adults without diabetes (non-DM) [2]. Atherosclerotic changes are known to begin in adolescence in the general population [3–5] and CVD occurs earlier in life and more frequently among people with T1D than in the general population [6]. Women with T1D have at least a four-fold increased risk of CVD compared to non-DM women, as opposed to a doubling of risk in men with T1D compared to non-DM men [7–9]. It is not clear how early in life CVD risk differences begin in females with T1D.

Several other factors have been identified as contributing to increased CVD risk in adults with T1D compared to non-DM including glycemic control and adiposity.

* Correspondence: paul.wadwa@ucdenver.edu
[2]Barbara Davis Center for Childhood Diabetes, University of Colorado Denver, 1775 Aurora Court, Mail Stop A140, Aurora, CO 80045, USA
Full list of author information is available at the end of the article

Intensive insulin therapy resulted in lower glycated hemoglobin (A1c), reduced CVD events and mortality in the Diabetes Control and Complications Trial (DCCT)/ Epidemiology of Diabetes Interventions and Complications (EDIC) study [10, 11]. However, in the DCCT more intensive glycemic control was associated with increased BMI, which was more pronounced in adolescents than in adults [12]. Similarly in adolescents, data from the SEARCH for Diabetes in Youth (SEARCH) study indicate that adolescents with T1D are frequently overweight and obese (22.1 % and 12.6 %, respectively) and were more likely to be overweight than non-diabetic children assessed by the National Health and Nutrition Survey (NHANES) [13]. While not explored in this study, more intensive insulin treatment is likely a contributor [13]. In a recent multinational comparison from the T1D Exchange and the DPV registry median BMI values in youth with T1D were greater than international and their respective national reference values [14].Thus, the added improvement of one major CVD risk factor (A1c) can lead to worsening of another (BMI). However, both weight and glycemic control can be especially difficult for girls with T1D, though it is unclear if increased BMI and A1c for girls during adolescence are the sole factors contributing to increased CVD risk, or if there are other possible risks in girls that are currently unaccounted for [15].

Therefore, our objective was to compare CVD risk factors – glycemic control, BMI, cholesterol, blood pressure, and inflammation - in girls compared to boys to determine how gender affects the relationship of diabetes status with CVD risk. Next, we sought to examine whether these differences are independent of differences in glycemic control and weight by gender and diabetes status.

Methods
Study subjects
A cross-sectional study design was used to assess CVD risk factors in youth with and without T1D. At enrollment, subjects were ages 12-19 years and those with T1D were diagnosed by a pediatric endocrinologist, treated with insulin, had diabetes duration over 5 years at entry into the study, and received care at the Barbara Davis Center for Childhood Diabetes (BDC). Non-diabetic control subjects were friends of study subjects or recruited from campus and community advertisements, and were required to be free from diagnosed diabetes. All had normal fasting glucose and HbA1c levels. No siblings or first-degree relatives of patients with T1D were included. Subjects were excluded for diabetes of any other type, or for a history of abnormal cardiac anatomy or arrhythmia that would preclude the subject from vascular function measurements. The study was approved by the Colorado Multiple Institution Review Board and

informed consent and assent (for subjects <18 years of age) was obtained in all subjects prior to participation in the study.

Study visit
All subjects fasted overnight (≥8 hours) and were asked to refrain from caffeine intake and smoking within 8 hours prior to study visit (to avoid potential effect on vascular measures). Tanner stage for all BDC patients was assessed by a clinician investigator or by the subject's BDC provider. Non-diabetic subjects were requested to have Tanner stage assessed by a clinician investigator with the option of self-assessment if the subject refused a physical exam. Medical history was obtained with standardized questionnaires including methods of insulin administration (injections vs. insulin pump use), dietary habits, and tobacco use. Blood pressure measurements were obtained after a 5 minute rest using a Dynapulse 5200A (PulseMetric, Inc., San Diego, CA) and 3 measurements were averaged. Height was measured by a wall-mounted stadiometer to the nearest 0.1 cm with shoes removed and weight by a Detecto scale to the nearest 0.1 kg [16, 17]. BMI Z-scores were calculated based on the 2000 Centers for Disease Control and Prevention age and gender specific standards [18].

Laboratory assays
A1c was measured using the DCA Vantage (Siemens, Malvern, PA) at the Children's Hospital Colorado (Aurora, CO) main clinical lab. Measurements for total cholesterol, triglycerides, and HDL- cholesterol were performed in the University of Colorado Hospital (UCH) Clinical and Translational Research Center (CTRC) Core lab using Olympus AU400e Chemistry. LDL- cholesterol was calculated using the Friedewald formula [19]. High-sensitivity C-reactive protein (hs-CRP) was measured at the Children's Hospital Colorado (Aurora, CO) CTRC core lab utilizing a multiplex assay platform Siemens (formally Dade Behring) BNII Nephelometer.

Statistical analysis
Participant characteristics were stratified by both diabetes status and gender and examined. Data are presented as means ± SD for continuous variables, geometric mean and range for continuous variables with non-normal distribution, or count and % for categorical variables. Triglycerides (Tg) and hs-CRP were log-transformed for analysis due to non-normal distribution and expressed as mean and range in Table 1. Because of multicollinearity between A1c and diabetes status, a centered A1c variable was calculated which represented absolute deviations from the mean A1c in both participants with and without T1D to allow for adjustment of A1c [20, 21]. Use of this statistical method to calculate deviation from the mean within a

Table 1 Unadjusted characteristics by sex and diabetes status

Variable	Non-diabetic controls N = 100		Type 1 diabetes subjects N = 300	
	Boys (n = 47)	Girls (n = 53)	Boys (n = 152)	Girls (n = 148)
Age, years[1]	14.9 ± 2.1	15.8 ± 2.0	15.6 ± 2.1	15.2 ± 2.1
Race-ethnicity, % NHW[3]	66 %	72 %	80 %	80 %
Type 1 diabetes duration, years	–	–	8.9 ± 2.9	8.6 ± 3.1
Current smoker, %[2]	2 %	9 %	11 %	3 %
Tanner stage, %[1,2]				
I	6 %	2 %	5 %	1 %
II	17 %	2 %	12 %	3 %
III	9 %	20 %	10 %	10 %
IV	34 %	21 %	20 %	35 %
V	34 %	55 %	53 %	51 %
A1c, %[2,3,4]	5.3 ± 0.3	5.3 ± 0.3	8.7 ± 1.5	9.2 ± 1.7
Centered A1c[2]	0.0 ± 0.3	0.0 ± 0.3	-0.3 ± 1.5	0.2 ± 1.7
BMI Z-score[2,3,4]	0.18 ± 1.14	0.39 ± 0.94	0.46 ± 0.78	0.76 ± 0.71
Total cholesterol, mg/dl[2,4]	142 ± 27	149 ± 29	148 ± 29	165 ± 36
Triglycerides[a], mg/dl	70(34-163)	82(43-235)	74(27-326)	78(28-394)
HDL-c, mg/dl[1,2,4]	46 ± 8	50 ± 10	49 ± 9	54 ± 11
LDL-c, mg/dl[2,4]	81 ± 23	81 ± 23	83 ± 22	94 ± 29
SBP, mmHg[1,2,3,4]	111 ± 9	107 ± 8	115 ± 9	112 ± 8
DBP, mmHg[2,3,4]	64 ± 6	64 ± 6	68 ± 7	69 ± 6
Hs-CRP[a], mg/dl[2,4]	0.31(0.03-5.85)	0.48(0.02-9.07)	0.46(0.05-9.2)	0.91(0.04-22)

[a]geometric mean (range)
NHW = non-Hispanic White
[1]$p < 0.05$ for boys vs. girls Non-DM
[2]$p < 0.05$ for boys vs. girls with type 1 diabetes
[3]$p < 0.05$ for Non-DM vs. type 1 diabetes boys
[4]$p < 0.05$ for Non-DM vs. type 1 diabetes girls

group allows for comparison of variability from the mean between 2 groups with non-overlapping distributions, which is expected for A1c in populations with and without T1D. Stratified two sample t-tests were used to look at differences across groups for continuous variables, and chi square tests were used to look for differences for categorical variables.

The relationship of gender and CVD risk factors were compared between youth with T1D and non-DM youth. Multivariable linear regression was used to calculate adjusted least square means to test the relationships of CVD risk factors by gender stratified by diabetes status. Interactions for the relationship between diabetes status and the CVD risk factors by gender were tested. Interactions with p-values less than 0.10 were considered significant. Pair-wise comparisons were made for CVD risk factors stratified by gender and diabetes status. CVD risk factors adjusted for Tanner stage, race/ethnicity, and smoking status were compared by gender for youth with and without T1D and also by diabetes status for each gender.

Secondary analyses were conducted to separately investigate the influence of A1c and BMI Z-score on CVD risk factors comparing youth with T1D to non-DM youth testing for adjusted least square means and interactions stratified by diabetes status and centered A1c and BMI Z-score. Statistical analyses were performed using SAS software, version 9.3 of the SAS System for Windows.

Results

A total of 400 participants enrolled in the study (T1D n = 300, Non-DM n = 100). Distributions for age, gender, current smoking status, and Tanner stage were similar between participants with and without T1D (Table 1). Participants with T1D had mean diabetes duration of 8.8 ± 3.0 years and 55 % were on insulin pumps.

Gender differences

When stratified by diabetes status and gender (Table 1), girls with T1D had higher A1c compared to boys with T1D ($p = 0.01$). Girls with T1D had higher

BMI Z-score ($p = 0.002$), total cholesterol ($p = <0.0001$), LDL-c ($p = <0.0001$), SBP ($p = 0.003$), DBP ($p = 0.04$) and hs-CRP ($p = <0.0001$) compared to boys with T1D. Girls with T1D also had higher HDL-c ($p = <0.0001$) than boys with T1D. In the non-DM participants, boys had higher SBP ($p = 0.008$) than girls and HDL-c ($p = 0.053$) was marginally lower, but there were no significant differences in BMI Z-score, total cholesterol, triglycerides, LDL-c, DBP, or hs-CRP.

Comparing CVD risk factors by diabetes status for each gender, girls with T1D had higher A1c ($p < 0.0001$), BMI Z-score ($p = 0.005$), total cholesterol ($p = 0.002$), LDL-c ($p = 0.001$), SBP ($p = 0.0006$), DBP ($p < 0.0001$), and hs-CRP ($p = 0.002$) compared to non-DM girls. Girls with T1D also had higher HDL-c ($p = 0.03$). In contrast, boys with T1D had higher A1c ($p < 0.0001$), BMI Z-score ($p = 0.04$), SBP ($p = 0.03$), and DBP ($p < 0.0001$), but had similar total cholesterol, triglycerides, HDL-c, LDL-c, and hs-CRP compared to non-DM boys.

Overall, 6.8 % of study participants reported that they were current smokers. Girls with T1D were less likely to be smokers than boys with T1D ($p = 0.02$), while the differences in smoking status between girls with and without T1D ($p = 0.08$), boys with and without T1D ($p = 0.07$), and non-DM boys and non-DM girls ($p = 0.12$) were not significantly different. Because the differences in smoking status reached or approached statistical significance in all comparisons, we adjusted for smoking in subsequent analyses.

Age was significantly different between non-DM boys and girls (non-DM boys: 14.9 ± 2.1 years vs. girls 15.8 ± 2.0 years, $p = 0.04$), while Tanner stage distribution was similar for boys with and non-DM ($p = 0.06$) as well as for girls with and non-DM ($p = 0.18$). As expected, the Tanner stage distribution was significantly different for boys compared to similar age girls with T1D ($p = 0.001$), as well as for non-DM participants in that girls had more advanced Tanner stage compared to boys, regardless of diabetes status (Table 1, $p = 0.01$). We adjusted for Tanner stage instead of age in order to account for any difference in pubertal status related to age difference between groups. There were no significant differences by diabetes status and gender with regards to race/ethnicity, except that a higher percentage of boys with T1D were NHW compared to non-diabetic boys (p = 0.04). Boys and girls with T1D also had similar diabetes duration ($p = 0.35$).

Mean levels for CVD risk factors (A1c, BMI Z-score, blood pressure, lipids, hs-CRP) adjusted for Tanner stage, race/ethnicity, and smoking status are shown by diabetes and gender status in Fig. 1. More atherogenic profiles were seen in univariate analysis in girls with T1D compared to both boys with T1D and non-DM girls. Specifically, girls with T1D had higher A1c, BMI Z-score, total cholesterol, LDL-c, DBP, and hs-CRP than

boys with T1D and non-DM girls ($p < 0.05$ for all). Additionally, girls with T1D had higher SBP than non-DM girls. Boys with T1D had a similar CVD risk profile compared to non-DM boys, except for higher A1c, BMI Z-score and DBP. Girls with T1D also had higher adjusted HDL-c than boys with T1D and non-DM girls. There were significant diabetes by gender interactions for total cholesterol (p = 0.04), LDL-c ($p = 0.02$), and hs-CRP ($p = 0.07$). These interactions indicate that for these specific CVD risk factors, differences were much greater between girls with and without T1D compared to the differences between boys with and without T1D.

To further investigate the more atherogenic CVD risk profile observed in girls with T1D, secondary analyses were performed with additional adjustment for BMI Z-score and centered A1c, to determine if the interactions by gender and diabetes were independent after accounting for the relationships between CVD risk factors and BMI and A1c (Table 2). Adjustment for centered A1c and BMI Z-score attenuated interactions between diabetes and gender for hs-CRP ($p = 0.25$) and total cholesterol ($p = 0.12$), while gender continued to be a significant effect modifier in the relationship between diabetes status and LDL-c ($p = 0.04$). In spite of the decline of significant interactions, the significant trends in increased least squared means CVD risk factors in girls with T1D that were observed in Table 1 and Fig. 1 remained after further adjustment for centered A1c or BMI Z-score, suggesting that girls with T1D have a worse CVD risk factor profile, independent of their increased BMI Z-score and A1c.

A1c and BMI differences

In a separate analysis, interactions with diabetes status and centered A1c as well as diabetes status and BMI Z-score (data not shown) were examined to assess how the relationship between diabetes status and CVD risk factors varied by A1c and BMI. The same CVD risk factors were considered and the models were adjusted for Tanner stage, race/ethnicity, and smoking status. None of the relationships between diabetes status and CVD risk factors varied by centered A1c, meaning there were no significant interactions. Similarly, the relationship between CVD risk factors and diabetes status did not vary by BMI Z-score, indicating that the relationship between diabetes status and CVD risk profile does not appear to be dependent on the BMI or A1c of the participants.

Discussion

In this study, adolescent girls with T1D had a significantly worse CVD risk profile compared to non-DM girls and boys with T1D. Specifically, girls with T1D had higher BMI Z-score, A1c, hs-CRP, total cholesterol, and LDL-c. In contrast, adolescent boys with T1D had a

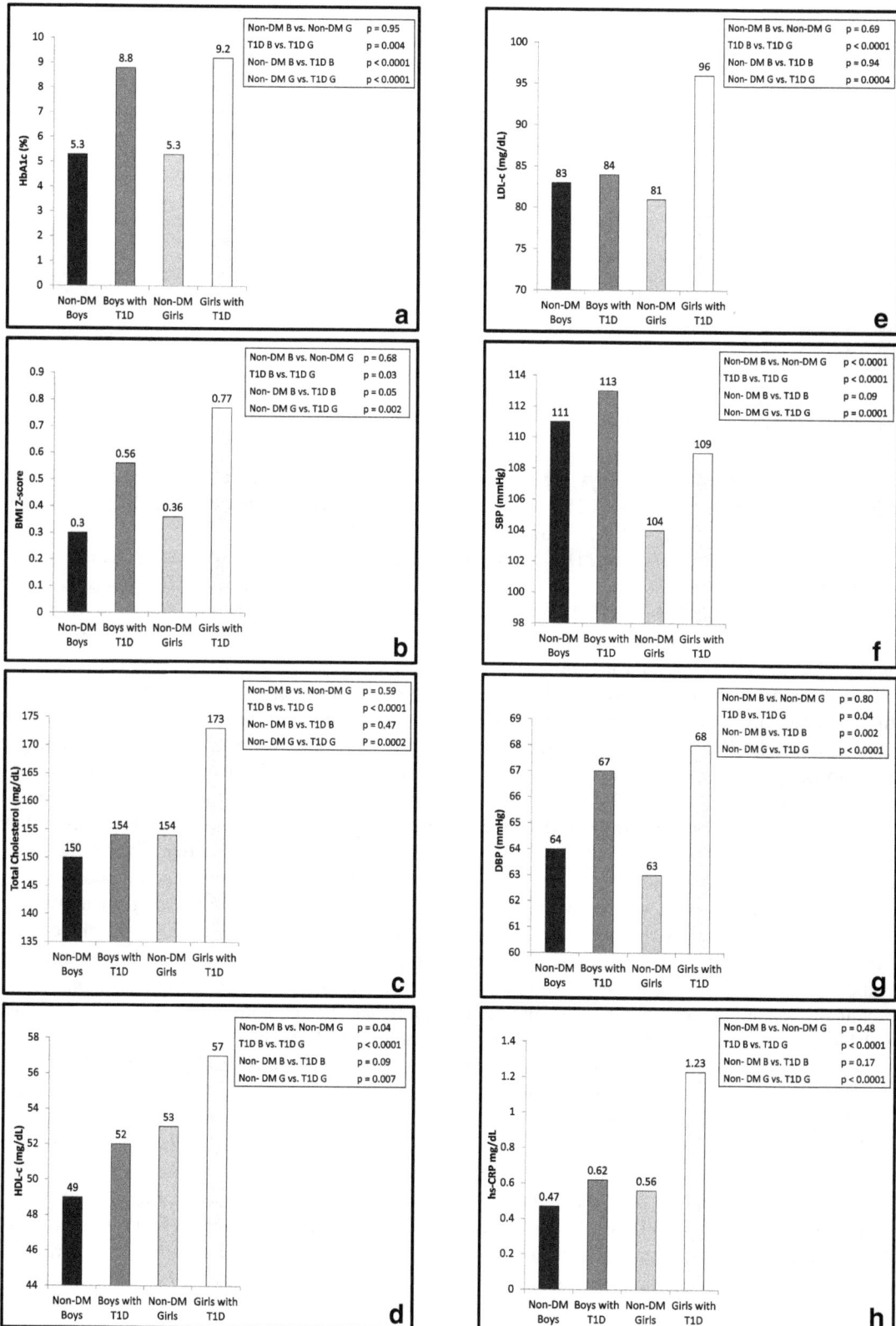

Fig. 1 a-h: Least Square Means for CVD risk factors stratified by gender and diabetes status and adjusted by Tanner stage, race/ethnicity, and smoking status. *P*-values for each respective pair-wise test are also presented in each panel. 1a-HbA1c, 1b-BMI z-score, 1c-total cholesterol, 1d-HDL-c, 1e-LDL-c, 1f-SBP, 1g-DBP, 1h-hs-CRP

Table 2 Cardiovascular disease risk factors by sex and diabetes status adjusted for mean centered A1c and BMI Z-score in addition to race/ethnicity, Tanner stage, and smoking status

Variable	Non-DM		Type 1 diabetes		P-value for interaction
Gender	Boys	Girls	Boys	Girls	All
Total cholesterol, mg/dl[2,4]	151 ± 6	154 ± 5	156 ± 5	171 ± 5	0.12
Triglycerides[a], mg/dl	82(70-96)	86(74-99)	83(73-95)	85(73-95)	0.62
HDL-c, mg/dl[1,2,3,4]	48 ± 2	53 ± 2	52 ± 2	57 ± 2	0.80
LDL-c, mg/dl[2,4]	84 ± 5	81 ± 4	85 ± 4	94 ± 4	0.04
SBP, mmHg[1,2,4]	112 ± 1	105 ± 1	113 ± 1	108 ± 1	0.26
DBP, mmHg[3,4]	64 ± 1	63 ± 1	67 ± 1	68 ± 1	0.30
hs-CRP[a], mg/dl[2,4]	0.52(0.34-0.80)	0.62(0.42-0.92)	0.64(0.45-0.91)	1.03(0.72-1.48)	0.25

Data are mean ± SE unless otherwise indicated
[1] $p < 0.05$ for non-DM boys vs. girls
[2] $p < 0.05$ for boys vs. girls with T1D
[3] $p < 0.05$ for Non-DM vs. T1D boys
[4] $p < 0.05$ for Non-DM vs. T1D girls
[a]denotes geometric least square mean and 95 % confidence interval

similar CVD risk profile to non-DM boys. The higher CRP and lipid levels observed in girls with T1D were not entirely explained by higher BMI and A1c when compared to both boys with T1D and non-DM girls. In addition, secondary analyses indicate that A1c and BMI do not modify the relationship between T1D status and the measured CVD risk factors, while gender appears to modify many of these relationships with more atherogenic CVD risk factors in adolescent girls with T1D. A recent study by Cree-Green et al. similarly found that female, but not male, adolescents with T1D had more atherogenic lipoprotein subfraction distribution which was correlated with insulin resistance [22].

Previous studies indicate that adults with T1D have shorter life expectancies compared to adults without diabetes where women with T1D lose nearly 13 years on average compared to non-diabetic women with 31 % of this difference attributed to heart disease [9, 23, 24]. Other studies have shown that girls with T1D have increased difficulty with maintaining a normal weight and glycemic control during adolescence [15, 25] and have worse lipid levels compared to their male counterparts [26]. The SEARCH for Diabetes in Youth Study found that girls with T1D showed a decrease in health-related quality of life as they aged through adolescence while boys saw an increase in their health-related quality of life during the same ages with physical activity and weight gain being major contributors to sex differences [27]. Other risk factors for increased CVD risk in adolescents with T1D have also been identified, such as increased consumption of sugary drinks [28], poor diet [29] and decreased physical activity [30]. In a previous analysis published on this cohort, we did not observe a difference in diet or physical activity between girls and boys with T1D indicating that these factors are likely not contributing to observed differences within adolescents with

T1D [5]. Though, some reports have shown a decrease in physical activity in girls with T1D compared to girls without diabetes [31].

However, the Coronary Artery Calcification in T1D (CACTI) study and other T1D cohorts have shown that adult women with T1D have similar BMI and A1c levels compared to men with T1D [7, 8]. Therefore, it is possible that even when women with T1D are able to improve their weight and glycemic control as adults, damage done during adolescence may still adversely affect their long-term CVD risk. Our findings suggest that women with T1D may have an increased risk for CVD events due to physiologic phenomenon that happens to girls during adolescence, in addition to exposure to higher A1c levels and other CVD risk factors even if these factors are improved in adulthood.

Other potential pathophysiologic pathways that may contribute to elevated early CVD risk in adolescent girls with T1D should be explored. For example, this study could indicate that there is an additional factor or factors that impact both increased CVD risk factors (including BMI) and glycemic control in women with T1D. We know that women and girls with T1D experience increased sex hormone and menstrual dysfunction compared to women and girls without T1D [32] including increased sex-hormone binding globulin and testosterone, as well as decreased estrogen [33, 34]. As a result, females with T1D also have a higher prevalence of polycystic ovarian syndrome [35], late menarche [36], irregular menstrual cycles, amenorrhea, and early menopause [37, 38]. Menstrual dysfunction can persist despite improved glycemic control [39–41]. Therefore, differences in hormones and pubertal processes and interactions with T1D and insulin treatment for the disease could contribute to difficulties achieving optimal glycemic control and weight management, in addition to increased inflammation, with worse effects in girls with T1D. Additionally, the loss of estrogen protection early in adolescence and greater insulin resistance could contribute to the increased dyslipidemia observed in this population [8, 42].

There are limitations to these data. The data for this analysis was collected cross-sectionally and participants with T1D and non-DM may not be representative of the underlying populations from which they were recruited. However, elevated BMI and A1c in adolescent girls with T1D have been observed elsewhere [15, 25]. Our findings expand upon those studies to highlight the increased CVD risk found in adolescent girls with T1D compared to boys with T1D or non-DM adolescent girls. Moreover, the increased CVD risk factors are independent of BMI and A1c.

Future research should focus more on girls with T1D to explore other factors that make this group especially susceptible to increased CVD risk. Additionally, the observed relationships should be investigated over time to understand at what stage in development the weight and glycemic control have more impact on development of CVD in adults with T1D and how gender and CVD risk in adolescence relates to CVD outcomes later in life. Finally, special clinical consideration and therapeutic interventions should be targeted towards young girls with T1D to address CVD risk factors in addition to achieving A1c targets and maintaining healthy weight to prevent later diabetic complications.

Conclusions

Adolescent girls with T1D have a worse CVD risk profile compared to non-DM girls and boys with T1D. In this study, we found that girls with T1D had higher BMI Z-score, A1c, hs-CRP, total cholesterol, and LDL-c. In contrast, adolescent boys with T1D had a similar CVD risk profile to non-DM boys. Interventions targeting CVD risk factors, lowering HbA1c and maintaining healthy BMI are needed for youth with T1D and may be especially important for adolescent girls with T1D.

Competing interests
The authors declare that they have no competing interests.

Authors' contributions
TLB analyzed data and wrote manuscript; DMM researched, contributed to discussion, and reviewed/edited the manuscript; FKB researched and reviewed/edited the manuscript; JKSB contributed to discussion and reviewed/edited the manuscript; RPW researched, contributed to the discussion and reviewed/edited the manuscript. All authors read and approved the final manuscript.

Acknowledgements
We would like to thank the study participants and their families as well as the staff of the Barbara Davis Center for Childhood Diabetes. Dr. Maahs was supported by a grant from NIDDK (DK075360), Dr. Snell-Bergeon by a Junior Faculty Award (1-10-JF-50) and Career Development Award (7-13-CD-10) from the American Diabetes Association and Dr. Wadwa by an early career award from the Juvenile Diabetes Research Foundation (11-2007-694). This project was supported by NIH//NCRR Colorado CTSI Grant Number UL1

RR025780, Children's Hospital Colorado, Pediatric CTRC M01-RR00069 and a grant from the Diabetes and Endocrinology Research Core P30 DK57516. Its contents are the authors' sole responsibility and do not necessarily represent official NIH views. The authors have no conflicts of interest to disclose.

Author details
[1]Colorado School of Public Health, 13001 East 17th Place, Aurora, CO 80045, USA. [2]Barbara Davis Center for Childhood Diabetes, University of Colorado Denver, 1775 Aurora Court, Mail Stop A140, Aurora, CO 80045, USA.

References
1. Rewers M. Why do people with diabetes die too soon? More questions than answers. Diabetes Care. 2008;31:830–2.
2. Secrest AM, Becker DJ, Kelsey SF, LaPorte RE, Orchard TJ. All-cause mortality trends in a large population-based cohort with long-standing childhood-onset type 1 diabetes: the Allegheny County type 1 diabetes registry. Diabetes Care. 2010;33:2573–9.
3. Berenson GS, Srinivasan SR, Bao W, Newman WP, Tracy RE, Wattigney WA. Association between multiple cardiovascular risk factors and atherosclerosis in children and young adults. The Bogalusa Heart Study. N Engl J Med. 1998;338:1650–6.
4. McGill HC, McMahan CA, Malcom GT, Oalmann MC, Strong JP. Effects of serum lipoproteins and smoking on atherosclerosis in young men and women. The PDAY Research Group. Pathobiological Determinants of Atherosclerosis in Youth. Arterioscler Thromb Vasc Biol. 1997;17:95–106.
5. Bishop FK, Wadwa RP, Snell-Bergeon J, Nguyen N, Maahs DM. Changes in diet and physical activity in adolescents with and without type 1 diabetes over time. Int J Pediatr Endocrinol. 2014;2014:17.
6. Laing SP, Swerdlow AJ, Slater SD, Burden AC, Morris A, Waugh NR, Gatling W, Bingley PJ, Patterson CC. Mortality from heart disease in a cohort of 23,000 patients with insulin-treated diabetes. Diabetologia. 2003;46:760–5.
7. Colhoun HM, Rubens MB, Underwood SR, Fuller JH. The effect of type 1 diabetes mellitus on the gender difference in coronary artery calcification. J Am Coll Cardiol. 2000;36:2160–7.
8. Dabelea D, Kinney G, Snell-Bergeon JK, Hokanson JE, Eckel RH, Ehrlich J, Garg S, Hamman RF, Rewers M, Coronary Artery Calcification in Type 1 Diabetes Study. Effect of type 1 diabetes on the gender difference in coronary artery calcification: a role for insulin resistance? The Coronary Artery Calcification in Type 1 Diabetes (CACTI) study. Diabetes. 2003;52:2833–9.
9. Livingstone SJ, Looker HC, Hothersall EJ, Wild SH, Lindsay RS, Chalmers J, Cleland S, Leese GP, McKnight J, Morris AD, Pearson DWM, Peden NR, Petrie JR, Philip S, Sattar N, Sullivan F, Colhoun HM. Risk of cardiovascular disease and total mortality in adults with type 1 diabetes: Scottish registry linkage study. PLoS Med. 2012;9:e1001321.
10. Nathan DM, Cleary PA, Backlund J-YC, Genuth SM, Lachin JM, Orchard TJ, Raskin P, Zinman B. Intensive diabetes treatment and cardiovascular disease in patients with type 1 diabetes. N Engl J Med. 2005;353:2643–53.
11. Orchard TJ, Nathan DM, Zinman B, Cleary P, Brillon D, Backlund J-YC, Lachin JM. Association between 7 years of intensive treatment of type 1 diabetes and long-term mortality. JAMA. 2015;313:45–53.
12. The DCCT Research Group. Weight gain associated with intensive therapy in the diabetes control and complications trial. Diabetes Care. 1988;11:567–73.
13. Liu LL, Lawrence JM, Davis C, Liese AD, Pettitt DJ, Pihoker C, Dabelea D, Hamman R, Waitzfelder B, Kahn HS. Prevalence of overweight and obesity in youth with diabetes in USA: the SEARCH for Diabetes in Youth study. Pediatr Diabetes. 2010;11:4–11.
14. DuBose SN, Hermann JM, Tamborlane WV, Beck RW, Dost A, DiMeglio LA, Schwab KO, Holl RW, Hofer SE, Maahs DM; T1D Exchange Clinic Network and Diabetes Prospective Follow-up Registry. Obesity in youth with type 1 diabetes in Germany, Austria and the United States. J Pediatr. 2015; 167(3): 627032.e1–4.
15. Meltzer LJ, Johnson SB, Prine JM, Banks RA, Desrosiers PM, Silverstein JH. Disordered eating, body mass, and glycemic control in adolescents with type 1 diabetes. Diabetes Care. 2001;24:678–82.
16. Maahs DM, Prentice N, McFann K, Snell-Bergeon JK, Jalal D, Bishop FK, Aragon B, Wadwa RP. Age and sex influence cystatin C in adolescents with and without type 1 diabetes. Diabetes Care. 2011;34:2360–2.

17. Specht BJ, Wadwa RP, Snell-Bergeon JK, Nadeau KJ, Bishop FK, Maahs DM. Estimated insulin sensitivity and cardiovascular disease risk factors in adolescents with and without type 1 diabetes. J Pediatr. 2013;162:297–301.

18. Centers for Disease Control and Prevention. A SAS Program for the 2000 CDC Growth Charts (ages 0 to <20 years). http://www.cdc.gov/nccdphp/dnpao/growthcharts/resources/sas.htm.

19. Friedewald WT, Levy RI, Fredrickson DS. Estimation of the concentration of low-density lipoprotein cholesterol in plasma, without use of the preparative ultracentrifuge. Clin Chem. 1972;18:499–502.

20. Berlin JA, Antman EM. Advantages and limitations of metaanalytic regressions of clinical trials data. Online J Curr Clin Trials. 1994;Doc No 134. PubMed PMID: 8199744.

21. Neter J, Kutner M, Nachtsheim C, Wasserman W. Applied Linear Statistical Models. Chicago: McGraw Hill College;1996.

22. Cree-Green M, Maahs DM, Ferland A, Hokanson JE, Wang H, Pyle L, Kinney GL, King M, Eckel RH, Nadeau KJ. Lipoprotein subfraction cholesterol distribution is more atherogenic in insulin resistant adolescents with type 1 diabetes. Pediatr Diabetes. 2015. doi: 10.1111/pedi.12277. [Epub ahead of print].

23. Livingstone SJ, Levin D, Looker HC, Lindsay RS, Wild SH, Joss N, Leese G, Leslie P, McCrimmon RJ, Metcalfe W, McKnight JA, Morris AD, Pearson DWM, Petrie JR, Philip S, Sattar NA, Traynor JP, Colhoun HM. Estimated life expectancy in a Scottish cohort with type 1 diabetes, 2008-2010. JAMA. 2015;313:37–44.

24. Lind M, Svensson A-M, Kosiborod M, Gudbjörnsdottir S, Pivodic A, Wedel H, Dahlqvist S, Clements M, Rosengren A. Glycemic control and excess mortality in type 1 diabetes. N Engl J Med. 2014;371:1972–82.

25. Bryden KS, Peveler RC, Stein A, Neil A, Mayou RA, Dunger DB. Clinical and psychological course of diabetes from adolescence to young adulthood: a longitudinal cohort study. Diabetes Care. 2001;24:1536–40.

26. Schwab KO, Doerfer J, Hungele A, Scheuing N, Krebs A, Dost A, Rohrer TR, Hofer S, Holl RW. Non-High-Density Lipoprotein Cholesterol in Children with Diabetes: Proposed Treatment Recommendations Based on Glycemic Control, Body Mass Index, Age, Sex, and Generally Accepted Cut Points. J Pediatr. 2015;167(6):1436–9.

27. Naughton MJ, Yi-Frazier JP, Morgan TM, Seid M, Lawrence JM, Klingensmith GJ, Waitzfelder B, Standiford DA, Loots B. Longitudinal associations between sex, diabetes self-care, and health-related quality of life among youth with type 1 or type 2 diabetes mellitus. J Pediatr. 2014;164:1376–83.e1.

28. Bortsov AV, Liese AD, Bell RA, Dabelea D, D'Agostino RB, Hamman RF, Klingensmith GJ, Lawrence JM, Maahs DM, McKeown R, Marcovina SM, Thomas J, Williams DE, Mayer-Davis EJ. Sugar-sweetened and diet beverage consumption is associated with cardiovascular risk factor profile in youth with type 1 diabetes. Acta Diabetol. 2011;48:275–82.

29. Liese AD, Bortsov A, Günther ALB, Dabelea D, Reynolds K, Standiford DA, Liu L, Williams DE, Mayer-Davis EJ, D'Agostino RB, Bell R, Marcovina S. Association of DASH diet with cardiovascular risk factors in youth with diabetes mellitus: the SEARCH for Diabetes in Youth study. Circulation. 2011;123:1410–7.

30. Centers for Disease Control and Prevention (CDC). Physical activity levels of high school students — United States, 2010. MMWR Morb Mortal Wkly Rep. 2011;60:773–7.

31. Schweiger B, Klingensmith G, Snell-Bergeon JK. Physical activity in adolescent females with type 1 diabetes. Int J Pediatr. 2010;2010:328318.

32. Codner E, Merino PM, Tena-Sempere M. Female reproduction and type 1 diabetes: from mechanisms to clinical findings. Hum Reprod Update. 2012;18(5):568–85.

33. Samara-Boustani D, Colmenares A, Elie C, Dabbas M, Beltrand J, Caron V, Ricour C, Jacquin P, Tubiana-Rufi N, Levy-Marchal C, Delcroix C, Martin D, Benadjaoud L,Jacqz Aigrain E, Trivin C, Laborde K, Thibaud E, Robert J-J, Polak M. High prevalence of hirsutism and menstrual disorders in obese adolescent girls and adolescent girls with type 1 diabetes mellitus despite different hormonal profiles. Eur J Endocrinol. 2012;166:307–16.

34. Snell-Bergeon JK, Sippl R, Brown T. The Role of Sex Hormones in Accelerated Vascular Disease Among Premenopausal Women With Type 1 Diabetes. Circulation. 2011;124:A14003–.

35. Codner E, Escobar-Morreale HF. Clinical review: Hyperandrogenism and polycystic ovary syndrome in women with type 1 diabetes mellitus. J Clin Endocrinol Metab. 2007;92:1209–16.

36. Schweiger BM, Snell-Bergeon JK, Roman R, McFann K, Klingensmith GJ. Menarche delay and menstrual irregularities persist in adolescents with type 1 diabetes. Reprod Biol Endocrinol. 2011;9:61.

37. Strotmeyer ES, Steenkiste AR, Foley TP, Berga SL, Dorman JS. Menstrual cycle differences between women with type 1 diabetes and women without diabetes. Diabetes Care. 2003;26:1016–21.

38. Dorman JS, Steenkiste AR, Foley TP, Strotmeyer ES, Burke JP, Kuller LH, Kwoh CK. Menopause in type 1 diabetic women: is it premature? Diabetes. 2001;50:1857–62.

39. Codner E, Cassorla F. Puberty and ovarian function in girls with type 1 diabetes mellitus. Horm Res. 2009;71:12–21.

40. Picardi A, Cipponeri E, Bizzarri C, Fallucca S, Guglielmi C, Pozzilli P. Menarche in type 1 diabetes is still delayed despite good metabolic control. Fertil Steril. 2008;90:1875–7.

41. Gaete X, Vivanco M, Eyzaguirre FC, López P, Rhumie HK, Unanue N, Codner E. Menstrual cycle irregularities and their relationship with HbA1c and insulin dose in adolescents with type 1 diabetes mellitus. Fertil Steril. 2010; 94:1822–6.

42. Göbl CS, Bozkurt L, Lueck J, El-Samahi M, Grösser P, Clodi M, Luger A, Kautzky-Willer A. Sex-specific differences in long-term glycemic control and cardiometabolic parameters in patients with type 1 diabetes treated at a tertiary care centre. Wien Klin Wochenschr. 2012;124:742–9.

21

Anti-Müllerian hormone as a marker of steroid and gonadotropin action in the testis of children and adolescents with disorders of the gonadal axis

Nadia Y. Edelsztein[1,2], Romina P. Grinspon[1], Helena F. Schteingart[1] and Rodolfo A. Rey[1,3*]

Abstract

In pediatric patients, basal testosterone and gonadotropin levels may be uninformative in the assessment of testicular function. Measurement of serum anti-Müllerian hormone (AMH) has become increasingly widespread since it provides information about the activity of the male gonad without the need for dynamic tests, and also reflects the action of FSH and androgens within the testis. AMH is secreted in high amounts by Sertoli cells from fetal life until the onset of puberty. Basal AMH expression is not dependent on gonadotropins or sex steroids; however, FSH further increases and testosterone inhibits AMH production. During puberty, testosterone induces Sertoli cell maturation, and prevails over FSH on AMH regulation. Therefore, AMH production decreases. Serum AMH is undetectable in patients with congenital or acquired anorchidism, or with complete gonadal dysgenesis. Low circulating levels of AMH may reflect primary testicular dysfunction, e.g. in certain patients with cryptorchidism, monorchidism, partial gonadal dysgenesis, or central hypogonadism. AMH is low in boys with precocious puberty, but it increases to prepubertal levels after successful treatment. Conversely, serum AMH remains at high, prepubertal levels in boys with constitutional delay of puberty. Serum AMH measurements are useful, together with testosterone determination, in the diagnosis of patients with ambiguous genitalia: both are low in patients with gonadal dysgenesis, including ovotesticular disorders of sex development, testosterone is low but AMH is in the normal male range or higher in patients with disorders of androgen synthesis, and both hormones are normal or high in patients with androgen insensitivity. Finally, elevation of serum AMH above normal male prepubertal levels may be indicative of rare cases of sex-cord stromal tumors or Sertoli cell-limited disturbance in the McCune Albright syndrome.

Keywords: Testis, Sertoli, Cryptorchidism, Puberty, Disorders of sex development

Background

In the adult male, the appraisal of the endocrine function of the gonadal axis usually relies on the assessment of serum levels of gonadotropins, testosterone and inhibin B. In pediatric ages, basal testosterone and gonadotropin levels may be largely uninformative. In fact, gonadotropin and testosterone secretion is active only during 3 to 6 months after birth in the male; thereafter, their serum levels remain very low or undetectable until the onset of puberty [1]. However, the use of non-classical biomarkers, like anti-Müllerian hormone (AMH), has become increasingly widespread since it not only informs about the activity of the male gonad without the need for dynamic tests but also reflects the action of FSH and androgens within the gonad [2]. This review will address the usefulness of AMH as a biomarker of testicular function in prepubertal and adolescent males, based on the knowledge of the endocrine regulation of testicular AMH secretion during pre- and post-natal development.

* Correspondence: rodolforey@cedie.org.ar
[1]Centro de Investigaciones Endocrinológicas "Dr. César Bergadá" (CEDIE), CONICET – FEI – División de Endocrinología, Hospital de Niños Ricardo Gutiérrez, Buenos Aires, Argentina
[3]Departamento de Biología Celular, Histología, Embriología y Genética, Facultad de Medicina, Universidad de Buenos Aires, Buenos Aires, Argentina
Full list of author information is available at the end of the article

Developmental physiology of the hypothalamic-pituitary-testicular axis

Testicular function is mainly regulated by the pituitary gonadotropins LH and FSH, which in turn depend on gonadotropin-releasing hormone (GnRH) action, from the hypothalamus. This hypothalamic-pituitary-gonadal axis evolves throughout development, from fetal life through adulthood. Specific maturational changes take place both in these organs as a whole and in the different cell types that make them up.

While sperm production has classically been the focus of adult reproductive function, somatic cells are crucial for the maintenance of spermatogenesis and gamete production. In the interstitial tissue, Leydig cells synthesize androgens and the insulin-like factor 3 (INSL3) [3], whereas in the seminiferous tubules, Sertoli cells regulate the nutrients and factors that reach the germ cells by means of the blood-testis barrier. Sertoli cells not only regulate the inflow of external substances, but also produce several substances which are critical to the proper progression of spermatogenesis [4]. Therefore, it appears evident that the assessment of gonadal function and the definition of male hypogonadism should rely on the understanding of normal testicular physiology resulting from the integrated function of the tubular and interstitial compartments, and its developmental changes from fetal life through maturity [5].

Sertoli cells as the most active population in the developing testis

Unlike the adult testis, where germ cells represent most of the gonadal size and Leydig cells are the most active endocrine cell population, in the prepubertal testis, Sertoli cells are the most numerous [6] and active testicular cell population [7, 8]. Even though Sertoli cells remain active during infancy and childhood, the testes have been erroneously considered as quiescent due to the reduced activity of the hypothalamic-gonadotrope axis. This activity is clearly reflected on the high levels of serum AMH and inhibin B.

Earlier in development, during fetal life and early infancy, the active hypothalamic-gonadotrope axis has effects on the seminiferous cords, reflected in the proliferation of both immature germ and Sertoli cells [9]. Sertoli cell proliferation, essentially dependent on FSH, results in a moderate increase in testicular volume, which cannot be detected by palpation [6, 10–12] but is clearly measurable by ultrasonography [13] (Fig. 1a).

It is around the onset of puberty that Sertoli cells undergo major morphological and physiological changes, leading to the switch from a proliferative, immature state, to a quiescent, mature one. Morphologically, there are changes in the nucleus and nucleolus [14]. The blood-testis barrier becomes distinct, creating two separate compartments within the tubules. Germ cells in the adluminal compartment become dependent on the function of the, now mature, Sertoli cells [15]. These maturational changes observed in Sertoli cells are induced essentially by an increase of intratesticular testosterone concentration early in pubertal development [14, 16]. Interestingly, Sertoli cells do not show maturational changes, in spite of the active androgen testicular production, during fetal and neonatal periods of life. This is due to the fact that before the age of 1 yr in humans [17, 18], the androgen receptor is not expressed in Sertoli cells (Fig. 1b), as experimentally confirmed in mice [19, 20].

AMH as a marker of prepubertal Sertoli cells: physiological concepts

AMH, also known as Müllerian Inhibiting Substance (MIS), is a glycoprotein dimer belonging to the transforming growth factor β (TGF-β) family [21, 22], which plays a major role in fetal sex differentiation by inducing the regression of the Müllerian ducts.

In the male, AMH expression begins when the seminiferous cords differentiate in the fetus [23], and remains high until puberty [23–26] (Fig. 1b and Table 1). The onset of AMH expression in fetal life is independent from gonadotropins, and involves several transcription factors. Initially, SOX9 binds to the AMH promoter [27, 28] and triggers its expression; subsequently, other transcription factors, such as SF1 [27, 29, 30], GATA4 [30, 31] and WT1 [32], further increase AMH production.

Because AMH is exclusively secreted into the circulation by Sertoli cells [33, 34], it has become one of the most useful markers to study testicular function during the prepubertal period in the male [35–37]. In the female, AMH is produced by ovarian granulosa cells of primary and small growing follicles up until transition to menopause [38–41].

AMH as a marker of FSH action in the testis

Once AMH expression is triggered independently of gonadotropins in fetal and postnatal life, FSH further increases testicular AMH output by inducing Sertoli cell proliferation and up-regulating AMH transcription (Fig. 2), which explains why patients with congenital central (hypogonadotropic) hypogonadism have low AMH serum levels that increase after treatment with exogenous FSH [42, 43]. These results clearly demonstrate that serum AMH is an adequate marker of FSH action in the prepubertal testis. The usefulness of serum AMH levels as an indicator of FSH action has also been studied in rodents: the absence of FSH stimulation during fetal and neonatal life results in low levels of AMH due to a decrease in Sertoli cell number and AMH expression, correlating also with smaller testes [44]. FSH administration to neonatal mice provokes an increase in

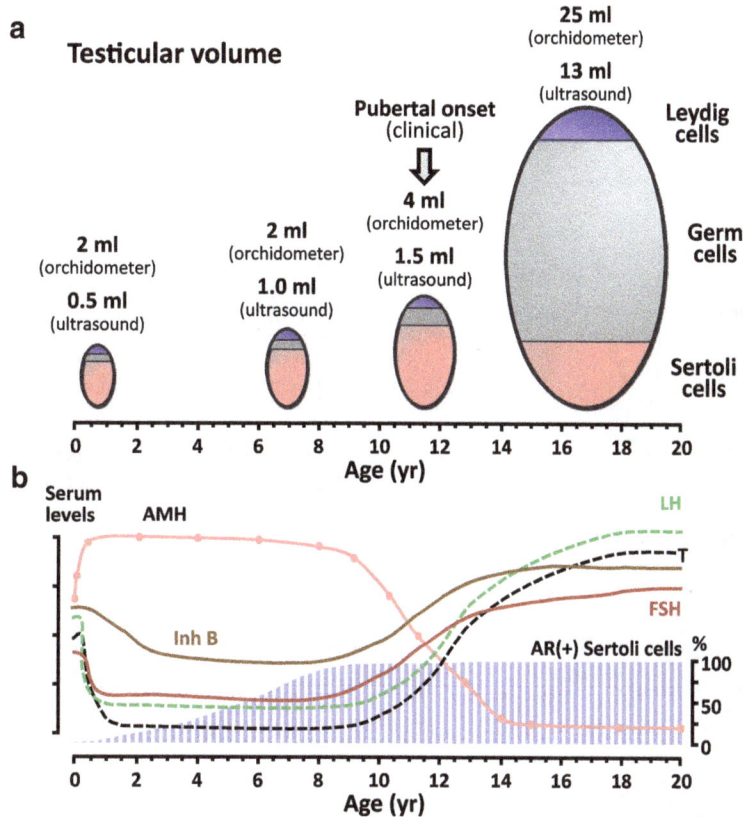

Fig. 1 Developmental physiology of the testis in postnatal life. **a**: Testicular volume increases slightly during infancy and childhood (from birth to the age of 8–10 yr), as measured by ultrasonography, mainly due to the increase of the Sertoli cell population. After pubertal onset, clinically defined by a testicular volume of 4 ml as measured by comparison with the orchidometer, testicular volume increases drastically due to the onset of pubertal spermatogenesis, which requires androgen-dependent Sertoli cell maturation. **b**: Schematic serum levels of gonadotropins (FSH and LH), testosterone (T), inhibin B (Inh B) and AMH from birth through adulthood (left axis) and percentage of Sertoli cells expressing the androgen receptor (AR, right axis). *Reprinted, with permission, from Rey et al. [85], copyright 2009 Wiley-Liss, Inc.*

Table 1 Serum AMH levels in normal boys

Age	Serum AMH	
	pmol/l[a]	ng/ml[a]
<14 days	250–1000	35–140
15 days – 6 months	400–1500	55–210
6 months – 2 years	600–2300	85–320
2–9 years	400–1800	55–250
9–18 years:		
Tanner 1	250–1400	35–200
Tanner 2	70–1000	10–140
Tanner 3	30–400	4–55
Tanner 4	30–160	4–22
Tanner 5	30–150	4–21
Adults	25–130	3–18

[a]Reference levels are taken from refs. [24, 25, 26]. For calculations, 1 ng/ml is equivalent to 7.14 pmol/l

testicular volume and in AMH transcription through the classical FSH receptor transduction pathway involving Gsα protein, adenylyl cyclase and stimulation of protein kinase A (PKA) activity, leading to the involvement of the aforementioned transcription factors SOX9, SF1, GATA4, and also of NFκB and AP2 [2, 20, 44, 45] (Fig. 2).

AMH as a marker of androgen action in the testis

At the onset of puberty, AMH serum levels start declining, as compared to prepubertal levels, and continue to decrease throughout puberty [46] (Fig. 1b and Table 1), as a consequence of the negative effect exerted by intra-testicular testosterone via the androgen receptor [20, 47] (Fig. 3). The androgen-mediated downregulation of AMH expression occurs concomitantly with the appearance of meiotic germ cells in the seminiferous tubules, indicating Sertoli cell maturation [20, 47, 48]. The inhibitory effect of androgens on AMH expression overrides the FSH-dependent stimulation in normal puberty (Fig. 3). The androgen-dependent inhibition of AMH

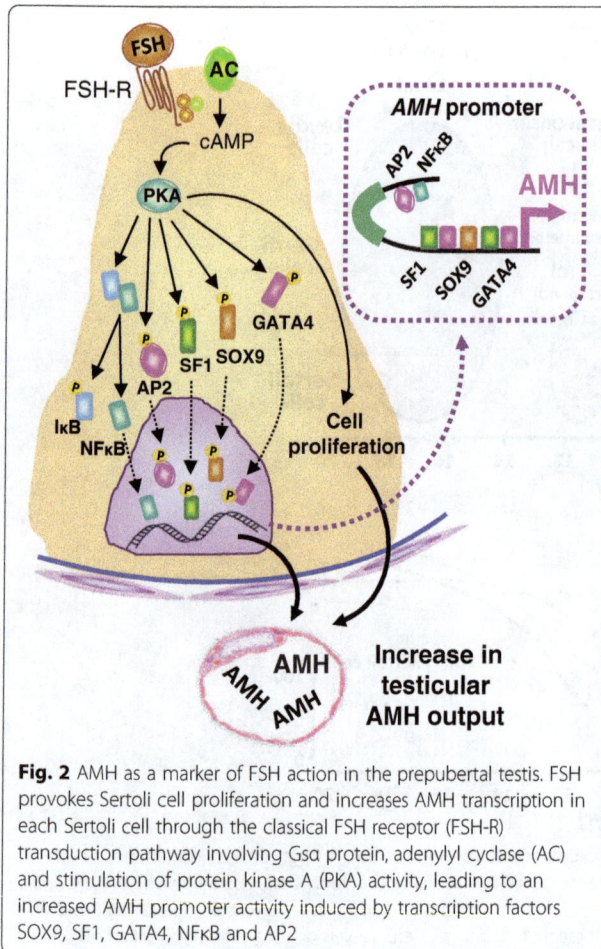

Fig. 2 AMH as a marker of FSH action in the prepubertal testis. FSH provokes Sertoli cell proliferation and increases AMH transcription in each Sertoli cell through the classical FSH receptor (FSH-R) transduction pathway involving Gsα protein, adenylyl cyclase (AC) and stimulation of protein kinase A (PKA) activity, leading to an increased AMH promoter activity induced by transcription factors SOX9, SF1, GATA4, NFκB and AP2

has also been observed in central precocious puberty and in male-limited gonadotropin-independent precocious puberty (testotoxicosis), clearly indicating that androgens are responsible for AMH down-regulation independently of gonadotropin levels [46]. Interestingly, the decline of AMH levels reflects an increase in intratesticular, and not necessarily circulating, testosterone concentration, as observed in the earliest stages of puberty [26, 46]. Conversely, in patients with central hypogonadism treated with exogenous testosterone, serum AMH remains high indicating that intratesticular androgen concentration is low [49]. This is in line with the lack of increase in testicular volume, since pubertal and adult spermatogenesis needs sufficient intratesticular androgen concentration to develop. Similarly, in cases of constitutional delay of puberty [50, 51] or of defective androgen production or sensitivity [20, 52, 53], the lack of androgen production or action results in the maintenance of high AMH levels (Fig. 3).

Androgen-mediated AMH down-regulation is also not observed in fetal life and during the first year of postnatal life (Fig. 3), even in patients with precocious puberty, owing to the above-mentioned physiological androgen

insensitivity of Sertoli cells, which is consequence of the lack of androgen receptor expression in Sertoli cells in those periods of life [17, 18, 54, 55].

Ever since Alfred Jost postulated the existence of AMH [56], it has been referred to as the fetal testicular hormone guiding the regression of the Müllerian ducts in the male fetus. The biological reasons for ongoing expression of AMH throughout childhood have been the source of many debates. Nonetheless, AMH detection in serum has become a very powerful tool in pediatrics. In the following part of this review, we aim to summarize the main conditions in which AMH can be used as a proper marker of Sertoli cell function in boys.

Serum AMH in the diagnosis of conditions affecting testicular function

Cryptorchidism

Cryptorchidism is a clinical sign with many different etiologies [57, 58]. It may be a consequence of primary (usually called hypergonadotropic) or central (hypogonadotropic) hypogonadism, or even result from anatomical defects of the inguinal region or the abdominal wall (i.e. not due to hypogonadism). Cryptorchidism may be associated with normal or impaired Sertoli cell function [59, 60] (Table 2). In boys with bilateral cryptorchidism, AMH is low in approximately 75 % of those with non-palpable gonads and 35 % of those with inguinal gonads, indicating Sertoli cell dysfunction [61].

Non-palpable gonads

In patients with non-palpable gonads, it is necessary to determine whether there is intraabdominal functional testicular tissue. The utility of gonadotropins, as indirect markers, is limited since they may be normal even in anorchid children [1]. Conversely, in boys with non-palpable gonads detectable serum AMH levels are highly predictive of the existence of testicular tissue while an undetectable AMH value is indicative of anorchidism [33, 34] (Table 2). An extremely rare exception is the Persistent Müllerian Duct Syndrome caused by *AMH* gene mutations, which may explain the finding of undetectable serum AMH in a boy with abdominal testes [62]. Vanishing or regression of testicular tissue occurring in the second half of fetal life does not preclude virilization, but micropenis and hypoplastic scrotum occur (Table 2). Serum AMH is low or undetectable, according to the amount of remaining functional testicular tissue [33, 34].

Monorchidism

Monorchidism is the presence of a solitary testis, which may undergo a compensatory volume increase. There is a dissociated capacity of the remaining testis to compensate for the absence of the other gonad: while Leydig cell

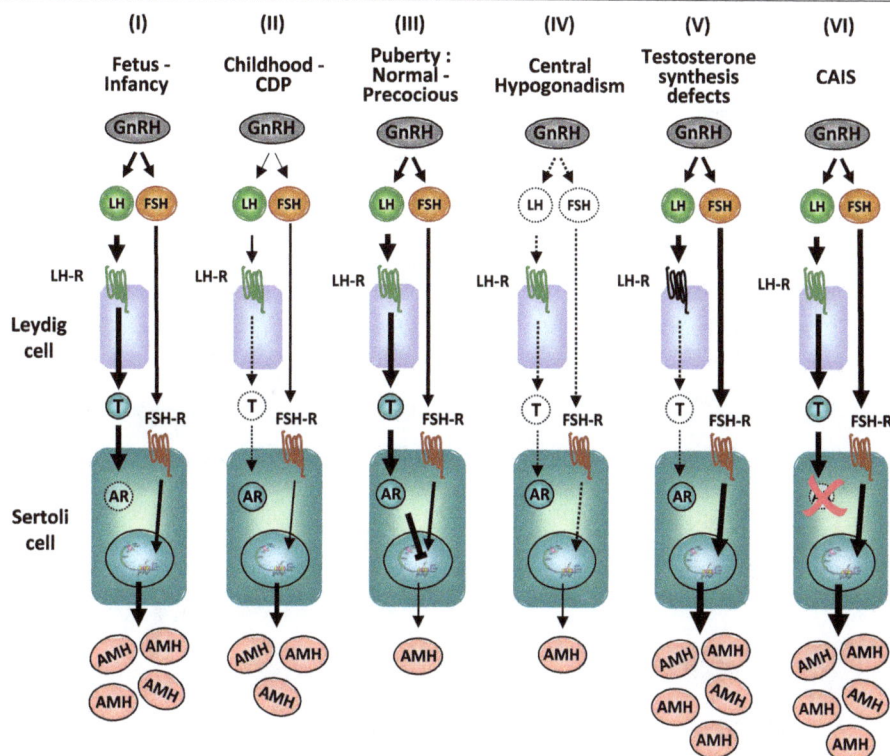

Fig. 3 Regulation of testicular AMH production by FSH and testosterone in normal and pathological conditions. Basal AMH production is independent of gonadotropins or androgens; however, FSH stimulates and testosterone inhibits AMH expression. In the *fetal period and during the first months of postnatal life (I)*, the hypothalamic-gonadotrope is active: FSH stimulates AMH production, whereas testosterone cannot inhibit it because Sertoli cells do not yet express the androgen receptor. During *childhood*, and in boys >14 years-old with *constitutional delay of puberty (II)*, the hypothalamic-gonadotrope is "quiescent", resulting in little or no effect on basal AMH production. In boys with *normal or precocious puberty (III)* with high intratesticular androgen concentrations (central precocious puberty, testotoxicosis, Leydig cell tumors), testosterone inhibition overrides FSH stimulation, resulting in a decrease in serum AMH. In patients with *central hypogonadism (IV)*, only basal AMH production is observed, with no further stimulation or inhibition. In patients with disorders of sex development due to *androgen synthesis defects (V)* or *androgen insensitivity (VI)*, the positive effect of FSH cannot be antagonized by testosterone, resulting in high AMH production in infancy and pubertal age. AR: androgen receptor; CAIS: complete androgen insensitivity syndrome; CDP: constitutional delay of puberty; FSH-R: FSH receptor; LH-R: LH receptor; T: testosterone

function is largely compensated, lower AMH and higher FSH in monorchid boys indicate that Sertoli cell proliferation and function is insufficient to fully compensate the function of the absent one [63].

Klinefelter syndrome

No overt signs of hypogonadism are evident before puberty in Klinefelter syndrome, a sex-chromosome aneuploidy with late-onset testicular dysgenesis. Serum AMH is normal during childhood and early puberty, in correlation with normal inhibin B and FSH, indicating that Sertoli cell function is preserved until advanced stages of puberty [64, 65]. At the onset of puberty, like in normal boys, androgens provoke a physiological decrease in serum AMH also in patients with Klinefelter syndrome. However, in the latter, Sertoli cell function deteriorates progressively from mid-puberty, resulting in extremely low or undetectable AMH, in coincidence with undetectable inhibin B, very high FSH levels and small testis volume. Germ cell degeneration has been described already

in early fetal development with a clear progression during postnatal life, mainly after pubertal onset [66].

Cryptorchidism and micropenis: suspicion of central hypogonadism

During the neonatal period and infancy, some clinical features associated with cryptorchidism, like micropenis and microorchidism, or the coexistence of anosmia or other pituitary hormone deficiencies are suggestive of central hypogonadism. Serum AMH is below the normal range in most cases of isolated central hypogonadism and of multiple pituitary hormone deficiency [42, 43, 49] (Table 2 and Fig. 3), although normal AMH levels do not rule out the diagnosis [67]. The lack of FSH stimulation during fetal and neonatal life is responsible for the decreased Sertoli cell numbers and low AMH expression in patients with congenital hypogonadotropic hypogonadism.[44, 45] The increase in serum AMH in those patients receiving FSH may be useful to monitor treatment efficacy [42, 43, 49].

Table 2 Serum AMH levels according to clinical presentation

Clinical sign	Serum AMH			
	Undetectable	Low	Normal	High
Cryptorchidism	Anorchidism (Testicular regression, bilateral gonadectomy) PMDS - *AMH* mutation	Primary hypogonadism (testicular dysgenesis syndrome) Central hypogonadism	Rules out testicular dysgenesis PMDS - *AMHR* mutation	--
Micropenis	Fetal testicular regression	Primary hypogonadism Central hypogonadism	Malformative micropenis	--
Absence of puberty	Testicular regression Bilateral gonadectomy	Primary hypogonadism Central hypogonadism	Constitutional delay of puberty	--
Precocious pubertal signs	--	Central Precocious Puberty Testotoxicosis Leydig cell tumor	Congenital adrenal hyperplasia Adrenal androgen-secreting tumors Exogenous androgen exposure	--
Prepubertal macro-orchidism	--	--	--	McCune-Albright syndrome Sex-cord stromal tumors
DSD	46,XY Complete gonadal dysgenesis	46,XY Partial gonadal dysgenesis Sex-chromosome gonadal dysgenesis Ovotesticular DSD	Androgen synthesis defects Androgen insensitivity 46,XY Malformative DSD 46,XX male (Testicular DSD)	Androgen synthesis defects Androgen insensitivity

Serum AMH levels are considered low, normal or high as compared to those expected for age in normal boys
AMH-R AMH receptor, *DSD* disorders of sex development, *PMDS* persistent Müllerian duct syndrome

Pubertal delay

Sertoli cells markers have been assessed to distinguish between constitutional delay of puberty and central hypogonadism. AMH is within normal prepubertal levels in boys with constitutional delay of puberty, reflecting a eugonadal state in these patients [51]. In untreated patients of pubertal age with congenital central hypogonadism, serum AMH levels are above those expected for age –reflecting that intratesticular testosterone is too low to inhibit AMH– but below those expected for Tanner stage 1, indicating that Sertoli cells have not been exposed to FSH [49, 68] (Table 2 and Fig. 3). Treatment with recombinant FSH provokes an increase in serum AMH, whereas further administration of hCG results in an elevation of intratesticular androgen levels and a decline in AMH [42, 49]. Conversely, down-regulation of AMH is less notorious when patients receive exogenous testosterone, probably due to the lower intratesticular androgen levels obtained with this treatment [49].

Precocious puberty

Like in normal puberty, serum AMH declines in boys with central or gonadotropin-independent precocious puberty, showing the well-known inhibition exerted by

androgens on Sertoli cell AMH production (Table 2 and Figs. 3 and 4). Low AMH together with increased testosterone levels for chronological age are suggestive of precocious testicular maturation.

Serum AMH determination may be particularly helpful in the diagnostic workup of boys with incipient signs of precocious puberty, e.g. testis volume increase from 2 to 3 ml with or without penile enlargement, in whom basal gonadotropin and testosterone levels are not yet informative. As already mentioned, the decline in serum AMH is an early biochemical sign of the increase in intratesticular testosterone concentration [69]. In infants below the age of 1 yr, AMH may not be useful (Figs. 3 and 4): serum levels are normal, owing to the lack of androgen receptor expression in Sertoli cells at that age, which makes this particular cell population of the testis transiently insensitive to androgens [18].

AMH may also be useful to monitor effectiveness during treatment with GnRH analogues, ketoconazole or anti-androgens. The decrease in testosterone production or action is reflected in the recovery of prepubertal AMH levels [18, 46]. Interestingly, lack of adherence to treatment resulting in intermittent inhibition of testosterone production can be suspected when AMH does not normalize [46].

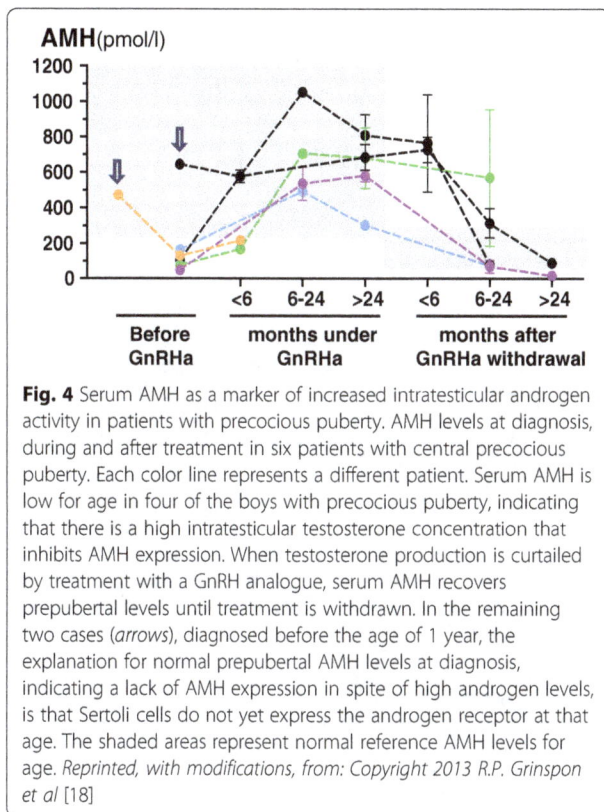

Fig. 4 Serum AMH as a marker of increased intratesticular androgen activity in patients with precocious puberty. AMH levels at diagnosis, during and after treatment in six patients with central precocious puberty. Each color line represents a different patient. Serum AMH is low for age in four of the boys with precocious puberty, indicating that there is a high intratesticular testosterone concentration that inhibits AMH expression. When testosterone production is curtailed by treatment with a GnRH analogue, serum AMH recovers prepubertal levels until treatment is withdrawn. In the remaining two cases (*arrows*), diagnosed before the age of 1 year, the explanation for normal prepubertal AMH levels at diagnosis, indicating a lack of AMH expression in spite of high androgen levels, is that Sertoli cells do not yet express the androgen receptor at that age. The shaded areas represent normal reference AMH levels for age. *Reprinted, with modifications, from: Copyright 2013 R.P. Grinspon et al* [18]

Prepubertal macro-orchidism

Although precocious puberty is one of the classic components of McCune-Albright syndrome, macro-orchidism in the absence of androgen-dependent secondary sexual characteristics has also been reported in boys [70, 71]. In some cases, increased Sertoli cell proliferation was detected by the presence of small hyperechogenic foci in ultrasound imaging [72]. The typical somatic activating mutation in the *GNAS1* gene, encoding for the Gsα protein involved in the FSH receptor transduction pathway, was present only in Sertoli cells, thus resulting in isolated Sertoli cell hyperfunction with Sertoli cell hyperplasia and increased AMH (Table 2), without activating Leydig cells [70].

Sex-cord stromal tumors

AMH immunohistochemistry is useful to identify the sex-cord stromal origin in testicular tumors. AMH expression has been shown in overt Sertoli cell tumors [73, 74], in large cell calcifying Sertoli cell tumors frequently associated with Peutz-Jeghers syndrome [74], in primary or metastatic granulosa cell tumors of the testis [73], and in intratubular Sertoli cell proliferations, which has been suggested to represent an "in situ" or early stage of Sertoli cell tumors [74]. Although a single determination of serum AMH may not be helpful to establish the initial diagnosis of the tumors in most of pediatric cases, because high

AMH is normally found in the prepubertal boy, increasing AMH levels may be suggestive of a progressive lesion.

Cancer survivors

Chemotherapy and radiotherapy affect primarily germ cells of the testis, while steroid secreting Leydig cells are less affected. Sertoli cell function has not been extensively studied in cancer survivors. Two reports including few patients treated with poly-chemotherapy or hematopoietic cell transplantation for medulloblastoma or posterior fossa ependymoma have shown AMH below normal range for age [75, 76], whereas our group could not demonstrate any decrease in serum AMH in a large series of patients with Acute Lymphoblastic Leukemia or Lymphoblastic Lymphoma who received poly-chemotherapy [77].

Ambiguous genitalia

When a 46,XY newborn is born with ambiguous or female genitalia, *i.e.* a 46,XY disorder of sex development (DSD), causes of insufficient virilization should be investigated [78]. 46,XY DSD may result from disorders affecting both tubular and interstitial testicular compartments, like gonadal dysgenesis, or from a condition affecting only the interstitial compartment, like Leydig cell aplasia or steroidogenic enzyme defects. While testosterone is low in both situations, serum AMH is helpful to establish a differential diagnosis since it is low in patients with gonadal dysgenesis but normal or high in patients with isolated androgen deficiency [53, 62, 78–80] (Table 2 and Fig. 3).

Alternatively, the action of androgen in target tissue may be affected in the androgen insensitivity syndrome. In these patients, both Sertoli and Leydig cell activity is preserved, as reflected by normal to elevated serum AMH and androgen levels [53, 62, 78–80] (Table 2 and Fig. 3).

In boys with isolated hypospadias, AMH and testosterone are usually normal, indicating that there is no testicular dysfunction, and a malformative DSD should be suspected. When hypospadias is associated with other clinical manifestations of undervirilization like cryptorchidism, a higher risk of abnormal hormone secretion by the gonads or androgen end-organ defects exists [81, 82].

The Persistent Müllerian Duct Syndrome is a rare form of 46,XY DSD usually diagnosed by the unexpected finding of Müllerian duct remnants during a surgical procedure for cryptorchidism. Serum AMH levels are useful to differentiate its etiology, with normal serum AMH in patients with AMH receptor mutations and extremely low or undetectable AMH levels in patients with AMH gene mutations [62] (Table 2).

In 46,XX DSD patients with ambiguous external genitalia, AMH levels above the normal female range exclude the diagnosis of congenital adrenal hyperplasia, aromatase defects or virilizing tumors, and are highly suggestive of an Ovotesticular DSD [53, 78, 83].

In fully virilized 46,XX DSD patients (XX males), AMH and testosterone are in the normal male range (Table 2), indicating that Leydig and Sertoli cells are not primarily affected [53, 78]. However, germ cells fail to progress through meiosis and undergo apoptosis at puberty, associated with low testicular volume [84].

Conclusions

Serum AMH is an extremely helpful marker for assessing testicular function in pediatric patients. In 46,XY patients with non-palpable gonads and in newborns with DSD, serum AMH is informative about the existence and functional capacity of testicular tissue. Serum AMH levels are commensurate with the amount of functional Sertoli cells present in prepubertal patients, including those with micro- or macro-orchidism, or ovotesticular DSD. Serum AMH is also a reliable marker of FSH action in the prepubertal testis, both in basal conditions to diagnose central hypogonadism and to monitor FSH treatment. Finally, declining serum AMH is indicative of effective androgen action within the seminiferous tubules, and therefore a useful marker in the diagnosis and follow-up of patients with precocious or delayed puberty.

Abbreviations
AMH: Anti-Müllerian hormone; AMH-R: AMH receptor; AR: Androgen receptor; CAIS: Complete androgen insensitivity syndrome; CDP: Constitutional delay of puberty; DSD: Disorders of sex development; FSH-R: FSH receptor; GnRHa: GnRH analogue; INSL3: Insulin-like factor 3; LH-R: LH receptor; MIS: Müllerian inhibiting substance; PKA: Protein kinase A; PMDS: Persistent Müllerian duct syndrome; T: Testosterone; TGFβ: Transforming growth factor β;

Acknowledgements
Not applicable.

Funding
This work was partially supported by grants PIP-11220120100279 of the Consejo Nacional de Investigaciones Científicas y Técnicas (CONICET), Argentina, to RAR and HFS, and PICT 2014-2490 of the Agencia Nacional de Promoción Científica y Tecnológica (ANPCYT), Argentina to RPG.

Authors' contributions
All authors participated in the conception and writing of the manuscript. Its final version was approved by all the authors.

Authors information
Not applicable.

Competing interests
RPG and RAR have received honoraria from the Consejo Nacional de Investigaciones Científicas y Técnicas (CONICET), Argentina, for technology services using the AMH ELISA. NYE and HFS declare that they have no competing interests.

Author details
[1]Centro de Investigaciones Endocrinológicas "Dr. César Bergadá" (CEDIE), CONICET – FEI – División de Endocrinología, Hospital de Niños Ricardo Gutiérrez, Buenos Aires, Argentina. [2]Departamento de Ecología, Genética y Evolución, Facultad de Ciencias Exactas y Naturales, Universidad de Buenos Aires, Buenos Aires, Argentina. [3]Departamento de Biología Celular, Histología, Embriología y Genética, Facultad de Medicina, Universidad de Buenos Aires, Buenos Aires, Argentina.

References
1. Grinspon RP, Ropelato MG, Bedecarrás P, et al. Gonadotrophin secretion pattern in anorchid boys from birth to pubertal age: pathophysiological aspects and diagnostic usefulness. Clin Endocrinol (Oxf). 2012;76:698–705.
2. Lasala C, Carré-Eusèbe D, Picard JY, et al. Subcellular and molecular mechanisms regulating anti-Mullerian hormone gene expression in mammalian and nonmammalian species. DNA Cell Biol. 2004;23:572–85.
3. Ivell R, Wade JD, Anand-Ivell R. INSL3 as a biomarker of Leydig cell functionality. Biol Reprod. 2013;88:147.
4. Petersen C, Söder O. The Sertoli cell - a hormonal target and 'super' nurse for germ cells that determines testicular size. Horm Res. 2006;66:153–61.
5. Rey RA, Grinspon RP, Gottlieb S, et al. Male hypogonadism: an extended classification based on a developmental, endocrine physiology-based approach. Andrology. 2013;1:3–16.
6. Nistal M, Abaurrea MA, Paniagua R. Morphological and histometric study on the human Sertoli cell from birth to the onset of puberty. J Anat. 1982;134:351–63.
7. Chemes HE. Infancy is not a quiescent period of testicular development. IntJAndrol. 2001;24:2–7.
8. Valeri C, Schteingart HF, Rey RA. The prepubertal testis: biomarkers and functions. Curr Opin Endocrinol Diabetes Obes. 2013;20:224–33.
9. Hadziselimovic F, Zivkovic D, Bica DTG, et al. The importance of mini-puberty for fertility in cryptorchidism. J Urol. 2005;174:1536–9.
10. Cassorla FG, Golden SM, Johnsonbaugh RE, et al. Testicular volume during early infancy. J Pediatr. 1981;99:742–3.
11. Main KM, Toppari J, Skakkebæk NE. Gonadal development and reproductive hormones in infant boys. Eur J Endocrinol. 2006;155:S51–7.
12. Kuiri-Hanninen T, Seuri R, Tyrvainen E, et al. Increased activity of the hypothalamic-pituitary-testicular axis in infancy results in increased androgen action in premature boys. J Clin Endocrinol Metab. 2011;96:98–105.
13. Joustra SD, van der Plas EM, Goede J, et al. New reference charts for testicular volume in Dutch children and adolescents allow the calculation of standard deviation scores. Acta Paediatr. 2015;104:e271–278.
14. Chemes HE, Dym M, Raj HG. Hormonal regulation of Sertoli cell differentiation. Biol Reprod. 1979;21:251–62.
15. Sharpe RM, McKinnell C, Kivlin C, et al. Proliferation and functional maturation of Sertoli cells, and their relevance to disorders of testis function in adulthood. Reproduction. 2003;125:769–84.
16. Rivarola MA, Pasqualini T, Chemes HE. Testicular testosterone and dihydrotestosterone during sexual development in humans. J Steroid Biochem. 1983;19:961–4.
17. Chemes HE, Rey RA, Nistal M, et al. Physiological androgen insensitivity of the fetal, neonatal, and early infantile testis is explained by the ontogeny of the androgen receptor expression in Sertoli cells. J Clin Endocrinol Metab. 2008;93:4408–12.
18. Grinspon RP, Andreone L, Bedecarrás P, et al. Male central precocious puberty: serum profile of anti-mullerian hormone and inhibin B before, during, and after treatment with GnRH analogue. Int J Endocrinol. 2013; 2013:823064. doi:10.1155/2013/823064.
19. Majdic G, Millar MR, Saunders PT. Immunolocalisation of androgen receptor to interstitial cells in fetal rat testes and to mesenchymal and epithelial cells of associated ducts. J Endocrinol. 1995;147:285–93.
20. Al-Attar L, Noël K, Dutertre M, et al. Hormonal and cellular regulation of Sertoli cell anti-Müllerian hormone production in the postnatal mouse. JClinInvest. 1997;100:1335–43.
21. Cate RL, Mattaliano RJ, Hession C, et al. Isolation of the bovine and human genes for Müllerian inhibiting substance and expression of the human gene in animal cells. Cell. 1986;45:685–98.
22. Josso N, Cate RL, Picard JY, et al. Anti-Müllerian hormone: the Jost factor. Recent ProgHormRes. 1993;48:1–59.

23. Josso N, Lamarre I, Picard JY, et al. Anti-Müllerian hormone in early human development. Early Hum Dev. 1993;33:91–9.

24. Bergadá I, Milani C, Bedecarrás P, et al. Time course of the serum gonadotropin surge, inhibins, and anti-Mullerian hormone in normal newborn males during the first month of life. J Clin Endocrinol Metab. 2006;91:4092–8.

25. Aksglæde L, Sorensen K, Boas M, et al. Changes in anti-Mullerian hormone (AMH) throughout the life span: a population-based study of 1027 healthy males from birth (cord blood) to the age of 69 years. J Clin Endocrinol Metab. 2010;95:5357–64.

26. Grinspon RP, Bedecarrás P, Ballerini MG, et al. Early onset of primary hypogonadism revealed by serum anti-Müllerian hormone determination during infancy and childhood in trisomy 21. Int J Androl. 2011;34:e487–98.

27. de Santa Barbara P, Bonneaud N, Boizet B, et al. Direct interaction of SRY-related protein SOX9 and steroidogenic factor 1 regulates transcription of the human anti-Müllerian hormone gene. Mol Cell Biol. 1998;18:6653–65.

28. Arango NA, Lovell-Badge R, Behringer RR. Targeted mutagenesis of the endogenous mouse Mis gene promoter: in vivo definition of genetic pathways of vertebrate sexual development. Cell. 1999;99:409–19.

29. Shen WH, Moore CC, Ikeda Y, et al. Nuclear receptor steroidogenic factor 1 regulates the Müllerian inhibiting substance gene: a link to the sex determination cascade. Cell. 1994;77:651–61.

30. Watanabe K, Clarke TR, Lane AH, et al. Endogenous expression of Mullerian inhibiting substance in early postnatal rat sertoli cells requires multiple steroidogenic factor-1 and GATA-4-binding sites. Proc Natl Acad Sci U S A. 2000;97:1624–9.

31. Viger RS, Mertineit C, Trasler JM, et al. Transcription factor GATA-4 is expressed in a sexually dimorphic pattern during mouse gonadal development and is a potent activator of the Müllerian inhibiting substance promoter. Development. 1998;125:2665–75.

32. Hossain A, Saunders GF. Role of wilms tumor 1 (WT1) in the transcriptional regulation of the mullerian-inhibiting substance promoter. Biol Reprod. 2003;69:1808–14.

33. Josso N. Paediatric applications of anti-Müllerian hormone research. Horm Res. 1995;43:243–8.

34. Lee MM, Donahoe PK, Silverman BL, et al. Measurements of serum Müllerian inhibiting substance in the evaluation of children with nonpalpable gonads. N Engl J Med. 1997;336:1480–6.

35. Grinspon RP, Rey RA. Anti-mullerian hormone and Sertoli cell function in paediatric male hypogonadism. Horm Res Paediatr. 2010;73:81–92.

36. Lindhardt Johansen M, Hagen CP, Johannsen TH, et al. Anti-mullerian hormone and its clinical use in pediatrics with special emphasis on disorders of sex development. Int J Endocrinol. 2013;2013:198698.

37. Josso N, Rey RA, Picard JY. Anti-müllerian hormone: a valuable addition to the toolbox of the pediatric endocrinologist. Int J Endocrinol. 2013;2013: 674105.

38. Vigier B, Picard JY, Tran D, et al. Production of anti-Müllerian hormone: another homology between Sertoli and granulosa cells. Endocrinology. 1984;114:1315–20.

39. Long WQ, Ranchin V, Pautier P, et al. Detection of minimal levels of serum anti-Müllerian hormone during follow-up of patients with ovarian granulosa cell tumor by means of a highly sensitive enzyme-linked immunosorbent assay. J Clin Endocrinol Metab. 2000;85:540–4.

40. Hagen CP, Aksglæde L, Sorensen K, et al. Serum levels of anti-Mullerian hormone as a marker of ovarian function in 926 healthy females from birth to adulthood and in 172 Turner syndrome patients. J Clin Endocrinol Metab. 2010;95:5003–10.

41. Broer SL, Eijkemans MJ, Scheffer GJ, et al. Anti-mullerian hormone predicts menopause: a long-term follow-up study in normoovulatory women. J Clin Endocrinol Metab. 2011;96:2532–9.

42. Young J, Chanson P, Salenave S, et al. Testicular anti-mullerian hormone secretion is stimulated by recombinant human FSH in patients with congenital hypogonadotropic hypogonadism. J Clin Endocrinol Metab. 2005;90:724–8.

43. Bougnères P, François M, Pantalone L, et al. Effects of an early postnatal treatment of hypogonadotropic hypogonadism with a continuous subcutaneous infusion of recombinant follicle-stimulating hormone and luteinizing hormone. J Clin Endocrinol Metab. 2008;93:2202–5.

44. Lukas-Croisier C, Lasala C, Nicaud J, et al. Follicle-stimulating hormone increases testicular Anti-Müllerian hormone (AMH) production through

sertoli cell proliferation and a nonclassical cyclic adenosine 5'-monophosphate-mediated activation of the AMH gene. Mol Endocrinol. 2003;17:550–61.

45. Lasala C, Schteingart HF, Arouche N, et al. SOX9 and SF1 are involved in cyclic AMP-mediated upregulation of anti-Mullerian gene expression in the testicular prepubertal Sertoli cell line SMAT1. Am J Physiol Endocrinol Metab. 2011;301:E539–547.

46. Rey R, Lordereau-Richard I, Carel JC, et al. Anti-müllerian hormone and testosterone serum levels are inversely related during normal and precocious pubertal development. J Clin Endocrinol Metab. 1993;77:1220–6.

47. Rey R. Endocrine, paracrine and cellular regulation of postnatal anti-Müllerian hormone secretion by Sertoli cells. Trends Endocrinol Metab. 1998;9:271–6.

48. Rey R, Al-Attar L, Louis F, et al. Testicular dysgenesis does not affect expression of anti-mullerian hormone by Sertoli cells in premeiotic seminiferous tubules. AmJ Pathol. 1996;148:1689–98.

49. Young J, Rey R, Couzinet B, et al. Antimüllerian hormone in patients with hypogonadotropic hypogonadism. J Clin Endocrinol Metab. 1999;84:2696–9.

50. Josso N, Legeai L, Forest MG, et al. An enzyme linked immunoassay for anti-Müllerian hormone: a new tool for the evaluation of testicular function in infants and children. J Clin Endocrinol Metab. 1990;70:23–7.

51. Adan L, Lechevalier P, Couto-Silva AC, et al. Plasma inhibin B and antimullerian hormone concentrations in boys: discriminating between congenital hypogonadotropic hypogonadism and constitutional pubertal delay. Med SciMonit. 2010;16:CR511–7.

52. Rey R, Mebarki F, Forest MG, et al. Anti-müllerian hormone in children with androgen insensitivity. J Clin Endocrinol Metab. 1994;79:960–4.

53. Rey RA, Belville C, Nihoul-Fékété C, et al. Evaluation of gonadal function in 107 intersex patients by means of serum antimüllerian hormone measurement. J Clin Endocrinol Metab. 1999;84:627–31.

54. Berensztein EB, Baquedano MS, Gonzalez CR, et al. Expression of aromatase, estrogen receptor alpha and beta, androgen receptor, and cytochrome P-450scc in the human early prepubertal testis. Pediatr Res. 2006;60:740–4.

55. Boukari K, Meduri G, Brailly-Tabard S, et al. Lack of androgen receptor expression in Sertoli cells accounts for the absence of anti-Mullerian hormone repression during early human testis development. J Clin Endocrinol Metab. 2009;94:1818–25.

56. Jost A. Problems of fetal endocrinology: the gonadal and hypophyseal hormones. Recent Prog Horm Res. 1953;8:379–418.

57. Toppari J, Rodprasert W, Virtanen HE. Cryptorchidism –disease or symptom? Ann Endocrinol (Paris). 2014;75:72–6.

58. Toppari J, Virtanen HE, Main KM, et al. Cryptorchidism and hypospadias as a sign of testicular dysgenesis syndrome (TDS): environmental connection. Birth Defects ResA ClinMolTeratol. 2010;88:910–9.

59. Zivkovic D, Hadziselimovic F. Development of Sertoli cells during mini-puberty in normal and cryptorchid testes. Urol Int. 2009;82:89–91.

60. Cortes D, Clasen-Linde E, Hutson JM, et al. The Sertoli cell hormones inhibin-B and anti Mullerian hormone have different patterns of secretion in prepubertal cryptorchid boys. J Pediatr Surg. 2016;51:475–80.

61. Misra M, MacLaughlin DT, Donahoe PK, et al. Measurement of Mullerian inhibiting substance facilitates management of boys with microphallus and cryptorchidism. J Clin Endocrinol Metab. 2002;87:3598–602.

62. Josso N, Rey R, Picard JY. Testicular anti-Mullerian hormone: clinical applications in DSD. Semin Reprod Med. 2012;30:364–73.

63. Grinspon RP, Habib C, Bedecarrás P, et al. Compensatory function of the remaining testis is dissociated in boys and adolescents with monorchidism. Eur J Endocrinol. 2016;174:399–407.

64. Bastida MG, Rey RA, Bergadá I, et al. Establishment of testicular endocrine function impairment during childhood and puberty in boys with Klinefelter syndrome. Clin Endocrinol (Oxf). 2007;67:863–70.

65. Aksglæde L, Christiansen P, Sorensen K, et al. Serum concentrations of Anti-Mullerian Hormone (AMH) in 95 patients with Klinefelter syndrome with or without cryptorchidism. Acta Paediatr. 2011;100:839–45.

66. Aksglæde L, Wikstrom AM, Rajpert-De Meyts E, et al. Natural history of seminiferous tubule degeneration in Klinefelter syndrome. Hum Reprod Update. 2006;12:39–48.

67. Vizeneux A, Hilfiger A, Bouligand J, et al. Congenital hypogonadotropic hypogonadism during childhood: presentation and genetic analyses in 46 boys. PLoS One. 2013;8:e77827.

68. Rohayem J, Nieschlag E, Kliesch S, et al. Inhibin B, AMH, but not INSL3, IGF1 or DHEAS support differentiation between constitutional delay of

growth and puberty and hypogonadotropic hypogonadism. Andrology. 2015;3:882–7.

69. Rey RA. Mini-puberty and true puberty: differences in testicular function. Ann Endocrinol (Paris). 2014;75:58–63.

70. Rey RA, Venara M, Coutant R, et al. Unexpected mosaicism of R201H-GNAS1 mutant-bearing cells in the testes underlie macro-orchidism without sexual precocity in McCune-Albright syndrome. Hum Mol Genet. 2006;15:3538–43.

71. Mamkin I, Philibert P, Anhalt H, et al. Unusual phenotypical variations in a boy with McCune-Albright syndrome. Horm Res Paediatr. 2010;73:215–22.

72. Wasniewska M, De Luca F, Bertelloni S, et al. Testicular microlithiasis: an unreported feature of McCune-Albright syndrome in males. J Pediatr. 2004;145:670–2.

73. Rey R, Sabourin JC, Venara M, et al. Anti-Mullerian hormone is a specific marker of sertoli- and granulosa-cell origin in gonadal tumors. Hum Pathol. 2000;31:1202–8.

74. Venara M, Rey R, Bergadá I, et al. Sertoli cell proliferations of the infantile testis: an intratubular form of Sertoli cell tumor? Am J Surg Pathol. 2001;25:1237–44.

75. Cuny A, Trivin C, Brailly-Tabard S, et al. Inhibin B and anti-Mullerian hormone as markers of gonadal function after treatment for medulloblastoma or posterior fossa ependymoma during childhood. J Pediatr. 2011;158:1016–1022 e1011.

76. Laporte S, Couto-Silva AC, Trabado S, et al. Inhibin B and anti-Mullerian hormone as markers of gonadal function after hematopoietic cell transplantation during childhood. BMCPediatr. 2011;11:20.

77. Grinspon R, Prada S, Sanzone M, et al. Sertoli cell function was not affected by chemotherapy in boys with acute lymphoblastic leukemia or lymphoblastic lymphoma. Horm Res Paediatr. 2014;82 Suppl 2:21.

78. Rey RA, Grinspon RP. Normal male sexual differentiation and aetiology of disorders of sex development. Best Pract Res Clin Endocrinol Metab. 2011;25:221–38.

79. Lee MM, Misra M, Donahoe PK, et al. MIS/AMH in the assessment of cryptorchidism and intersex conditions. Mol Cell Endocrinol. 2003;211:91–8.

80. Hagen CP, Aksglaede L, Sorensen K, et al. Clinical use of anti-Mullerian hormone (AMH) determinations in patients with disorders of sex development: importance of sex- and age-specific reference ranges. Pediatr Endocrinol Rev. 2011;9 Suppl 1:525–8.

81. Grinspon RP, Rey RA. When hormone defects cannot explain it: malformative disorders of sex development. Birth Defects Res C Embryo Today. 2014;102:359–73.

82. Rey RA, Codner E, Iñíguez G, et al. Low risk of impaired testicular Sertoli and Leydig cell functions in boys with isolated hypospadias. J Clin Endocrinol Metab. 2005;90:6035–40.

83. Grinspon RP, Nevado J, Mori Alvarez ML, et al. 46,XX ovotesticular DSD associated with a SOX3 gene duplication in a SRY-negative boy. Clin Endocrinol (Oxf). 2016;85(4):673–5.

84. Aksglæde L, Jorgensen N, Skakkebæk NE, et al. Low semen volume in 47 adolescents and adults with 47, XXY Klinefelter or 46, XX male syndrome. Int J Androl. 2009;32:376–84.

85. Rey RA, Musse M, Venara M, Chemes HE. Ontogeny of the androgen receptor expression in the fetal and postnatal testis: its relevance on Sertoli cell maturation and the onset of adult spermatogenesis. Microsc Res Tech. 2009;72:787–95.

22

Association of immunohistochemical markers with premalignancy in Gonadal Dysgenesis

Bonnie McCann-Crosby[1*], Sheila Gunn[1], E. O'Brian Smith[2], Lefkothea Karaviti[1] and M. John Hicks[3]

Abstract

Background: Gonadal dysgenesis (GD) is associated with increased risk of gonadal malignancy. Determining a patient's risk and appropriate timing of gonadectomy is challenging, but immunohistochemical markers (IHM) may help establish the diagnosis of malignant germ cell tumors (GCT). Our objective was to identify the prevalence of specific IHM expression in patients with GD and determine if the patterns of expression can help identify malignancy versus pre-malignancy state. We evaluated the published literature using the Grading of Recommendation, Assessment, Development, and Evaluation (GRADE) system to provide recommendations on the predictive role of IHM in the detection of germ cell malignancy.

Methods: The data for this retrospective study included karyotype, gonadal location, external masculinization score, age at time of gonadectomy or biopsy, microscopic description and diagnosis of gonadal tissue, and immunohistochemical staining, including octamer binding transcription factor (OCT) 3/4, placental-like alkaline phosphatase (PLAP), β-catenin, alpha-fetoprotein (AFP), and stem cell factor receptor CD117 (c-KIT). Patients with complete or partial GD who had undergone gonadectomy or gonadal tissue biopsy were included.

Results: The study included 26 patients with GD, 3 of whom had evidence of GCT (11.5 %, gonadoblastoma, dysgerminoma): 2 had Swyer syndrome, 1 had 46,XY partial GD. One patient with XY partial GD had gonadoblastoma-like tissue. All 4 patients (15 %) had strong expressions of 4 tumor markers (OCT 3/4, PLAP, β-catenin, CD117), as did 5 other patients (19 %, ages 2–14 months) without GCT: 4 had XY GD, 1 had 46,XX GD. β-catenin was expressed in 96 % of patients in a cytoplasmic pattern, CD117 in 78 %, OCT 3/4 in 55 %, PLAP in 37 %, and AFP in 1 patient (4 %). Tumor marker expression was not specific for ruling out malignancy in patients <1 year.

Conclusions: In patients older than 1 year, expression of all three markers (OCT 3/4, PLAP, CD117) may be instrumental in the decision-making process for gonadectomy, even in the absence of overt germ cell malignancy. Our literature review suggests that OCT 3/4 expression is most helpful in predicting risk of malignancy. Additional criteria are needed to stratify risk in patients younger than 1 year of age, as these markers are not reliable in that age group.

Keywords: Gonadal dysgenesis, Germ cell tumor, Gonadectomy, Immunohistochemical markers

Background

Gonadal dysgenesis (GD), a condition with interrupted gonadal development leading to gonadal dysfunction, is a subset of disorders of sexual differentiation (DSD). Dysgenetic gonads are characterized by varying degrees of immaturity or dysfunction which can present with a wide range of genital ambiguity. Depending on the gonadal morphology, GD can be classified as either complete (CGD) or partial (PGD) [1]. CGD is characterized by a

* Correspondence: mccann@bcm.edu
[1]Division of Pediatric Endocrinology, Baylor College of Medicine, Texas Children's Hospital, Houston, TX 77030, USA
Full list of author information is available at the end of the article

lack of testicular development, presenting as phenotypic females with bilateral streak gonads. In contrast, PGD is characterized by partial testicular development and often presents with ambiguous genitalia. The gonadal histology in PGD typically consists of hypoplastic testicular tubules intermixed with areas of ovarian-like stroma [2]. Patients with GD who have Y-chromosome material are at increased risk for the development of type II germ cell tumors (GCT), including dysgerminoma (DG) and seminoma arising from their precursor lesions gonadoblastoma (GB) and carcinoma *in situ* (CIS)/intratubular germ cell neoplasia unclassified (ITGCNU), respectively [3]. Early gonadectomy has been recommended for patients with GD who have a Y-chromosome component to prevent the development of malignancy, but recommendations for the timing of the gonadectomy remain controversial. Although gonadectomy is effective in preventing gonadal malignancy, it leads to infertility and requires a lifelong commitment to taking hormone-replacement therapy. Guidelines for a more conservative approach than exclusively performing gonadectomy are lacking.

Determining a patient's risk for development of gonadal malignancy is necessary in the decision-making process for performing a gonadectomy. Certain factors, including the underlying etiology of the GD, location of the gonads, degree of virilization, and certain tumor marker expression in gonadal tissue, are known to influence the risk of developing gonadal malignancy. The risk of developing gonadal malignancy in patients with 46, XY complete GD (CGD; i.e., Swyer syndrome) has been reported to be 15-45 %, whereas the risk is reported to be 15-40 % in patients with partial GD (PGD) who have 45,X/46,XY and other chromosomal variants [4–7]. Gonads that are located intra-abdominally are at higher risk of developing tumors compared to those that are located in the scrotum. Studies also have shown that a correlation exists between the degree of virilization of the external genitalia and the risk of developing gonadal malignancy, with the lowest risk seen in normally virilized males and the highest risk in patients with ambiguous genitalia, reflective of the degree of testicular function [8].

Immunohistochemical markers including octamer binding transcription factor (OCT) 3/4, stem cell factor receptor CD117 (C-KIT), testis-specific protein on the Y chromosome (TSPY) gene, alpha-fetoprotein (AFP), placental-like alkaline phosphatase (PLAP), and β-catenin have been established as markers of germ cell malignancy. Several studies have investigated the use of these markers to assess for early neoplastic changes. OCT 3/4 is a transcription factor that is essential for the maintenance of pluripotentiality of embryonic stem cells and primordial germ cells [9]. Abnormal regulation of OCT 3/4 leads to inappropriate cell survival and has been shown to be present in precursor cells of type II GCTs. β-catenin is involved in regulating cell differentiation and may interact with OCT 3/4 in the transformation of GB into seminoma/DG [10]. CD 117 is the receptor for stem cell factor (SCF), and is responsible for proper migration of primordial germ cells during development. It is present only in immature germ cells and is highly expressed in early stages of germ cell development [11]. Placental-like alkaline phosphatase (PLAP) is a marker for primordial germ cells and is present in CIS and GB [12]. The TSPY gene is thought to act as an oncogene in the context of a dysgenetic gonad, leading to the development of GB [13]. AFP is a well-known marker for GCTs with yolk sac differentiation [14].

The objective of our study was to analyze the premalignant and malignant gonadal pathology findings in patients with GD and to determine the prevalence of specific immunohistochemical marker expressions. Our findings prompted us to evaluate the literature using the Grading of Recommendation, Assessment, Development, and Evaluation (GRADE) system on risk factors that are predictive of malignancy, as this is a major concern for pediatric endocrinologists and urologists when they must decide which patients require gonadectomy, and which may benefit from a more conservative approach with retention of the gonads.

Methods
The protocol for this study was approved by Institutional Review Board at Baylor College of Medicine, Houston, Texas.

Tissue collection and clinical data
Gonadectomy or gonadal biopsy samples from 26 patients with GD were retrieved from the archives of the pathology department at Texas Children's Hospital, Houston, Texas. All samples were reviewed by M.J.H., an American Board of Pathology (Tampa, FL, USA) certified anatomic pathologist experienced in germ cell malignancy and gonadal histology, in order to confirm the diagnosis and determine if adequate tissue from the lesions was available for immunohistochemical evaluation. A patient was considered to have XY GD if there was an XY karyotype and histologic evidence of deficient testicular development. A patient was considered to have XX GD if there was an XX karyotype and histologic evidence of testicular development and ambiguous genitalia. Patients who had complete absence of testicular tissue with a female phenotype were considered to have CGD, whereas patients who had some testicular tissue and ambiguous genitalia were considered to have PGD. Additional clinical data were obtained retrospectively from the medical records and included the patients' karyotype, age at time of gonadectomy or gonadal biopsy, location of gonads, sex assignment, and the external masculinization score (EMS). The EMS is an objective measure of the degree of virilization of the genitalia and takes into account individual features including the presence or absence of scrotal fusion, location of the urethral meatus, penile length, and the location of each gonad [15]. The scores range from 0–12, with a score of 0 representing a phenotypic female and a score of 12 representing a normally virilized male. Patients with lack of detailed external phenotype descriptions or insufficient gonadal tissues for staining and review were excluded.

Immunohistochemical staining

Tissue sections were prepared from formalin-fixed embedded paraffin tissue blocks for hematoxylin-eosin (H&E) staining for routine microscopic examination and for immunohistochemical staining. All routine H&E and immunohistochemical staining were performed in an anatomic pathology laboratory certified by the College of American Pathologists (CAP) (Northfield, IL, USA), using procedures certified by the CAP with appropriate positive and negative controls and using automated H&E (Leica Microsystems, Inc., Buffalo, IL, USA) and immunohistochemical (Leica Bond III Automated Immunohistochemical and *In Situ* Hybridization Biosystem, Leica Microsystems) staining systems that have undergone inspection by the CAP. Automated immunohistochemical staining was performed using proprietary citrate-buffered and surfactant reagents (Novocastra Bond Epitope Retrieval System 1, Leica Microsystems, Inc.) and proprietary antibody kits (Novacastra-Leica Microsystems, Inc.) titrated for OCT 3/4 (clone: NCL-L-OCT3/4), PLAP (clone: NCL-L-PLAP-8A9), β-catenin (clone: NCL-L-B-CAT), CD117 (clone: (c-kit) (clone: YR145 Rab)), and AFP (clone: NCL-L-AFP). Appropriate positive and negative controls for each antibody were utilized. All tissue sectioning, routine H&E staining, and immunohistochemical staining were performed by histotechnologists certified by the American Society of Clinical Pathology (ASCP) (Chicago, IL, USA).

Microscopic examinations of the immunohistochemical staining with each antibody were reviewed concurrently by two examiners (MJH, BMC) in a blinded fashion. The tissue sections from each specimen were evaluated based upon strength of immunoreactivity (negative = 0; weak +; strong ++), origin of tissue immunoreacting (ovarian, testicular), and the cytologic component immunoreacting (cytoplasmic or nuclear).

Statistical analysis

The prevalence of germ cell neoplasia was calculated for each subgroup of GD (XY CGD, XY PGD, and XX GD). Sensitivity and specificity for each immunohistochemical marker were calculated with 95 % confidence intervals. The positive predictive value for each immunohistochemical marker was calculated using Bayes rule, given the reported prevalence of germ cell neoplasia in GD as 15-40 %.

Evaluation of the literature

We identified a clinically relevant question to be answered from the evidence for the management of patients with GD:

In patients with gonadal dysgenesis, is there a predictive role of immunohistochemical markers in the detection of germ cell malignancy?

We searched databases for research-based articles on pediatric patients with GD and immunohistochemical staining. The databases included Pub Med, Cochrane Collaboration, and Google Scholar. We included only articles published in English and studies that included more than five patients. Specific keywords and terms used included: immunohistochemistry, XY gonadal dysgenesis, germ cell tumor, GB, and DG. The GRADE system was used to evaluate the literature and provide recommendations [16]. The quality of the evidence was evaluated as "very-low quality," "low quality," "moderate quality," or "high quality." The recommendations provided were either "strong" or "weak".

Results

The clinical data for the 26 cases included in this study are shown in Table 1. Patient 14 had a right gonadectomy at age 12 months and a left testicular biopsy at 33 months, thus a total of 27 gonadal samples were reviewed in this study. Twenty patients had XY PGD, four patients had XX PGD, and two patients had XY CGD. The age at the time of gonadectomy or gonadal biopsy ranged from 2 months to 18 years (median, 20 months). Three patients (11.5 %) had evidence of GCT, two of whom had XY CGD and one who had XY PGD. Both of the XY CGD patients had both a GB (Fig. 1) and DG (Fig. 2), whereas the patient with XY PGD had only a GB. An additional patient with XY PGD had tissue resembling a GB (Fig. 3) and was classified as having *in-situ* neoplasia.

The immunohistochemical findings are summarized in Table 1 according to the type of gonadal tissue that was encountered (streak gonad, ovarian and testicular components, testicular tissue, GB-like, GB, and DG). The three patients with a GCT and the one patient with GB-like tissue all showed strong expression of four tumor markers (OCT 3/4, PLAP, β-catenin, and CD117). Five additional patients (patients 10, 13, 14a, 16, and 21) who did not have evidence of GCT on microscopy also showed strong expression of the same four markers. Four of these five additional patients (age ranges, 2–12 months) had XY PGD and one (aged 14 months) had XX PGD. The overall expression of the immunohistochemical markers from all cases was as follows: β-catenin in 96 % of total samples, CD117 in 78 %, OCT 3/4 in 55 %, PLAP in 37 %, and AFP in 4 %.

The sensitivity, specificity, and positive predictive value (given the prevalence of gonadal malignancy in GD as reported in the literature at 15-40 %) were calculated for each immunohistochemical marker individually, as well as the combination of OCT 3/4, PLAP, and CD117 and are shown in Table 2. Positive staining for all three markers (OCT 3/4, PLAP, and CD117) as well as positive staining alone for PLAP showed the highest sensitivity (100 %, 95 % CI 40.2-100 %), specificity (73.9 %,

Table 1 Clinical characteristics and immunohistochemical staining results

Patient	Age	Diagnosis	Sex assignment (M/F)	Karyotype	Gonadal location	EMS out of 12	Malignancy	Gonadal tissue type	OCT 3/4	PLAP	B-Catenin	AFP	CD117
1	6 y	XY PGD	F	45,X[16]/46,X + mar[4], SRY positive	Abdomen	1	No	Streak	-	-	++C	-	+C
2	11 y	XY PGD	F	45,X/46,XY	Abdomen	1	No	Streak	-	-	++C	-	+C
3	12 y	XY PGD	F	45,X/46,XY	Abdomen	1	No	Streak	-	-	++C	-	-
4	16 y	XY PGD	F	45,X[11]/46, X, idic (Y) (q11.21)	Abdomen	1	No	Streak	-	-	++N	-	-
5	7 m	XY PGD	M	45, X/46, XY	L- abdomen R- scrotum	8.5	No	Streak	-	-	++C	-	-
6	7 m	XY PGD	M	45, X/46, XY	L-Scrotum R-abdomen	11.5	No	Streak	-	-	++C	-	-
7	4 m	XX PGD	M	46, XX	Inguinal	3	No	O/T	+C, T & O	-	++C, T & O	-	+C, T
8	6 m	XX PGD	M	46, XX	Inguinal	4	No	O/T	+C, T & O	-	++C, T & O	-	++C, O
9	2 y	XX PGD	M	46, XX	Inguinal	5	No	O/T	+C, T & O	-	-T	-	-T
10	5 m	XY PGD	M	46, XX/46, XXY	L-scrotum R- abdomen	6	No	O/T	++N, T +C, O	++C, T -O	++C, O ++C, T & O	-	++C, O ++C, T & O
11	8 m	XY PGD	M	46, XY with mosaicism for 45, X/46, XY in 40 % of cells	L- abdomen R- scrotum	6.5	No	O/T	-	-	++C	++C	+C
12	9 y	XY PGD	M	46, XY/47, XXY/45,X	Abdomen	8	No	O/T	-	-	++C	-	-T
13	14 m	XX PGD	M	46, XX	L- inguinal R- scrotum	8.5	No	O/T	++N	++C	++C	-	+C, O
14a	12 m	XY PGD	M	45, X/46, XY	R abdomen	8	No	O/T	++N	++C	++C	-	++C
14b	33 m	XY PGD	M	45, X/46, XY	L-scrotal	8	No	Dysgenetic Testis	+N	-	++C	-	+C
15	15 y	XY PGD	F	46, XY and gain of chrom 16p11.2	Inguinal	2	No	Dysgenetic Testis	-	-	+C	-	-
16	2 m	XY PGD	F	45, X/46, XY	Abdomen	4	No	Dysgenetic Testis	++N	++C	++C	-	++C
17	22 m	XY PGD	F	45, X/46, XY	Inguinal	5	No	Dysgenetic Testis	++N	++C	++C	-	+C
18	4 y	XY PGD	F	46, XY with gain of chrom 2q14.1	Inguinal	5	No	Dysgenetic Testis	-	-	++C	-	-

Table 1 Clinical characteristics and immunohistochemical staining results (*Continued*)

Patient	Age	Diagnosis	Sex assignment (M/F)	Karyotype	Gonadal location	EMS out of 12	Malignancy	Gonadal tissue type	OCT 3/4	PLAP	B-Catenin	AFP	CD117
19	16 y	XY PGD	F	46, XY	Inguinal	5	No	Dysgenetic Testis	+C	-	++C	-	+C
20	11 m	XY PGD	M	46, XY	Inguinal	6	No	Dysgenetic Testis	-	-	-	-	-
21	6 m	XY PGD	M	46, XY	L-scrotum R-abdomen	9	No	Dysgenetic Testis	++N	++C	++C	-	++C
22	20 m	XY PGD	M	45, X/46, XY	Inguinal	9	No	Dysgenetic Testis	-	-	++C	-	-
23	7 m	XY PGD	F	46, XY, t(11;16)(q22.1;q12.2)	Abdomen	1	GB-like	GB-like arising from immature testicular tissue	++N	++C	++C	-	++C
24	11 m	XY PGD	M	46, XY	L- abdomen R- scrotum	9.5	L gonad- GB	GB arising from streak-like ovarian tissue	++N	++C	++C	-	++C
25	17 y	XY CGD	F	46, XY	Abdomen	1	GB with DG	DG and GB arising from steak gonad with Ovarian stroma	++N	++C	++C	-	++C
26	18 y	XY CGD	F	46, XY	Abdomen	1	R ovary- GB & DG L ovary- GB	GB and DG arising from streak gonad with Ovarian stroma	++N	++C	++C	-	++C

PGD Partial Gonadal Dysgenesis, *CGD* Complete Gonadal Dysgenesis, *O/T* Ovarian and Testicular Components, *DG* Dysgerminoma, *GB* Gondadoblastoma, - negative staining, + weakly positive, ++ strongly positive, *C* cytoplasm, *N* nuclei, *T* testicular tissue, *O* ovarian tissue

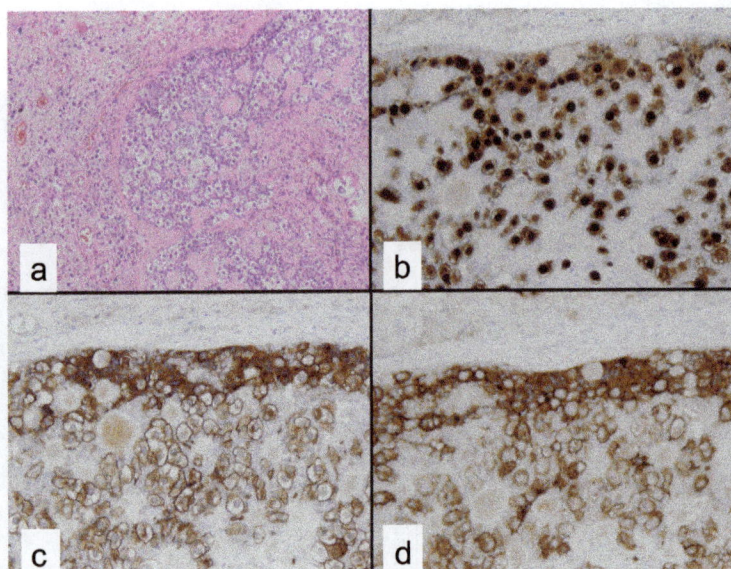

Fig. 1 Gonadoblastoma arising within Gonadal Dysgenesis: **a** Gonadoblastoma with large germ cells with vesicular nuclei, prominent nucleoli and abundant cytoplasm and hyaline globules infiltrating adjacent gonad (H&E stain); **b** Nuclear immunoreactivity with OCT3/4; **c** CD117 (c-Kit) cytoplasmic immunoreactivity; **d** Placental alkaline phosphatase (PLAP) cytoplasmic immunoreactivity

95 % CI 51–89.7 %), and positive predictive value (40.3-71.9 %).

With respect to gonadal location, all samples with germ cell neoplasia originated from abdominal gonads. Three of the four patients with germ cell neoplasia were phenotypic females with an EMS score of 1 (Patient 23 had clitoromegaly and a single introitus which is not accounted for using the EMS scoring system as there is no additional score for clitoromegaly alone), whereas one patient with XY PGD was phenotypically male and had an EMS score of 9.5.

Literature review: evidence and recommendations

In patients with GD, is there a predictive role of immunohistochemical markers in the detection of germ cell malignancy?

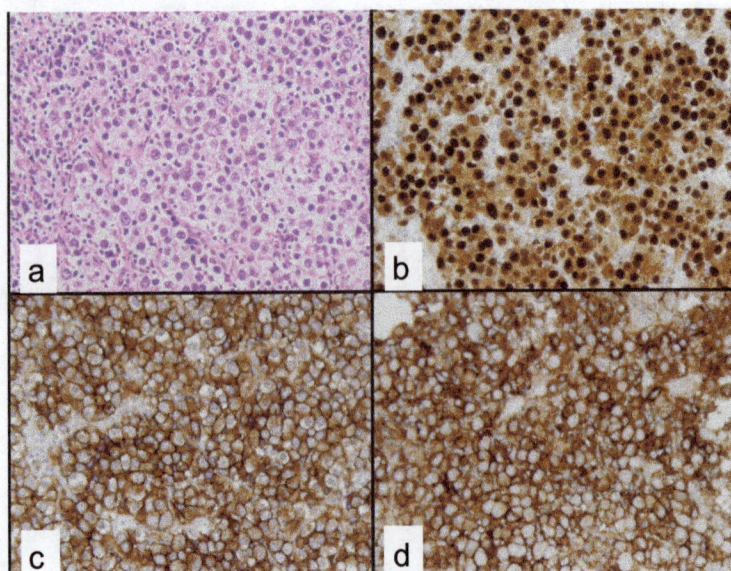

Fig. 2 Dysgerminoma arising within Gonadal Dysgenesis: **a** Dysgerminoma with sheets of round large uniform tumor cells with granular cytoplasm and with lymphocytes in background (H&E stain); **b** Nuclear immunoreactivity with OCT3/4; **c** CD117 (c-Kit) cytoplasmic immunoreactivity; **d** Placental alkaline phosphatase (PLAP) cytoplasmic immunoreactivity

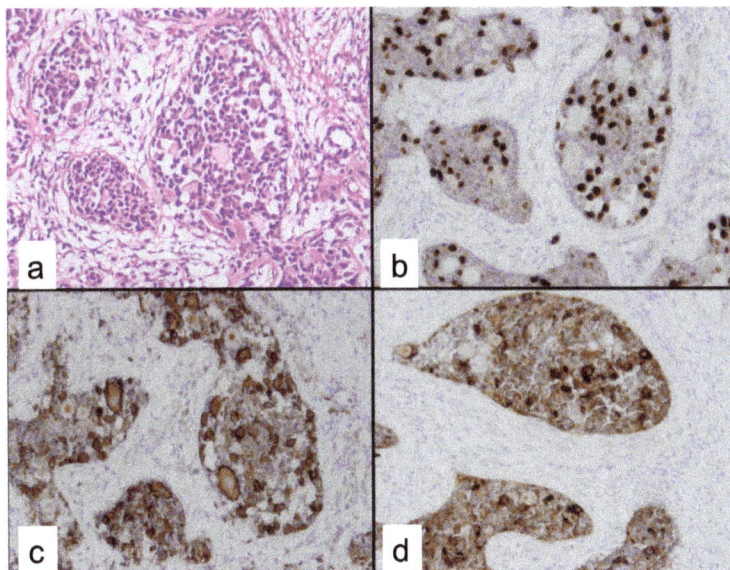

Fig. 3 *In Situ* gonadoblastoma arising within Gonadal Dysgenesis: **a** Several noninvasive gonadoblastoma-like nests comprised of large germ cells with vesicular nuclei, prominent nucleoli, and abundant cytoplasm and hyaline globules (H&E stain); **b** Nuclear immunoreactivity with OCT3/4; **c** CD117 (c-Kit) cytoplasmic immunoreactivity; **d** Placental alkaline phosphatase (PLAP) cytoplasmic immunoreactivity

Evidence

Seven observational studies published between 2001 and 2013 were identified that assisted in answering this question [10, 17–22]. The GRADE tool was used to evaluate the evidence and provide recommendations. These studies are summarized in Table 3.

Among all the immunohistochemical markers evaluated, OCT 3/4 had the most consistent staining intensity for GB and DG, with PLAP and CD 117 showing less consistent expression. Several studies have shown expression of OCT 3/4, PLAP, and CD 117 in undifferentiated gonadal tissue adjacent to GB nests. Multiple studies have suggested that OCT 3/4 -positive immature germ cells in dysgenetic testes or undifferentiated gonadal tissue are at high risk for development of GB [19–21].

The location of OCT 3/4-positive cells has been shown to be important in differentiating between an *in-situ* neoplasia and maturation delay. In one study, all children younger than 9 months old had OCT 3/4-positive cells that were found centrally in the seminiferous tubules, whereas in three older patients with CIS, OCT 3/4-positive cells were located along the basal lamina [20]. The presence of OCT 3/4-positive cells in testicular parenchyma of patients who are younger than 1 year of age is thought to be due to germ cell maturation delay and, thus, cannot be used to diagnose CIS [11].

Recommendations

1. In patients who are older than 1 year of age, the presence of OCT 3/4-positive immature germ cells located along the basal lamina in dysgenetic testes or undifferentiated gonadal tissue confers a high risk for development of germ cell neoplasia and should lead to gonadectomy.

Evidence Quality: Low
Strength of Recommendation: Strong

Table 2 Sensitivity, specificity, and positive predictive value for tumor markers (n = 26)

Tumor markers	Sensitivity (95 % CI)	Specificity (95 % CI)	Positive predictive value given prevalence of gonadal malignancy as 15-40 %
OCT 3/4, PLAP, and CD117 combined	100 % (40.2-100 %)	73.9 % (51.6-89.7 %)	40.3-71.9 %
OCT 3/4	100 % (40.2-100 %)	52.2 % (30.6-73.1 %)	26.9-58.2 %
PLAP	100 % (40.2-100 %)	73.9 % (51.6-89.7 %)	40.3-71.9 %
B-catenin	100 % (40.2-100 %)	4.4 % (0.7-22.0 %)	15.6-41.1 %
CD117	100 % (40.2-100 %)	34.8 % (16.4-57.3 %)	21.3-50.6 %
AFP	0 % (0-59.8 %)	95.7 % (78.0-99.3 %)	0 %

Calculations based on the total case number of 26

Table 3 GRADE evaluation of literature for immunohistochemical markers that can be used to determine high risk of malignancy in GD

Author	Study design and objective	Design limitations / Inconsistency of results / Indirectness of evidence	Sample	Results/Conclusions	Quality
Palma (2013)	Retrospective Observational Study	Insufficient sample size	18 gonadal samples from 15 pediatric patients with 45,X/46,XY PGD	1 patient had GB, 1 patient had DG	Low
	To determine whether OCT 3/4 and β-Catenin are expressed in dysgenetic gonads before GB development and whether TSPY participates in malignant invasive behavior	No inconsistencies	Ages not specified	14/18 samples stained + for OCT 3/4	
		Head-to-Head comparison in correct population		Only 3 samples stained + for β-catenin	
				-Seen in Dysgenetic testes, UGT, GB, and DG, not + in streak tissue or mature germ cells	
				Tissue expressing OCT 3/4 and TSPY is associated with a high risk for GB development.	
				Suggest that β-catenin is not involved in dysgenetic gonad progression to GB, participates after GB is established.	
Barros (2011)	Retrospective Observational Study	Insufficient sample size	32 gonadal samples from 16 patients with Turner Syndrome and Y chromosome material	19 % had + nuclear OCT4 staining, suggesting the presence of germ cell tumor cells (likely GB or CIS)	Low
	To investigate the frequency of gonadal tumors among patients with Turner syndrome and Y-chromosome material	No inconsistencies	Ages 8–18 yrs.	OCT4 immunohistochemistry is more sensitive than conventional H&E staining to indicate the risk of development of germ cell tumors in TS patients	
		Head-to-Head comparison in correct population			
Palma (2008)	Retrospective Observational Study	Insufficient sample size	7 patients with PGD and GB	OCT 3/4 was + in the nuclei of immature germ cells in GB	Low
	To evaluate the participation of β-catenin and OCT 3/4 in the oncogenic pathways involved in the transformation of GB into seminoma/DG	No inconsistencies	Ages 2–33 m	B-catenin was overexpressed in immature germ cells in GB	
		Head-to-Head comparison in correct population		B-catenin and OCT 3/4 co-localized in immature germ cells in GB nests in all cases	
				The proliferation of immature germ cells in GB may be due to an interaction between OCT 3/4 and accumulated β-Catenin in the nuclei of the immature germ cells	
Cools (2006)	Retrospective Observational Study	Insufficient sample size	60 gonadal samples from 43 patients with GD	Incidence of GCTs was 35 %	Low
	To define the histological origin of GB, allowing the identification of high-risk patients	No inconsistencies	Ages 1 m–25 yrs.	Germ cells within GB were + for OCT 3/4, c-KIT, PLAP, and TSPY	
		Head-to-Head comparison in correct population		In UGT found adjacent to GB, OCT 3/4, PLAP, and c-KIT + germ cells were found	
				A gonadal biopsy revealing the presence of UGT with OCT 3/4+ cells on the basal lamina contains high risk for GCT and should lead to gonadectomy.	

Table 3 GRADE evaluation of literature for immunohistochemical markers that can be used to determine high risk of malignancy in GD *(Continued)*

Quality assessment			Summary of findings		Quality
Author	Study design and objective	Design limitations / Inconsistency of Results / Indirectness of Evidence	Sample	Results/Conclusions	
Cools (2005)	Retrospective Observational Study. To distinguish germ cells with maturation delay from those with CIS	Insufficient sample size; Different populations (not looking specifically at GD patients)	58 gonadal samples from 30 patients with undervirilization syndromes. Ages 1 m–23 yrs.	OCT 3/4 was found in all patients <9 m of age. -In young patients and controls, OCT 3/4 + cells were found centrally in the tubule. -In 3 older patients with CIS, OCT 3/4 + cells were found along the basal lamina. Expression of PLAP and c-KIT was similar to OCT 3/4, but less consistent. The presence of germ cells + for OCT 3/4, PLAP, or c-KIT in patients < 1 yr is in accordance with expected maturation delay and is insufficient for the diagnosis of CIS. The location of OCT 3/4 positive cells is important in differentiating between CIS and maturation delay	Low
Kersemaekers (2005)	Retrospective Observational Study. To investigate the pathogenesis of GB and evaluate its relationship to CIS.	Insufficient sample size; No inconsistencies; Head-to-Head comparison in correct population	6 gonads from 5 patients with GD containing GB. Ages 14–21 yrs.	4 patients had DG arising from GB. c-KIT was the least consistent marker. PLAP was + in all GBs and adjacent invasive components. Most of the tumor cells in invasive DG were weakly + or – for PLAP. OCT 3/4 was + in all GBs and DGs. Seen in more immature cells, not mature cells. The development of an invasive germ cell tumor seems to involve selection and clonal expansion of an immature germ cell + for OCT 3/4 and TSPY	Low
Slowikowska-Hilczer (2001)	Retrospective Observational Study. To investigate the appearance of CIS in patients with 46,XY testicular dysgenesis in different ages and in adult patients from other groups	Insufficient sample size; No inconsistencies; Head-to-Head comparison in correct population	23 patients with XY GD. Ages 3 m–7 yrs.	On the basis of PLAP expression, CIS was detected in 10 cases (43.5 %) with GD. GB was found in 4 cases of GD and DG was found in 1 patient with GD (17 years old). Results showed a high prevalence of CIS in XY GD, indicating the importance of early histopathological evaluation of the gonads in these patients	Low

2. In patients who are younger than 1 year of age, caution should be taken in interpreting positive OCT 3/4 cells, as this finding can be reflective of normal delay of germ cell maturation.

Evidence Quality: Low
Strength of Recommendation: Weak

Discussion

We studied 27 gonadectomy and gonadal biopsy samples in 26 patients with GD to investigate pre-malignant and malignant characteristics and identify factors that might be useful in predicting the development of germ cell malignancy and, thus, guide the decision-making process for performing a gonadectomy. Our findings as compared to what has been reported in the literature are summarized in Table 4.

The overall prevalence of GCTs found in the 26 patients with GD included in this series was 11.5 % (n = 3), with an additional patient having evidence of *in-situ* GB-like tissue. Invasive GCTs were found in 7.7 % (n = 2). Excluding the four patients with XX GD, the prevalence of GCTs becomes 13.6 %, which is slightly lower than the prevalence of 15-40 % seen in patients with XY GD as reported in previous studies. An important limitation in interpreting the prevalence of GCT in our study compared to previous studies is our small sample size. All patients in our series with a GCT had abdominal gonads, consistent with previous studies reporting the highest risk of malignancy in abdominal gonads and the lowest risk in scrotal gonads. The age of the patients in our study with *in-situ* or invasive germ cell neoplasia ranged from 7 months to 18 years, with the two older patients (ages 17 and 18 years) having invasive germ cell neoplasia. GB has been described in patients with XY GD younger than 1 year of age [23, 24].

OCT 3/4, CD117, and PLAP are established markers of germ cell malignancy, and these three markers were easily identified in all patients in our series with either *in-situ* or invasive GCTs. Whereas all the immunohistochemical markers besides AFP provided high sensitivity for GCTs, PLAP showed the highest specificity in our study. β-Catenin was identified in 96 % of the samples and, thus, was the least specific for germ cell neoplasia. Consistent with what has been seen in other studies, OCT 3/4 showed robust, nuclear staining and was easily identifiable [25]. Our data suggest that in patients with GD who are older than 1 year of age, the simultaneous expression of OCT 3/4, PLAP, and CD117 should be an indication for performing gonadectomy, as these markers are highly sensitive for germ cell malignancy and pre-invasive lesions. In patients reared as males with mild undervirilization and gonads that can be repositioned surgically into the scrotum, gonadal biopsy with staining for these markers should be considered at the time of orchidopexy to evaluate the malignant potential.

Although OCT 3/4, CD117, and PLAP are highly sensitive, their low specificity renders their use in clinical practice difficult in ruling out germ cell malignancy, particularly when evaluating patients who are younger than 1 year of age. A study looking at these markers in normal fetal testicular development showed that OCT 3/4, CD 117, and PLAP can be present in the germ cells of neonates as germ cell maturation delay or block is expected, and they are unreliable in detecting CIS/ITGCNU in very young children [11]. As seen in our study, two patients younger than 1 year of age had evidence of GB (age, 11 months) or *in-situ* GB-like tissue (age, 7 months); hence, further criteria are needed to identify patients at risk for malignancy in this age group. In these younger patients, surrogate measures including location of gonads, morphology of gonadal tissue, function of testicular tissue

Table 4 Comparison of features between the present study and previous studies

	Present study	Previous studies
Prevalence of germ cell tumor in GD population	11.5 %	15-40 %
Age	7 m - 18 y	Wide age range at presentation. GB has been identified in cases < 1 yr of age.
Location of gonads in patients with malignancy	100 % in abdomen	Abdominal gonads have been shown to have highest risk of malignant transformation.
Degree of virilization in patients with malignancy	3 of 4 pts were phenotypic female.	Low risk: Normally virilized males
	1 pt was ambiguous.	Intermediate Risk: Mild undervirilization
		High Risk: Ambiguous genitalia
Gross pathology findings	3 pts had GB arising from streak gonad with ovarian stroma.	Low Risk: Streak gonad without germ cells, ovary, testis without immature germ cells
	1 pt had GB arising from immature testicular tissue.	High Risk: Undifferentiated gonadal tissue, dysgenetic testicle
Immunohistochemistry	All pts with GCT had strong expression of OCT 3/4, PLAP, β-catenin, and CD117	OCT 3/4, PLAP, β-catenin, and CD117 are established markers of germ cell malignancy.

as determined by hormonal studies, and degree of virilization should be evaluated to determine risk for developing malignant transformation. Future outcomes studies are needed to determine the usefulness of these additional measures in determining the potential for development of a malignancy.

Conclusions

We analyzed our data and used a systematic method to evaluate the literature to provide recommendations for the usefulness of immunohistochemical markers in detecting premalignant and malignant germ cell tumors in gonadal dysgenesis. Our findings are consistent with the literature with regards to the usefulness of OCT 3/4 as a marker that is highly reliable for germ cell malignancy and pre-invasive lesions in patients older than 1 year of age. Our data also demonstrate the usefulness of PLAP and CD117 in addition to OCT 3/4 in assessing premalignant potential. Additional criteria seen in both our study and the literature including abdominal gonads and undervirilization are important risk factors for germ cell malignancy in patients with XY gonadal dysgenesis. It is critical to identify each patient's individual risk for malignancy and careful consideration is required before gonadal biopsy and/or gonadectomy are recommended. As seen in our study, patients younger than 1 year of age can present with germ cell malignancy, however, the use of immunohistochemical markers is not reliable in assessing premalignancy in this age group. Thus, to prevent unnecessary gonadectomy in these younger patients, further studies are needed to evaluate surrogate measures that can be used to predict risk of malignancy. In summary, we have set the stage for evaluation of malignancy risk and the decision-making process for gonadectomy in patients with GD using immunohistochemistry; an approach confirmed by our literature review. We have indicated that surrogate measures need to be elaborated to determine which patients require gonadal biopsy and/or gonadectomy. This paper offers a preliminary overview of the available evidence and what risk factors need to be assessed in anticipation of gonadectomy. A more standardized approach is needed for the management of these patients.

Abbreviations

GD: Gonadal dysgenesis; CGD: Complete gonadal dysgenesis; PGD: Partial gonadal dysgenesis; MGD: Mixed gonadal dysgenesis; GB: Gonadoblastoma; DG: Dysgerminoma; CIS: Carcinoma *in situ*; TSPY: Testis-specific protein-Y; DSD: Disorders of sex development; ITGCNU: Intratubular germ cell neoplasia unclassified; GCT: Germ cell tumor; PLAP: Placental-like alkaline phosphatase; OCT (3/4): Octamer binding transcription factor; AFP: Alpha fetoprotein; SCF: Stem cell factor; EMS: External masculinization score; IHM: Immunohistochemical markers.

Competing interests

The authors declare that they have no competing interests.

Authors' contributions

BMC collected the patient data, reviewed the immunohistochemical staining, performed statistical analysis, performed the literature review, used the GRADE tool to evaluate the literature, and drafted the manuscript. SG critically reviewed the manuscript and made key changes with respect to the design and intellectual content. ES assisted with statistical methods and analysis of data. LK was involved in the initial conception and study design as well as critical review and key changes to the intellectual content. JH participated in the study design, performed immunohistochemical staining and reviewed the pathology, critically reviewed the manuscript and made key changes to the intellectual content. All authors read and approved the final manuscript.

Authors' information

BMC is a third year-pediatric endocrinology fellow at Baylor College of Medicine, Texas Children's Hospital.
SG is an associate professor of pediatric endocrinology & metabolism at Baylor College of Medicine, Texas Children's Hospital.
ES is a professor of statistics at Baylor College of Medicine, Children's Nutrition Research Center.
LK is a professor of pediatric endocrinology & metabolism at Baylor College of Medicine, Texas Children's Hospital.
MJH is a professor of pathology at Baylor College of Medicine, Texas Children's Hospital.

Acknowledgements

The authors thank Dr. B. Lee Ligon, Center for Research, Innovation and Scholarship (CRIS), Dept. of Pediatrics, BCM, for editorial assistance. They also thank several members of the Gender Medicine Team at Texas Children's Hospital for their support of this project: Dr. Jennifer Dietrich, associate professor and chief of pediatric and adolescent gynecology at Baylor College of Medicine; Dr. David Roth, a professor and chief of pediatric urology at Baylor College of Medicine; and Dr. Laurence McCullough, a professor of medicine and medical ethics and chair for medical ethics and health policy at Baylor College of Medicine. Finally, the authors thank Dr. Jake Kushner, Chief of Pediatric Diabetes and Endocrinology at Baylor College of Medicine for his support of this paper.

Author details

¹Division of Pediatric Endocrinology, Baylor College of Medicine, Texas Children's Hospital, Houston, TX 77030, USA. ²Department of Pediatrics, Children's Nutrition Research Center, Baylor College of Medicine, Houston, TX 77030, USA. ³Department of Pathology, Baylor College of Medicine, Texas Children's Hospital, Houston, TX 77030, USA.

References

1. Ostrer H. 46,XY Disorder of Sex Development and 46,XY Complete Gonadal Dysgenesis. In: Pagon RA, Adam MP, Ardinger HH, Wallace SE, Amemiya A, Bean LJH, Bird TD, Dolan CR, Fong CT, Smith RJH, Stephens K, editors. Seattle (WA): GeneReviews(R); 1993.
2. Berkovitz GD, Fechner PY, Zacur HW, Rock JA, Snyder 3rd HM, Migeon CJ, et al. Clinical and pathologic spectrum of 46, XY gonadal dysgenesis: its relevance to the understanding of sex differentiation. Medicine. 1991;70(6):375–83.
3. Verp MS, Simpson JL. Abnormal sexual differentiation and neoplasia. Cancer Genet Cytogenet. 1987;25(2):191–218.
4. Cools M, Drop SL, Wolffenbuttel KP, Oosterhuis JW, Looijenga LH. Germ cell tumors in the intersex gonad: old paths, new directions, moving frontiers. Endocr Rev. 2006;27(5):468–84. doi:10.1210/er.2006-0005.
5. Pleskacova J, Hersmus R, Oosterhuis JW, Setyawati BA, Faradz SM, Cools M, et al. Tumor risk in disorders of sex development. Sex Dev. 2010;4(4–5):259–69. doi:10.1159/000314536.
6. Rocha VB, Guerra-Junior G, Marques-de-Faria AP, de Mello MP, Maciel-Guerra AT. Complete gonadal dysgenesis in clinical practice: the 46, XY karyotype accounts for more than one third of cases. Fertil Steril. 2011;96(6):1431–4. doi:10.1016/j.fertnstert.2011.09.009.

7. Michala L, Goswami D, Creighton SM, Conway GS. Swyer syndrome: presentation and outcomes. BJOG. 2008;115(6):737–41. doi:10.1111/j.1471-0528.2008.01703.x.

8. Cools M, Pleskacova J, Stoop H, Hoebeke P, Van Laecke E, Drop SL, et al. Gonadal pathology and tumor risk in relation to clinical characteristics in patients with 45, X/46, XY mosaicism. J Clin Endocrinol Metab. 2011;96(7):E1171–80. doi:10.1210/jc.2011-0232.

9. Nichols J, Zevnik B, Anastassiadis K, Niwa H, Klewe-Nebenius D, Chambers I, et al. Formation of pluripotent stem cells in the mammalian embryo depends on the POU transcription factor Oct4. Cell. 1998;95(3):379–91.

10. Palma I, Pena RY, Contreras A, Ceballos-Reyes G, Coyote N, Erana L, et al. Participation of OCT3/4 and beta-catenin during dysgenetic gonadal malignant transformation. Cancer Lett. 2008;263(2):204–11. doi:10.1016/j.canlet.2008.01.019.

11. Honecker F, Stoop H, de Krijger RR, Chris Lau YF, Bokemeyer C, Looijenga LH. Pathobiological implications of the expression of markers of testicular carcinoma in situ by fetal germ cells. J Pathol. 2004;203(3):849–57. doi:10.1002/path.1587.

12. Jacobsen GK, Norgaard-Pedersen B. Placental alkaline phosphatase in testicular germ cell tumours and in carcinoma-in-situ of the testis. An immunohistochemical study. Acta pathologica, microbiologica, et immunologica Scandinavica Section A. Pathology. 1984;92(5):323–9.

13. Li Y, Vilain E, Conte F, Rajpert-De Meyts E, Lau YF. Testis-specific protein Y-encoded gene is expressed in early and late stages of gonadoblastoma and testicular carcinoma in situ. Urol Oncol. 2007;25(2):141–6. doi:10.1016/j.urolonc.2006.08.002.

14. Talerman A, Haije WG, Baggerman L. Serum alphafetoprotein (AFP) in diagnosis and management of endodermal sinus (yolk sac) tumor and mixed germ cell tumor of the ovary. Cancer. 1978;41(1):272–8.

15. Ahmed SF, Khwaja O, Hughes IA. The role of a clinical score in the assessment of ambiguous genitalia. BJU Int. 2000;85(1):120–4.

16. Atkins D, Best D, Briss PA, Eccles M, Falck-Ytter Y, Flottorp S, et al. Grading quality of evidence and strength of recommendations. BMJ. 2004;328(7454):1490. doi:10.1136/bmj.328.7454.1490.

17. Palma I, Garibay N, Pena-Yolanda R, Contreras A, Raya A, Dominguez C, et al. Utility of OCT3/4, TSPY and beta-catenin as biological markers for gonadoblastoma formation and malignant germ cell tumor development in dysgenetic gonads. Dis Markers. 2013;34(6):419–24. doi:10.3233/DMA-130972.

18. Barros BA, Moraes SG, Coeli FB, Assumpcao JG, De Mello MP, Maciel-Guerra AT, et al. OCT4 immunohistochemistry may be necessary to identify the real risk of gonadal tumors in patients with Turner syndrome and Y chromosome sequences. Hum Reprod. 2011;26(12):3450–5. doi:10.1093/humrep/der310.

19. Cools M, Stoop H, Kersemaekers AM, Drop SL, Wolffenbuttel KP, Bourguignon JP, et al. Gonadoblastoma arising in undifferentiated gonadal tissue within dysgenetic gonads. J Clin Endocrinol Metab. 2006;91(6):2404–13. doi:10.1210/jc.2005-2554.

20. Cools M, van Aerde K, Kersemaekers AM, Boter M, Drop SL, Wolffenbuttel KP, et al. Morphological and immunohistochemical differences between gonadal maturation delay and early germ cell neoplasia in patients with undervirilization syndromes. J Clin Endocrinol Metab. 2005;90(9):5295–303. doi:10.1210/jc.2005-0139.

21. Kersemaekers AM, Honecker F, Stoop H, Cools M, Molier M, Wolffenbuttel K, et al. Identification of germ cells at risk for neoplastic transformation in gonadoblastoma: an immunohistochemical study for OCT3/4 and TSPY. Hum Pathol. 2005;36(5):512–21. doi:10.1016/j.humpath.2005.02.016.

22. Slowikowska-Hilczer J, Walczak-Jedrzejowska R, Kula K. Immunohistochemical diagnosis of preinvasive germ cell cancer of the testis. Folia Histochem Cytobiol. 2001;39(2):67–72.

23. Dumic M, Jukic S, Batinica S, Ille J, Filipovic-Grcic B. Bilateral gonadoblastoma in a 9-month-old infant with 46, XY gonadal dysgenesis. J Endocrinol Invest. 1993;16(4):291–3.

24. Haddad NG, Walvoord EC, Cain MP, Davis MM. Seminoma and a gonadoblastoma in an infant with mixed gonadal dysgenesis. J Pediatr. 2003;143(1):136. doi:10.1016/S0022-3476(03)00132-X.

25. de Jong J, Stoop H, Dohle GR, Bangma CH, Kliffen M, van Esser JW, et al. Diagnostic value of OCT3/4 for pre-invasive and invasive testicular germ cell tumours. J Pathol. 2005;206(2):242–9. doi:10.1002/path.1766.

Permissions

List of Contributors

Peter A Lee
Department of Pediatrics, Milton S. Hershey Medical Center, Penn State College of Medicine, Hershey, PA, USA

John Germak, Robert Gut and Naum Khutoryansky
Novo Nordisk Inc, Princeton, NJ, USA

Judith Ross
Department of Pediatrics, Thomas Jefferson University duPont Hospital for Children, Philadelphia, PA, USA

Maria Isabel Hernandez, Andrea Castro, Ketty Bacallao, Leon Trejo, Germán Iñiguez, Ethel Codner and Fernando Cassorla
Institute of Maternal and Child Research (IDIMI), Faculty of Medicine, University of Chile, Santa Rosa 1234, 2nd floor IDIMI, Casilla, 226-3 Santiago, Chile

Alejandra Avila
Institute of Maternal and Child Research (IDIMI), Faculty of Medicine, University of Chile, Santa Rosa 1234, 2nd floor IDIMI, Casilla, 226-3 Santiago, Chile
Departments of Pediatrics, Hospital Clínico San Borja Arriarán, Santiago, Chile

Aníbal Espinoza
Department of Radiology, Hospital Clínico San Borja Arriarán, Santiago, Chile

Amy M Vedin
Center for Endocrinology, Diabetes, and Metabolism, Children's Hospital Los Angeles, 4650 Sunset Boulevard, Mailstop #61, Los Angeles, CA 90027, USA

Mitchell E Geffner
Center for Endocrinology, Diabetes, and Metabolism, Children's Hospital Los Angeles, 4650 Sunset Boulevard, Mailstop #61, Los Angeles, CA 90027, USA
Saban Research Institute of Children's Hospital Los Angeles, 4650 Sunset Boulevard, Los Angeles, CA 90027, USA

Hanna Karlsson
Pfizer Inc., Pfizer Endocrine Care, KIGS/KIMS/ACROSTUDY, SE-191 90 Sollentuna, Sweden

Cassandra Fink
The Vision Center, Children's Hospital Los Angeles, 4650 Sunset Boulevard, Mailstop #88, Los Angeles, CA 90027, USA

Mark Borchert
The Vision Center, Children's Hospital Los Angeles, 4650 Sunset Boulevard, Mailstop #88, Los Angeles, CA 90027, USA
Saban Research Institute of Children's Hospital Los Angeles, 4650 Sunset Boulevard, Los Angeles, CA 90027, USA

Jill Hamilton and Farid H Mahmud
Divisions of Endocrinology, The Hospital for Sick Children Research Institute, University of Toronto, Toronto, Canada
Department of Pediatrics, The Hospital for Sick Children Research Institute, University of Toronto, Toronto, Canada
Physiology and Experimental Medicine Program, The Hospital for Sick Children Research Institute, University of Toronto, Toronto, Canada

Clodagh S O'Gorman
Divisions of Endocrinology, The Hospital for Sick Children Research Institute, University of Toronto, Toronto, Canada
Department of Pediatrics, The Hospital for Sick Children Research Institute, University of Toronto, Toronto, Canada
Physiology and Experimental Medicine Program, The Hospital for Sick Children Research Institute, University of Toronto, Toronto, Canada
Department of Paediatrics, Graduate Entry Medical School, University of Limerick, Limerick, Ireland

Tim Bradley
Divisions of Cardiology, The Hospital for Sick Children Research Institute, University of Toronto, Toronto, Canada
Department of Pediatrics, The Hospital for Sick Children Research Institute, University of Toronto, Toronto, Canada

Catriona Syme
Physiology and Experimental Medicine Program, The Hospital for Sick Children Research Institute, University of Toronto, Toronto, Canada

Christopher P Houk
Medical College of Georgia, 1120 15th Street, Room BG1007, Augusta, GA 30912, USA

Peter A Lee
Penn State College of Medicine, Milton S. Hershey Medical Center, Hershey, PA 17033-0850, USA

Indiana University School of Medicine, The Riley Hospital for Children, 702 Barnhill Dr, Indianapolis, IN 46202, USA

David H Geller
Division of Pediatric Endocrinology, Cedars-Sinai Medical Center, David Geffen-UCLA School of Medicine 8700 Beverly Blvd., Rm 4220, Los Angeles, CA 90048, USA

Danièle Pacaud
Division of Pediatric Endocrinology, Alberta Children's Hospital, University of Calgary, 2888 Hospital Drive NW, Calgary, Alberta T2N 4Z6, Canada

Catherine M Gordon
Divisions of Adolescent Medicine and Endocrinology, Children's Hospital and Harvard Medical School, 300 Longwood Avenue, 333 Longwood-6, Boston, MA 02115, USA

Madhusmita Misra
Pediatric Endocrine Unit, Mass General Hospital for Children and Harvard Medical School, 55 Fruit Street, Boston, MA 02114, USA

Juan F Sotos
Nationwide Children's Hospital, The Ohio State University – College of Medicine, 700 Children's Drive, Columbus, OH 43205, USA

Naomi J Tokar
Nationwide Children's Hospital, 700 Children's Drive, Columbus, OH 43205, USA

Karl Hager, Kori Jennings and Seiyu Hosono
JS Genetics, Inc, 2 Church St. South, B-05, New Haven, CT 06519, USA

Susan Howell and Nicole R Tartaglia
Children's Hospital Colorado, Aurora, CO 80045, USA

Jeffrey R Gruen
Yale Child Health Research Center, Yale University School of Medicine, New Haven, CT 06520, USA
Department of Pediatrics, Yale University School of Medicine, New Haven, CT 06520, USA
Department of Genetics, Yale University School of Medicine, New Haven, CT 06520, USA
Investigative Medicine Program, Yale University School of Medicine, New Haven, CT 06520, USA

Scott A Rivkees
Yale Child Health Research Center, Yale University School of Medicine, New Haven, CT 06520, USA
Department of Pediatrics, Yale University School of Medicine, New Haven, CT 06520, USA

Department of Pediatrics, University of Florida, Gainesville, FL 32610, USA

Henry M Rinder
Department of Laboratory Medicine, Yale University, New Haven, CT 06510, USA

Franziska K Bishop, R Paul Wadwa, Janet Snell-Bergeon, Nhung Nguyen and David M Maahs
Barbara Davis Center for Childhood Diabetes, University of Colorado Denver, 1775 Aurora Ct, MS F527, 80045 Aurora, CO, USA

Therese A Wiegers
Netherlands institute for health services research (NIVEL), 3500 BN Utrecht, The Netherlands

Sarita A Sanches
Netherlands institute for health services research (NIVEL), 3500 BN Utrecht, The Netherlands
VU Medical Centre, department of Rehabilitation Medicine, room PK -1 Y 158, De Boelelaan 1118, 1081 HZ, The Netherlands

Barto J Otten and Hedi L Claahsen-van der Grinten
Department of Paediatric Endocrinology, Radboud University Nijmegen Medical Centre, 6500 HB Nijmegen, The Netherlands

Peter A Lee
The Milton S. Hershey Medical Center, College of Medicine, Pennsylvania State University, Hershey, PA 17033, USA
Section of Pediatric Endocrinology and Diabetology, James Whitcomb Riley Hospital for Children, School of Medicine, Indiana University, Indianapolis, IN 46202, USA

John Fuqua
Section of Pediatric Endocrinology and Diabetology, James Whitcomb Riley Hospital for Children, School of Medicine, Indiana University, Indianapolis, IN 46202, USA

E Kirk Neely
Division of Pediatric Endocrinology and Diabetes, Room G313, Stanford University Medical Center, Stanford, CA 94305, USA

Di Yang, Lois M Larsen, Cynthia Mattia-Goldberg and Kristof Chwalisz
Abbott Laboratories, 200 Abbott Park Road, Abbott Park, IL 60064, USA

Lulu Wang
School of Medicine, Vanderbilt University, Nashville, TN, USA

Ashley H Shoemaker
Monroe Carell Jr. Children's Hospital at Vanderbilt University, Nashville, TN 37232-9170, USA

Vanessa A Curtis
Department of Pediatrics, University of Iowa Carver College of Medicine, 200 Hawkins Drive, 2859 JPP, Iowa City, IO 52242-1083, USA

Aaron L Carrel and David B Allen
Department of Pediatrics, University of Wisconsin School of Medicine and Public Health, Madison, WI, USA

Jens C Eickhoff
Department of Biostatistics and Medical Informatics, University of Wisconsin, Madison, WI, USA

Jill H Simmons, Miranda Raines and Randon Hall
Department of Pediatrics, Division of Endocrinology and Diabetes, Vanderbilt Children's Hospital, Nashville, TN, USA

Kathryn D Ness
Department of Pediatrics, Division of Pediatric Endocrinology, Seattle Children's Hospital, Seattle, WA, USA

Tebeb Gebretsadik
Department of Biostatistics, Vanderbilt University Medical Center, Nashville, TN, USA

Subburaman Mohan4
Musculoskeletal Disease Center, Jerry L Pettis VA Medical Center, and Departments of Medicine and Biochemistry, Loma Linda University, Loma Linda, CA, USA

Anna Spagnoli
Department of Pediatrics, Division of Pediatric Endocrinology, University of North Carolina at Chapel Hill, Chapel Hill, NC, USA

Andreas Bieri, Monika Oser-Meier, Marco Janner, Chantal Cripe-Mamie, Kathrin Pipczynski-Suter, Primus E Mullis and Christa E Flück
Pediatric Endocrinology, Diabetology and Metabolism, University Children's Hospital, Inselspital, Freiburgstrasse 15, CH - 3010 Bern, Switzerland

Josephine Ho, Carol Huang and Danièle Pacaud
Department of Pediatrics, University of Calgary, Calgary, T3B 6A8, Canada

Alberto Nettel-Aguirre
Department of Pediatrics, University of Calgary, Calgary, T3B 6A8, Canada

Department of Community Health Sciences, University of Calgary, Calgary, T3B 6A8 Canada

Meghan Slattery
Neuroendocrine Unit, Massachusetts General Hospital and Harvard Medical School, BUL 457B, Neuroendocrine Unit, 55 Fruit Street, MGH, Boston, MA 02114, USA

Madhusmita Misra
Neuroendocrine Unit, Massachusetts General Hospital and Harvard Medical School, BUL 457B, Neuroendocrine Unit, 55 Fruit Street, MGH, Boston, MA 02114, USA
Pediatric Endocrine Unit, Massachusetts General Hospital for Children and Harvard Medical School, Boston, MA 02114, USA

Miriam A Bredella and Martin Torriani
Department of Radiology, Massachusetts General Hospital and Harvard Medical School, Boston, MA 02114, USA

Takara Stanley
Pediatric Endocrine Unit, Massachusetts General Hospital for Children and Harvard Medical School, Boston, MA 02114, USA

Christine E. Cherella and Ari J. Wassner
Division of Endocrinology, Boston Children's Hospital, Harvard Medical School, 300 Longwood Avenue, Boston, MA 02115, USA

Mia Elbek Sømod, Kurt Kristensen and Niels Holtum Birkebæk
Department of Pediatrics, Aarhus University Hospital, Skejby, Palle Juul Jensens Boulevard 99, DK-8200 Aarhus N, Denmark

Esben Thyssen Vestergaard
Medical Research Laboratory, Aarhus University, Nørrebrogade 44 building 3B, DK-8000 Aarhus C, Denmark
Department of Pediatrics, Randers Regional Hospital, DK-8930 Randers, Denmark

Talia L. Brown
Colorado School of Public Health, 13001 East 17th Place, Aurora, CO 80045, USA
Barbara Davis Center for Childhood Diabetes, University of Colorado Denver, 1775 Aurora Court, Mail Stop A140, Aurora, CO 80045, USA

David M. Maahs, Franziska K. Bishop, Janet K. Snell-Bergeon and R. Paul Wadwa
Barbara Davis Center for Childhood Diabetes, University of Colorado Denver, 1775 Aurora Court, Mail Stop A140, Aurora, CO 80045, USA

Romina P. Grinspon and Helena F. Schteingart
Centro de Investigaciones Endocrinológicas "Dr. César Bergadá" (CEDIE), CONICET – FEI – División de Endocrinología, Hospital de Niños Ricardo Gutiérrez, Buenos Aires, Argentina

Nadia Y. Edelsztein
Centro de Investigaciones Endocrinológicas "Dr. César Bergadá" (CEDIE), CONICET – FEI – División de Endocrinología, Hospital de Niños Ricardo Gutiérrez, Buenos Aires, Argentina
Departamento de Ecología, Genética y Evolución, Facultad de Ciencias Exactas y Naturales, Universidad de Buenos Aires, Buenos Aires, Argentina

Rodolfo A. Rey
Centro de Investigaciones Endocrinológicas "Dr. César Bergadá" (CEDIE), CONICET – FEI – División de Endocrinología, Hospital de Niños Ricardo Gutiérrez, Buenos Aires, Argentina

Departamento de Biología Celular, Histología, Embriología y Genética, Facultad de Medicina, Universidad de Buenos Aires, Buenos Aires, Argentina

Bonnie McCann-Crosby, Sheila Gunn and Lefkothea Karaviti
Division of Pediatric Endocrinology, Baylor College of Medicine, Texas Children's Hospital, Houston, TX 77030, USA

E. O'Brian Smith
Department of Pediatrics, Children's Nutrition Research Center, Baylor College of Medicine, Houston, TX 77030, USA

M. John Hicks
Department of Pathology, Baylor College of Medicine, Texas Children's Hospital, Houston, TX 77030, USA

Index

www.ingramcontent.com/pod-product-compliance
Lightning Source LLC
Chambersburg PA
CBHW080641200326
41458CB00013B/4695